DEJA REVIEW™

Emergency Medicine

NOTICE

Medicine is an ever-changing science. As new research and clinical experience broaden our knowledge, changes in treatment and drug therapy are required. The authors and the publisher of this work have checked with sources believed to be reliable in their efforts to provide information that is complete and generally in accord with the standards accepted at the time of publication. However, in view of the possibility of human error or changes in medical sciences, neither the authors nor the publisher nor any other party who has been involved in the preparation or publication of this work warrants that the information contained herein is in every respect accurate or complete, and they disclaim all responsibility for any errors or omissions or for the results obtained from use of the information contained in this work. Readers are encouraged to confirm the information contained herein with other sources. For example and in particular, readers are advised to check the product information sheet included in the package of each drug they plan to administer to be certain that the information contained in this work is accurate and that changes have not been made in the recommended dose or in the contraindications for administration. This recommendation is of particular importance in connection with new or infrequently used drugs.

DEJA REVIEW™

Emergency Medicine

Second Edition

David H. Jang, MD

Medical Toxicology Fellowship
New York University
New York, New York

Emergency Medicine Residency
University of Pittsburgh Medical Center
Pittsburgh, Pennsylvania

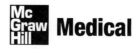

New York   Chicago   San Francisco   Lisbon   London   Madrid   Mexico City
Milan   New Delhi   San Juan   Seoul   Singapore   Sydney   Toronto

Déjà Review™: Emergency Medicine, Second Edition

1 2 3 4 5 6 7 8 9 0   DOC/DOC   15 14 13 12 11

ISBN 978-0-07-171518-8
MHID 0-07-171518-5

This book was set in Palatino by Glyph International.

The editors were Kirsten Funk and Cindy Yoo.

The production supervisor was Catherine Saggese.

Project management was provided by Shruti Vasishta, Glyph International.

RR Donnelley was printer and binder.

This book is printed on acid-free paper.

Library of Congress Cataloging-in-Publication Data

Jang, David H., author.
    Deja review. Emergency medicine / David H. Jang, MD.—Second Edition.
        p. ; cm.—(Deja review)
    Emergency medicine
    Includes index.
    ISBN-13: 978-0-07-171518-8 (pbk. : alk. paper)
    ISBN-10: 0-07-171518-5 (pbk. : alk. paper)   1. Emergency medicine—Examinations, questions, etc.   I. Title.   II. Title: Emergency medicine.   III. Series: Deja review.
    [DNLM: 1. Emergency Treatment—Examination Questions.   2. Emergency Medicine—Examination Questions.   WB 18.2]
    RC86.9.J36   2011
    616.02′5—dc22
                                                                                          2010050480

Contents

Contributors

Peter H. Adler, MD
Emergency Physician
University of Pittsburgh Medical Center
Shadyside Hospital
Pittsburgh, Pennsylvania
Gastrointestinal Emergencies

Amy E. Betz, MD
Acting Instructor
Division of Emergency Medicine
Harborview Medical Center
University of Washington Medical Center
Seattle, Washington
Trauma
Pediatric Emergencies

Jason M. Biggs, MD
Attending Physician
Department of Emergency Medicine
St. Clair Hospital
Pittsburgh, Pennsylvania
Genitourinary Emergencies
Behavioral Emergencies

Isaac S. Bruck, MD, PhD
Resident
Department of Emergency Medicine
Metropolitan Hospital Center
New York, New York
Infectious Diseases

Alan Lo, MD
Inova Fairfax Hospital
Department of Emergency Medicine
Associate Professor of Emergency Medicine
Virginia Commonwealth University School
    of Medicine
Falls Church, Virginia
Ophthalmologic Emergencies
ENT and Dental Emergencies

Reviewers

Matthias Barden
Medical Student, M3
University of Southern California
Keck School of Medicine
Class of 2011

Nicole H. Campfield
Medical Student, M4
University of Medicine & Dentistry
  of New Jersey
Class of 2010

Adam Darnobid
Medical Student, M4
SUNY Upstate Medical College
Syracuse, New York
Class of 2009

Erica Katz, MD
PGY-1
Stony Brook University Medical Center
Department of Emergency Medicine
Stony Brook, New York

Matthew LaPorta, DO, RN
Resident
Department of Surgery
Inova-Fairfax Hospital
Falls Church, Virginia

Tina Nguyen, MD
PGY-1
Harbor-UCLA Emergency Medicine Program
Torrance, California

Preface

This second edition of *Deja Review* Emergency Medicine has been designed to allow you to review the essential facts needed to excel in the Emergency Medicine clerkship. In order to do well both on the wards and on the USMLE Step 2CK exam, you must have a solid foundation in the core clerkship competencies. This guide has been written as a high-yield resource, to endorse the rapid recall of the essential facts in a well-organized and efficient manner.

The first chapter introduces the basic principles of the subject. Then the chapters move through defined sub-topics within emergency medicine as an organ-based approach. There are two main additions to this second edition. To represent a growing area in Emergency Medicine, we have added an Orthopedics chapter. The other addition is the stimulus chapter at the end of the book. The stimulus chapter is very similar to what is seen on the EM boards and is very applicable on a EM rotation. Very often a diagnosis and management must be made based on a radiographic finding or an ECG.

ORGANIZATION

The *Deja Review* series is a unique resource that has been designed to allow you to review the essential facts and determine your level of knowledge on the subjects tested on your clerkship shelf exams, as well as the United States Medical Licensing Examination (USMLE) Step 2CK. All concepts are presented in a question and answer format that covers key facts on commonly tested topics during the clerkship.

This question and answer format has several important advantages:

* It provides a rapid, straightforward way for you to assess your strengths and weaknesses.
* Prepares you for "pimping" on the wards
* It allows you to efficiently review and commit to memory a large body of information.
* It serves as a quick, last-minute review of high-yield facts.
* Compact, condensed design of the book is conducive to studying on the go.

At the end of each chapter, you will find clinical vignettes. These vignettes are meant to be representative of the types of questions tested on national licensing exams to help you further evaluate your understanding of the material just presented in the chapter. The clinical vignettes seen in this EM review book are "classic" presentations but patients rarely present in that fashion, however are nonetheless important for learning.

HOW TO USE THIS BOOK

This book is intended to serve as a tool during your emergency medicine clerkship. Remember, this text is not intended to replace comprehensive textbooks, course packs, or lectures. It is simply intended to serve as a supplement to your studies during your emergency medicine rotation and throughout your preparation for Step 2CK. This text was thoroughly reviewed by a number of medical students and interns to represent the core topics tested on shelf examinations. For this reason, we encourage you to begin using this book early in your clinical years to reinforce topics you encounter while on the wards. You may use the book to quiz yourself or classmates on topics covered in recent lectures and clinical case discussions. A bookmark is included so that you can easily cover up the answers as you work through each chapter. The compact, condensed design of the book is conducive to studying on the go. Carry it in your white coat pocket so that you can access during any downtime throughout your busy day.

However you choose to study, I hope you find this resource helpful throughout your preparation for shelf examinations, the USMLE Step 2CK, and throughout your clinical years.

David H. Jang, MD

Acknowledgments

To the love of my life, Min Young, for her support and patience with all things in life; the residents and attendings at the University of Pittsburgh Affiliated Residency in Emergency Medicine, who all have been excellent and continue to push me to help others better.

I also extend my appreciation to the staff and excellent teaching that I have also received at the New York University for my fellowship training in medical toxicology.

CHAPTER 1

Introduction to Emergency Medicine

EMERGENCY MEDICAL SERVICES

What was the significance of the Highway Safety Act of 1966 to the development of Emergency Medical Services (EMS) in the United States?

This act authorized the Department of Transportation to provide funding for improvement of ambulance service and prehospital provider training, as well as the development of highway safety programs and EMS standards.

Which paper helped to bring about the Highway Safety Act of 1966?

Accidental Death and Disability: The Neglected Disease of Modern Society, which highlighted the dangerous conditions of emergency care in the United States.

What important advancements in EMS occurred in the First National Conference on EMS in 1969?

Development of a curriculum, certification process, and national register for the emergency medical technician (EMT)—ambulance

In what year was the emergency medical technician (EMT) recognized as an occupational specialty by the Department of Labor?

1972

What are the 15 elements of an EMS system as defined by the Emergency Medical Services Act of 1973?

1. Personnel
2. Training
3. Communications
4. Transportation
5. Facilities
6. Critical care units
7. Public safety agencies
8. Consumer participation
9. Access to care
10. Transfer to care
11. Standardization of patient's records
12. Public information and education
13. Independent review and evaluation
14. Disaster linkage
15. Mutual aid agreement

What are the five types of EMS service systems?

1. Public Service (often provided by the fire department)
2. Hospital-based
3. "Third Service" model, usually a separate division of the local government
4. "Public Utility" model (a private ambulance company)
5. Volunteer model

What determines which service system is appropriate for a given community?

The type of EMS system depends on the needs and the resources of the community.

What are the two general categories of care provided by EMS systems?

1. Basic life support (BLS): is a level of medical care which is used for patients with life-threatening illness or injury until the patient can be given full medical care. It can generally be provided without any medical equipment.
2. Advanced cardiac life support (ACLS): ACLS is an extension of BLS. Requires extensive knowledge and training when compared to BLS. Important distinctions include use of medication, early defibrillation, and interpretation of an ECG.

Name three main methods of patient transport:

1. Ground transportation—ambulance
2. Rotary wing transportation—helicopter
3. Fixed wing transportation—jet

What is the average cost of an ambulance transport?

$180 to $600

Can a patient refuse EMS treatment and/or transport?

Yes. A competent, conscious adult patient may refuse treatment or transport, but the patient must be informed of risks when refusing. The medical director should be informed of the situation as well.

What are the four levels of EMS training and some specific skill sets?

First responder. Requires approximately 60 classroom hours of training: initial scene and patient evaluation; cardiopulmonary resuscitation (CPR); basic airway skills; hemorrhage control; spinal immobilization

EMT—Basic. Requires 100 classroom hours as well as 10 clinical hours: skills of the first responder; triage and patient assessment; AED use; assist patient in taking medications

EMT—Intermediate. Requires 300 to 400 hours of classroom and clinical training: advanced patient assessment; intravenous line placement; manual defibrillation; administration of a limited number of medications

EMT—Paramedic. Requires 1000 to 1200 hours of classroom training plus a clinical internship: electrocardiogram (ECG) interpretation; needle decompression of a tension pneumothorax; needle and surgical cricothyrotomy; transthoracic cardiac pacing; administration of selected medications

What advancement in communication significantly improved the public's access to emergency medical services?

911

What are the responsibilities of the emergency medical dispatcher?

Answering, triaging, and prioritizing all calls

Alerting and dispatching the appropriate unit

Providing pre-arrival instructions to EMS providers

Define unique characteristics of an EMS medical director.

They provide essential medical leadership, system quality improvement, system oversight, and coordination of guideline development for routine and disaster care, and research.

What is the definition of a disaster?

A disaster is an incident that overwhelms the response capacities of a community. This occurs when the number or severity of patients presenting to the emergency medical response system in a given period of time overwhelms the available resources.

What are the three phases of a disaster plan?

Activation. This includes the initial response by EMS and the organization of an incident command center

Implementation. Components include search and rescue, triage, and transport of patients

Recovery

What are the two phases of a disaster operation?

1. Prehospital
2. Hospital

List the components of the prehospital phase of a disaster operation:

Triage of patients

Scene control

Communications

Public health considerations

The second phase of a disaster operation focuses on hospital preparedness. List the six components that must be considered during this phase.

1. Development of a central control center
2. Activation of the disaster plan
3. Designation of treatment areas
4. Organization of documentation
5. Mobilization of security
6. Designation of waiting areas

What is the definition of triage?

Triage is the process of classifying injured patients into groups according to the priority for treatment. The goal is to do the most good for the largest number of potential survivors.

Describe the four patient triage categories:

Dead or unsalvageable.

Critical. These patients are severely injured but salvageable and require immediate medical attention

Serious. These patients have no immediate life-threatening injuries

Minor. Often these patients are referred to as the walking wounded

AIRWAY MANAGEMENT

Table 1-1

Sedative/Induction	Dosage	Onset	Duration
Etomidate	0.3-0.4 mg/kg IV	1 min	3-6 min
Fentanyl	0.5-2 ug/kg IV	1 min	30-60 min
Ketamine	1-2 mg/kg IV	1 min	15 min
Midazolam	0.2-0.4 mg/kg IV	30 s	15-20 min
Propofol	1-2 mg/kg IV	30 s	3-5 min
Neuromuscular Blocking Agents	**Dosage**	**Onset**	**Duration**
Succinylcholine	1-2 mg/kg IV	<1 min	3-5 min
Rocuronium	1 mg/kg IV	<1 min	>30 min
Vecuronium	0.1 mg/kg IV	2-3 min	30-60 min

IV, intravenous.

What are some reasons a patient may need airway management?	Oxygenation Prevention/overcoming airway obstruction Protection against aspiration Assisted ventilation
What are some important things to do prior to any airway procedure?	Inspect the patient's oropharynx Assess for possible cervical spine injury Listen for any airway problems (ie, stridor) Suction any secretions prior to procedures
List some important causes of airway obstruction.	Foreign bodies Trauma (expanding hematoma) Infections (epiglottis) Congenital (tracheomalacia)
What is a complication of the inability to secure an airway in a timely fashion?	Hypoxia with irreversible brain damage

What are some important points for each of the following airway devices?

Oral airway

C-shaped rigid instrument placed into the mouth; placed to create a patent airway by supporting soft tissue structures; used to prevent tongue from falling posterior; used in patients with no gag reflex

Nasal airway

A nasopharyngeal tube placed into a nostril; typically used to bypass obstructing tongue; used in somnolent patient with a gag reflex

Bag valve mask (BVM)

The mainstay of airway management; inflating bag with a non-rebreathing valve; critical to airway management; two-person use is optimal to avoid air leak

Esophageal tracheal combitube (ETC)

Plastic twin-lumen tube with inflatable cuffs; placed blindly into the oropharynx; commonly used as a backup airway to endotrachial tube (ETT); typically used in the prehospital setting

Laryngeal mask airway (LMA)

Tubular oropharyngeal airway; contains a distal laryngeal mask; inserted blindly into the oropharynx; commonly used as backup airway to ETT

Endotracheal tube (ETT)

Cuffed-tube placed into the larynx; placed normally by direct laryngoscopy; considered the gold standard for airway management; often protects from aspiration

What is rapid sequence intubation (RSI)?

The use of special drugs to rapidly sedate and paralyze a patient to allow ETT placement. This is as opposed to standard intubation which is used by anesthetists in the controlled environment of the OR.

What is the primary reason for the use of RSI medications?

It allows optimal conditions to secure an airway by relaxing the oropharynx to allow better visualization.

What is a disadvantage of RSI?

If unable to intubate, it can result in complete loss of airway control.

What is the most important thing to keep in mind while performing RSI?

Always have a back-up airway ready! Back-up airways include an LMA, or in case that all else fails, a surgical airway kit.

What are the seven Ps of RSI?

Prepare. Have different sized tubes and blades ready; ensure cuff works; have back-up airway ready.

Preoxygenate. Preoxygenate for about 2 to 5 min; hypoxia develops faster in children and pregnant women.

Position. Flexion of lower neck; extension at the atlantooccipital joint; this allows direct visualization of the larynx; bad positioning common reason for failure.

Premedicate (induction). Induce a deep level of unconsciousness; agent depends on situation such as trauma.

Paralyze. Administer neuromuscular blocking agent; succinylcholine most preferred agent.

Place ETT. Visualization of vocal cords is critical.

Prove Placement. Look for tube condensation; bilateral chest rise; auscultate stomach and lung; capnography is considered the gold standard for confirmation.

What is the Sellick's maneuver?

The application of external cricoid pressure to help prevent aspiration as well as aid in direct visualization of vocal cords.

What are some reasons that succinylcholine is used most often in RSI?

Rapid onset of action

Brief duration of action

What are some adverse side effects to keep in mind about the use of succinylcholine?

Increases intraocular/intracranial pressure

Avoid in hyperkalemic states such as crush injuries or burns

Avoid in patients with history of paralysis

In rare cases can cause malignant hyperthermia

List some alternative paralytics that can be used if succinylcholine is contraindicated:

Non-depolarizing paralytics, such as:
Rocuronium or
Vecuronium

What are some critical points to be aware of when considering the following?

Cricothyrotomy

The primary surgical back-up airway; placement of trach/ETT through a surgical incision in the neck and cricoid membrane; contraindicated in children less than 8 years of age

Tracheotomy

Longer to perform than cricothyrotomy; preferred in children; also used in patients with tracheal injury

Digital intubation

Index/middle fingers to palpate epiglottis; typically used in a comatose patient; success rate is lower than RSI

Retrograde intubation

Use of a guide wire via the cricoid membrane; the guide wire guides the tube via the cord; not commonly used in the prehospital setting

SHOCK

What is the definition of shock?

It is a clinical syndrome that is characterized by the body's inability to meet the demands of tissue/organ perfusion resulting in decreased venous oxygen content and lactic acidosis. Although commonly assessed with the use of hemodynamic parameters, the actual condition depends on the sufficiency of perfusion, rather than any given set of hemodynamic criteria.

What is the initial step in management for any patient who presents with possible shock?

Airway

Breathing

Circulation

What are four categories of shock?

1. Cardiogenic (including MI, arrhythmias, valvular disease, direct trauma)
2. Hypovolemic (including hemorrhagic, volume depletion secondary to emesis/diarrhea)
3. Distributive (including septic, adrenal insufficiency, allergic)
4. Obstructive (including cardiac tamponade, tension pneumothorax, pulmonary embolism)

What are some autonomic responses that occur with shock?	Increase in heart rate and contractility of heart (not in cardiogenic)
	Constriction of venous capacity vessels (not in distributive)
	Arteriolar vasoconstriction
	Release of vasoactive hormones
	Activation of renin-angiotensin system
What are some important vasoactive hormones that are released during a state of shock?	Dopamine
	Norepinephrine
	Epinephrine
	Cortisol
Name two critical organs to which the autonomic system tries to preserve blood flow:	1. Brain
	2. Heart
What are some common metabolic derangements that can occur with shock?	Metabolic acidosis (lactic acidosis)
	Hyponatremia
	Hyperkalemia
	Prerenal azotemia
What are some important elements from the history that should be considered in determining the likely etiology of the shock state?	Medications (ie, anaphylaxis)
	History of heart disease
	History of volume depletion (ie, emesis)
	Neurologic disease
	Mechanism of trauma
What is an important way to assess shock as well as evaluate therapeutic intervention?	Hemodynamic monitoring
What are some components of hemodynamic monitoring?	ECG
	Pulse oximetry
	Central venous pressure (CVP)
	Arterial line
Name some important early interventions to consider in a state of shock:	Airway control (intubate if necessary)
	Mechanical ventilation (decreases work of breathing)
	Aggressive fluid resuscitation
	Ensure oxygen delivery (pressors if needed)
What is the normal circulating volume of blood in a normal adult?	5 L

What is the hallmark response for each of the following categories of hemorrhage?

Class I (about 750 mL or 15% blood loss)

Usually no response in a healthy person

Class II (750-1500 mL or up to 30% blood loss)

Tachycardia and narrowed pulse pressure; mild hypotension; subtle change in mental status

Class III (>1500 mL or up to 40% blood loss)

Tachycardia and pronounced hypotension; decline in mental status; peripheral hypoperfusion

Class IV (>2 L or greater than 40% blood loss)

Hemodynamic decompensation is common; aggressive resuscitation is required

What is important to know about children and athletes who have acute hemorrhage?

They compensate very well (no tachycardia or hypotension), but can decompensate very rapidly without any warnings.

What other etiologies of hypotension besides hemorrhage should be considered in the setting of trauma?

Tension pneumothorax

Cardiac tamponade

Why are two large-bore IV lines more effective than long narrow IV lines?

Infusion rate of fluids is much faster through short and wide tubes (According to Poiseuille's law, the fluid's resistance to flow increases with length, and decreases with an increase in the diameter of the cylinder).

What are commonly used large-bore IVs?

13- or 14-gauge needles

What are some options for fluid resuscitation?

Isotonic crystalloids (most common)

Colloids (Expensive and no different from crystalloids, used in liver failure patients with hypoalbuminemia)

Blood

Name two commonly used isotonic crystalloid fluids used for resuscitation:

1. Normal saline (NS)
2. Lactated ringers (LR)

What are the general guidelines for the infusion of blood products in the setting of trauma?

Minimal response to 2 to 3 L of fluids

Obvious loss of blood

Hematocrit of less than 16

What are some issues to consider with the use of blood products?

Transfusion reaction

Availability

Infections

Limited storage life

Name some examples of blood products that are available:	Whole blood Packed red blood cells (PRBC) Fresh-frozen plasma (FFP) Platelets
What is the definition of anaphylaxis?	Severe hypersensitivity reaction with multisystem involvement that commonly includes airway compromise and hypotension.
What is a hypersensitivity reaction?	Inappropriate immune response to an antigen.
What is an anaphylactoid reaction?	Reaction that presents similar to anaphylaxis, but is not IgE mediated and does not require prior sensitization. It is mediated by mast cell degranulation usually caused by iatrogenic agents.
List some common causes of anaphylactoid reactions:	Radiocontrast dye Medications Muscular depolarizing agents
List three common causes of anaphylactic reactions:	1. Medication 2. Foods 3. Insects
What are the most common foods associated with allergic reactions?	Nuts Milk Shellfish
What is the most common drug class implicated in allergic reactions?	Penicillin
What is the recurrence rate of anaphylaxis for penicillin upon re-exposure?	Less than 25%
What is the cross-reactivity of a penicillin allergy to cephalosporins?	Less than 10%
What is the pathophysiology of anaphylaxis?	Mast cell and basophil degranulation due to IgE cross-linking, direct activation, and complement activation.
What are some clinical features of anaphylaxis?	Diffuse urticaria, rhinorrhea, conjunctivitis, nausea, angioedema, airway compromise such as stridor, and hypotension.

How is anaphylaxis diagnosed?   Clinically—special attention to airway and blood pressure

What is the mainstay in the treatment of suspected anaphylaxis?   Epinephrine

List some commonly used agents for the treatment of general allergic reactions:

Antihistamines

Corticosteroids

Asthma medications (Beta-2 selective agonists)

What is the definition of cardiogenic shock?   Inadequate tissue perfusion due to decrease in cardiac output despite adequate circulating volume.

What is a common cause of cardiogenic shock?   Myocardial infarction

What are some other causes of cardiogenic shock?

Mechanical obstruction

Sepsis

Myocarditis

Right ventricular infarct

What are some signs and symptoms of cardiogenic shock?

Evidence of volume overload (ie, rales)

Hypotension

Mental status change

Cool/clammy skin

Diaphoresis

Jugular venous distension

What are some important points for each of the diagnostic tests commonly used to evaluate cardiogenic shock:

   ECG

Cornerstone test to diagnose ischemia

Can also detect arrhythmias, drug toxicity, and electrolyte derangements

Also to detect right ventricular infarct as well as MI in general

   Chest radiograph

May show pulmonary edema/effusion

Normal chest does not rule out shock

   Echocardiography

Used to assess left-ventricular function

Color flow doppler can assess mechanical cause such as valvular disease

Readily available as a bedside test

What are some laboratory tests to consider in cardiogenic shock?

Cardiac enzyme

Brain natriuretic peptide (BNP)

Arterial blood gas

Serum lactate

What are some important things to know about sepsis?

Up to 50% mortality of those who develop refractory shock

Gram −/+ often common cause of sepsis

Sepsis is more common in older adults

What are the most frequent sites of infection that can lead to sepsis?

Genitourinary tract

Abdomen

Lung

What are co-morbid conditions that can predispose one to sepsis?

Burns

Diabetes mellitus

Immunosuppressive agents

What is the definition of bacteremia?

Presence of bacteria in the blood

Name the criteria of systemic inflammatory response syndrome (SIRS):

Temperature: <36°C or >38°C

Tachycardia: >90 beats/min

Tachypnea: > 20 breaths/min

WBC: >12,000 cells/mm³, <4000 cells/mm³ or >10% bands

What is sepsis?

Systemic response to infection that meet the criteria for systemic inflammatory response syndrome (SIRS).

What is severe sepsis?

Hypotension with inadequate organ perfusion induced by sepsis with another metabolic dysfunction such as lactic acidosis.

What is septic shock?

Severe sepsis with refractory hypotension despite adequate fluid resuscitation.

What are some clinical features of sepsis in the following organ systems?

Respiratory

Acute respiratory distress system (ARDS); pneumonia

Cardiovascular

Myocardial depression and tachycardia; poor response to fluid administration

Renal

Acute renal failure due to renal ischemia; oliguria

Hepatic	Cholestatic jaundice; elevated liver function tests; elevated bilirubin
Endocrine	Hyperglycemia is common; elevated cortisol and glucagon; insulin resistance and decreased insulin
Hematology	Neutrophilia or neutropenia; thrombocytopenia; disseminated intravascular coagulation
What are some general management considerations in sepsis?	ABCs (aggressive fluid resuscitation)
	Not atypical for patients to require greater than 6 L of fluids
	Inotropes and/or vasoconstrictors if not responsive to fluids
	Empiric antibiotic coverage is the cornerstone
	Evaluate the patient for a source of infection

FLUIDS

What percent of the total body weight is comprised of water?	60% (42 L in a 70 lb patient)
Of the total body water, what percent makes up the intracellular and extracellular compartments?	2/3 Intracellular (28 L in a 70 lb patient)
	1/3 Extracellular (14 L in a 70 lb patient)
What makes up the extracellular compartment?	Interstitial fluid and plasma
What proportion of the extracellular fluid is contained in each compartment?	3/4 interstitial (11 L in a 70 lb patient
	1/4 plasma (3 L in a 70 lb patient)
Define the following terms in regards to water regulation:	
Osmosis	Net movement of water across a selectively permeable membrane driven by a difference in solute concentrations on the two sides of the membrane.
Osmolality	Total number of particles in solution.
Semipermeable membrane	Allows passage of the solvent, but not solute (cell membranes).
What is the normal serum osmolality?	280 to 295 mOsm/L

Name some important solutes that contribute to serum osmolality:	Chloride, sodium, bicarbonate, and glucose.
What is the equation used to calculate the serum osmolarity?	$2\,[Na^+] + Glucose/18 + BUN/2.8$
What is the osmolal gap?	Difference between the measured osmolality and calculated osmolarity, indicating that osmolytes other than Na, glu, BUN are present in the serum.
List some causes of an increased osmol gap:	Uremia Increase in serum sodium (no gap) Alcohol ingestion Ketoacidosis
How much water does an average human adult require each day?	2 to 4 L
Name two hormones involved in the regulation of free water:	1. Aldosterone 2. Antidiuretic hormone (ADH)
What are the two primary triggers for the release of ADH?	Acute volume depletion Increased serum osmolality
Does aldosterone play a significant role in maintaining serum osmolality?	No

ELECTROLYTES

Hyponatremia

What is the plasma sodium concentration in hyponatremia?	$[Na^+] <135\ mEq/L$
What is the plasma sodium concentration in severe hyponatremia?	$[Na^+] <120\ mEq/L$
What are some signs and symptoms of hyponatremia?	Primarily neurologic: headaches, confusion, and seizures, but can be asymptomatic depending on rate of change.
What is an important complication of severe hyponatremia?	Cerebral edema

Name the two common causes of hyponatremia:

1. Syndrome of inappropriate antidiuretic hormone secretion (SIADH)
2. Decrease in effective circulating volume

What is the primary hormone that regulates free water in the body?

Antidiuretic hormone (ADH)

What are two triggers that result in increased secretion of ADH?

Increase in serum osmolality

Decrease in circulating volume

Name an area of the body that mediates ADH release in response to circulating volume:

Secreted from posterior pituitary in response to baroreceptors in the carotid sinus.

Name some conditions that can result in a decrease in effective circulating volume resulting in ADH secretion:

True volume depletion (GI bleeding)

Exercise-associated hyponatremia

Heart failure

Cirrhosis

Thiazide diuretics

What is the mechanism by which hyponatremia occurs in patients with congestive heart failure (CHF) even though they may have a marked increase in plasma volume?

The carotid sinus will sense a reduced pressure from fall in cardiac output and increase ADH release.

What is the mechanism by which hyponatremia occur in patients with cirrhosis?

Peripheral vasodilation in cirrhosis that will result in decreased return of venous blood with a resultant drop in cardiac output (increased ADH secretion).

What are some conditions that may be associated with SIADH?

Lung cancer

Drugs

Infections (ie, brain abscess)

Traumatic brain injury

Name two other conditions in which hyponatremia can also occur:

1. Adrenal insufficiency
2. Hypothyroidism

What are two disorders in which hyponatremia can occur despite normal/low ADH levels?

1. Primary polydipsia
2. Advanced renal failure

Name two causes of primary polydipsia:

1. Psychogenic
2. Hypothalamic lesions

Name cause of hyponatremia with high plasma osmolality.

Hyperglycemia

Pseudohyponatremia (increased plasma lipid or protein content)

What are some elements to keep in mind in the history and physical of a patient with hyponatremia?

History of fluid loss

Signs of volume overload

Signs/symptoms suggestive of adrenal insufficiency or hypothyroidism

History that may point to SIADH such as small cell carcinoma

History of traumatic brain injury

What are three important laboratory tests to consider in differentiating hyponatremia?

1. Urine osmolality
2. Plasma osmolality
3. Urine sodium concentration

What is the plasma osmolality in most hyponatremic patients?

Reduced (<275–290 mOsm/L)

What is the primary use of urine sodium concentration in elevating hyponatremia?

Helps to distinguish between effective volume depletion and other causes

What is the initial treatment in patients who are asymptomatic and have a plasma sodium concentration above 120 mEq/L?

Gradual correction with water restriction or administration of isotonic saline.

What are four things to consider when managing patients with hyponatremia?

1. Assessing risk of osmotic demyelination
2. Appropriate rate of correcting hyponatremia to avoid demyelination
3. Determine the best method to raise $[Na^+]$
4. Estimate the sodium deficit if giving sodium

What can lead to the development of central pontine myelinolysis?

Rapid correction of severe hyponatremia

What are some signs and symptoms of central pontine myelinolysis?

Dysphagia

Dysarthria

Quadriparesis

Lethargy

Coma

Death

At what rate should hyponatremia be corrected each day?

No more than 10 mEq/L per day

What are some indications for aggressive treatment of hyponatremia?

Acute hyponatremia with severe neurologic symptoms such as seizures.

Hypernatremia

What is the plasma sodium concentration in hypernatremia?	$[Na^+] > 145$ mEq/L
What is the plasma sodium concentration in severe hypernatremia?	$[Na^+] > 155$ mEq/L

What are some causes of hypernatremia in the following groups:

Sodium gain	Excessive saline/hypertonic bicarbonate administration
	Hypertonic dialysis
	Hypertonic feedings
Water loss	Decreased water intake or excessive free water restriction
	Osmotic diuresis (ie, diabetes mellitus)
	Diabetes insipidus (central and nephrogenic causes)
What is the most likely cause of hypernatremia in the emergency department?	Volume loss
What is the urine output of a healthy patient with decreased volume status (dehydration)?	Low urine output (<20 mL/h) and high urine osmolality (>1000 mOsm/Kg)
What is diabetes insipidus (DI)?	Condition characterized by excessive thirst and excretion of large amounts of severely diluted urine.
Name two types of DI and define them:	Neurogenic DI: failure of ADH release from the posterior pituitary gland
	Nephrogenic DI: insensitivity of the kidneys to ADH
What are some characteristic findings in the urine of patients with DI?	Low urine osmolality (200-300 mOsm/Kg); Low urine sodium (60-100 mEq/kg)
What are some causes of central DI?	Pituitary surgery
	Traumatic brain injury
	Neoplasm
What are some important considerations in the management of central DI?	Identify and correct underlying cause
	Sodium restriction
	May require vasopressin

What are some causes of nephrogenic DI?	Renal disease
	Malnutrition
	Hypokalemia
	Chronic lithium use (used as a mood stabilizer)
What is the treatment of nephrogenic DI?	Sodium restriction
	May require dialysis
What are some signs and symptoms of hypernatremia?	Altered mental status such as confusion, dehydration, and seizures.
What is the cornerstone of treatment for hypernatremia due to volume depletion?	Volume repletion
What is the formula to estimate body water deficit (BWD)?	$BWD = TBW \times ([Na^+]/140 - 1)$ (TBW is based on weight × estimated percent water)
What is important to remember with volume-replacement for hypernatremia?	Avoid overly rapid correction due to potential for cerebral edema.

Hypokalemia

What is the plasma potassium concentration in hypokalemia?	$[K^+] < 3.5$ mEq/L
What is the plasma potassium concentration in severe hypokalemia?	$[K^+] < 2.5$ mEq/L
Name three toxic ingestions associated with significant hypokalemia:	1. Chronic toluene use (an industrial solvent)
	2. Methylxanthines (bronchodilators)
	3. Barium
What are some important causes of hypokalemia in the following conditions:	
Renal	Types I and II renal tubular acidosis
	Diuretics
	Cushing syndrome
	Hypomagnesemia

GI condition	Emesis
	Starvation
	Diarrhea
	Laxative abuse
Other	Hypothyroidism and intracellular shift

What are some signs and symptoms of hypokalemia, especially if <2.5 mEq/L?	Pronounced weakness
	Hyporeflexia
	Ileus
	Paralysis
	Dysrhythmias
What are some characteristic ECG changes of hypokalemia?	Flat T-waves, U-waves, ST depression, and prolonged QT interval
What is a potential concern in a patient with a history of congestive heart failure who has hypokalemia?	Potentiates digoxin toxicity
What are some considerations in the management of chronic/subacute hypokalemia?	Oral replacement of potassium preferred; correction of any magnesium deficits
What are some considerations in the management of acute hypokalemia?	Acute hypokalemia can be life-threatening
	About 40 mEq will raise $[K^+]$ by 1 mEq/L

Hyperkalemia

What is the plasma potassium concentration in hyperkalemia?	$[K^+]$ >4.5 mEq/L
What is the plasma potassium concentration in severe hyperkalemia?	$[K^+]$ >6.5 mEq/L
What are some important causes of hyperkalemia in the following conditions:	
Renal	Renal failure
	Aldosterone insufficiency
	Potassium-sparing diuretics
	Type IV renal tubular acidosis

Decreased cellular uptake	Drugs (ie, beta-blockers)
	Diabetic ketoacidosis
Increased potassium level	Hemolysis
	GI bleeding
	Cellular breakdown such as trauma and rhabdomyolysis

What are some signs and symptoms of hyperkalemia?

Lethargy

Weakness

Hypotension

Dysrhythmias

Paralysis

What is the most important diagnostic test to order in suspected hyperkalemia?

ECG

What are some ECG changes associated with the following degree of hyperkalemia?

Table 1-2

Hyperkalemia Level (mEq/L)	ECG Changes
5.5-6.5	Peaked/large amplitude T-waves
6.5-8.0	QRS widening
	PR interval prolongation
	P-wave flattening
>8.0	Ventricular fibrillation
	Sine wave appearance

What is the intervention of choice in any ECG changes suggestive of hyperkalemia?

Calcium (chloride or gluconate)

What are some treatment options for hyperkalemia?

Table 1-3

Treatment Method	Mechanism	Dose	Onset
Albuterol	Cellular shifting	10-20 mg (inhaler)	20-30 min
Insulin and glucose	Cellular shifting	0.1 units/kg of regular insulin	20-30 min
		50 g of glucose	
Sodium bicarbonate	Cellular shifting	1 mEq/kg IV	10 min
Kayexalate	Excretion	15-30 g PO	1-2 h
Furosemide	Excretion	40 mg IV	
Hemodialysis	Excretion		
Calcium gluconate	Membrane antagonism/ stabilization	10-30 cc IV	1-2 min

Hypocalcemia

What is the plasma calcium concentration in hypocalcemia?	$[Ca^{2+}]$ <8.5 mg/dL
What is the plasma calcium concentration in severe hypocalcemia?	$[Ca^{2+}]$ <7 mg/dL
What are some causes of hypocalcemia?	Hypomagnesemia Rhabdomyolysis Hypoparathyroidism Acute pancreatitis with fat necrosis Vitamin D deficiency Renal failure
What are some signs and symptoms of hypocalcemia?	Typically neuromuscular irritability: Paresthesias Carpopedal spasms Hyperreflexia Seizures Positive Chvostek or Trousseau sign
What is the Chvostek sign?	Tapping of facial nerve that results in tetany

What is the Trousseau sign?	Carpal spasm that may be elicited by occluding the brachial artery (ie, BP cuff)
What are some considerations in the management of hypocalcemia?	Identify and treat the underlying cause
	CaCl$_2$ (10% solution) over 20 min if acutely symptomatic

Hypercalcemia

What is the plasma calcium concentration in hypercalcemia?	[Ca^{2+}] >10.5 mg/dL
What is the plasma calcium concentration in severe hypercalcemia?	[Ca^{2+}] >12 mg/dL
What are some causes of hypercalcemia?	Malignancy
	Vitamin D toxicity
	Acute osteoporosis
	Hyperparathyroidism
	Granulomatous disease, including sarcoidosis
What are some signs and symptoms of hypercalcemia?	"Moans, groans, stones, and bones, with psychic overtones." This describes various manifestations such as nausea, abdominal pain, kidney stones, bone pain, and altered mental status.
What are some ECG changes that can be seen with hypercalcemia?	Short QT interval, widening of the T-wave, and heart block.
What are some considerations in the management of hypercalcemia?	Identify and treat the underlying cause
	Assess volume status: fluids are often first line therapy
	Decrease bone reabsorption with bisphosphonates
	Furosemide with normal saline (NS)
	Avoid thiazide diuretics (loop diuretics excrete calcium, thiazides reabsorbed calcium)

Hypomagnesemia

What is the plasma magnesium concentration in hypomagnesemia?	$[Mg^{2+}]$ <1.4 mEq/L
What is the plasma magnesium concentration in severe hypomagnesemia?	$[Mg^{2+}]$ <0.5 mEq/L
What are some important causes of hypomagnesemia?	Pancreatitis Chronic ethanol use Malnutrition Endocrine disorder (hypoaldosteronism) Drugs (Thiazide or loop diuretics)
What are some signs and symptoms of hypomagnesemia?	Similar to hypocalcemia: tetany, tremors, dysrhythmias, and hypokalemia.
What are some ECG findings that can be seen in hypomagnesemia?	Prolongation of PR and QT interval, ST depression, and wide QRS complex.
What are some considerations in the management of hypomagnesemia?	Identify and treat the underlying cause Check serum potassium and calcium Magnesium sulfate replacement

Hypermagnesemia

What is the serum magnesium level in hypermagnesemia?	$[Mg^{2+}]$ >2.2 Eq/L
What is the serum magnesium level is severe hypermagnesemia?	$[Mg^{2+}]$ >3 m Eq/L
What are some important causes of hypermagnesemia?	Renal failure Iatrogenic Adrenal insufficiency
What are some signs and symptoms of hypermagnesemia?	Hyporeflexia Weakness Respiratory depression Bradycardia and hypotension
What are some ECG findings that can be seen in hypermagnesemia?	Extreme ST elevation and T-waves along with prolonged PR and QT interval.

What are some considerations in the management of hypermagnesemia?	Identify and treat the underlying cause
	Hemodialysis for very high concentrations
	Calcium gluconate for conduction problems

Hypochloremia

What is the plasma chloride concentration in hypochloremia?	[Cl⁻] <100 mEq/L
What is the plasma chloride concentration in severe hypochloremia?	[Cl⁻] <70 mEq/L
What are some causes of hypochloremia?	GI loss such as diarrhea and emesis
	Hypochloremic alkalosis
What are some considerations in the management of hypochloremia?	Identify and treat the underlying cause
	NaCl for severe hypochloremia

Hyperchloremia

What is the plasma chloride concentration in hyperchloremia?	[Cl⁻] >110 mEq/L
What is the plasma chloride concentration in severe hyperchloremia?	[Cl⁻] >120 mEq/L
What are some causes of hyperchloremia?	Bicarbonate loss
	Dehydration
What are some considerations in the management of hyperchloremia?	Restore volume status with normal saline for GI bicarbonate loss
	Bicarbonate for renal bicarbonate loss

Acid and Base Balance

Name three types of acid the body handles to maintain acid-base balance:	1. Exogenous acid
	2. Abnormal metabolic pathway (anaerobic glycolysis)
	3. Fixed acids (non-volatile acids produced via the breakdown of fats/carbohydrates/protein)

Name two organs that are crucial for maintaining acid-base balance:

1. Lungs
2. Kidneys

How much volatile acids does the lung excrete each day?

15,000 mg in the form of CO_2

How much non-volatile acids does the kidney excrete each day?

70 mEq/L

What are three mechanisms by which the kidneys excrete non-volatile acid?

1. Excretion with ammonia
2. Excretion with urinary buffers
3. Direct hydrogen excretion

What maintains regulation of hydrogen ion concentration on a minute-to-minute basis?

Bicarbonate-carbonic acid system

What are important things to consider in the history of a patient who presents with an abnormal acid-base status?

Respiratory status

Volume status

Medication

Illicit drug use

Briefly give some causes for the following acid-base disturbance:

   Respiratory acidosis

   Opioids; respiratory failure; sedative-hypnotics

   Respiratory alkalosis

   Liver failure; salicylates; heart failure

   Anion gap metabolic acidosis

   Hypoxia; sepsis; seizures

   Normal anion gap acidosis

   Renal tubular acidosis; elevated chloride

   Metabolic alkalosis

   Volume depletion; hyperaldosteronism

What else is important to consider in an acid-base disturbance?

Existence of a mixed acid-base disturbance (calculate expected compensation, and compare to measured values).

Name two characteristic laboratory findings in metabolic acidosis:

1. pH <7.35
2. HCO_3^- <20 mEq/L

What is a common cause of metabolic acidosis in the emergency setting?

Lactic acidosis (tissue hypoperfusion such as sepsis)

What are some causes of normal anion gap acidosis (>Cl$^-$)?

Renal tubular acidosis

Diarrhea

Extensive fluid resuscitation

Adrenal insufficiency

What are some causes of an anion gap acidosis (MUD PILES):	Methanol, metformin
	Uremia
	Diabetes ketoacidosis/alcoholic ketoacidosis/starvation ketoacidosis
	Paraldehyde, phenformin
	Iron, Isoniazid
	Lactic acidosis (cyanide/hydrogen sulfide)
	Ethylene glycol
	Salicylates, strychnine
What is the treatment for metabolic acidosis?	Identify and treat the underlying cause
	Consider use of sodium bicarbonate if pH is less than 7.1 or bicarbonate is less than 5 mEq/L
Name two characteristic laboratory finding in metabolic alkalosis:	1. pH >7.45 2. HCO_3^- <26 mEq/L
How can one characterize metabolic alkalosis even further?	Chloride-sensitive versus chloride-resistant
What are some causes of chloride-sensitive alkalosis?	Diuretics
	Emesis
	Nasogastric suction
What is the treatment of choice for chloride-sensitive alkalosis?	Normal saline
What are some causes of chloride-resistant alkalosis?	Mineralocorticoid excess
	Primary reninism
	Chronic potassium depletion
What is the treatment of choice for chloride-resistant alkalosis?	Correction of hypovolemia
	Acetazolamide may help
	Administer potassium as a chloride salt
Name two characteristic laboratory findings in respiratory acidosis:	1. pH <7.40 2. CO_2 >45 mm Hg
What are some causes of respiratory acidosis?	Neuromuscular disease
	CNS depression
	Chronic obstructive pulmonary disease (COPD)
	Decreased tidal volume secondary to pain

How long before full renal compensation occurs?

48 hours of steady-state alteration

What are some considerations in the treatment of respiratory acidosis?

Identify and treat the underlying cause

Bronchodilators for COPD/bronchospasms

Assisting and increasing ventilation

Oxygen therapy (reduces pulmonary HTN)

Name two characteristic laboratory findings in respiratory alkalosis:

1. pH >7.4
2. CO_2 <35 mm Hg

What are some causes of respiratory alkalosis?

CNS (ie, anxiety)

Drugs (ie, salicylates)

Hypoxemia

What are some considerations in the treatment of respiratory alkalosis?

Identify and treat the underlying cause

Respiratory alkalosis is rarely life-threatening

Avoid rapid correction of $PaCO_2$

CHAPTER 2

Neurologic Emergencies

HEADACHES

Cluster Headaches

What is the definition of a cluster headache?	Clustering of painful headaches occurring about once a day over a period of many weeks, peaks in about 5 min, and may last for an hour.
What are some factors associated with the development of cluster headaches?	Male gender Smoking Ethanol use Stress
What are some signs and symptoms of a cluster headache?	Burning headache on unilateral side Lacrimation and flushing Often rapid onset Up to 20 to 30% of patients may exhibit a partial Horner syndrome
What is Horner syndrome?	Deficiency of sympathetic activity in the unilateral face, also known as oculosympathetic palsy.
What are some physical findings in Horner syndrome?	Ptosis—eyelid drooping Anhidrosis—lack of sweating Miosis—constricted pupil Enophthalmos—inward deviation of eyeball Loss of ciliospinal reflex (pupil dilation in response to painful ipsilateral neck stimuli) *Typically all unilateral on affected side

Name some commonly used medications for abortive therapy:	Sumatriptan (selective 5-HT$_{1B \text{ and } 1D}$ receptor agonist)
	High-flow oxygen
	Dihydroergotamine (vasoactive ergot derivative has many adverse reactions)
Name some commonly used medications for prophylactic treatment:	Beta-blockers
	Tricyclic antidepressants
	Calcium channel blockers

Migraine

List some defining features of migraine:	Severe headache that afflicts millions
	Can be characterized by autonomic dysfunction
	It is more prevalent in women
	Often chronic and recurrent
What are some signs and symptoms of a migraine?	Pulsating, severe, unilateral headache often associated with nausea, emesis, and photophobia/phonophobia
What are some of the proposed mechanisms by which a migraine may occur?	Vascular structure involvement (constriction)
	Serotonergic involvement
	Involvement of the trigeminal nerve
List two major categories of migraines:	Common
	Classic (also known as a migraine with an aura)
What are some features of an aura?	Commonly manifested as a visual phenomena (scintillating scotoma)
	Can have motor/sensory disturbances (may mimic a stroke)
	Often precedes a migraine
	Fully reversible and lasts for about 10 to 20 min
	Present in about 15% of migraines
What are some factors that may provoke or exacerbate a migraine?	Physical activity
	Changes in sleep cycle
	Menstruation
	Particular foods (ie, chocolate)

What is the definition of status migrainous?	It is a severe migraine lasting for over 72 hours that often require admission to relieve the pain.
List other differential causes for a migraine which may be life-threatening:	Cerebrovascular disease Giant cell arteritis Subarachnoid hemorrhage Intracranial mass lesions
Is neuroimaging such as a non-contrast CT of the head required?	No—but it is important to rule out other considerations in the following situations: 1. "Worse headache of their life" 2. Associated neurologic abnormalities such as seizures
What are some classes of medication used as prophylaxis?	Beta-blockers (such as timolol, propranolol) Tricyclic antidepressants (such as amitriptyline, nortriptyline) Calcium channel blockers (such as verapamill) Serotonin receptor agonists (such as sumatriptan) Ergotamines (such as dihydroergotamine) NSAIDS (such as naproxen)
What are some commonly used abortive therapies for migraines?	Metoclopramide/prochlorperazine Non-steroidal anti-inflammatory drugs such as toradol (ketorolac) Opioids (typically less effective than other treatments)

Giant Cell Arteritis (Temporal Arteritis)

What is giant cell arteritis?	Autoimmune inflammation of one or more branches of the external carotid artery, particularly the medium and large vessels that branch from the neck.
Name three branches of the carotid artery that are commonly affected by giant cell arteritis:	1. Temporal artery 2. Posterior ciliary artery 3. Ophthalmic artery

What are some important things to know about giant cell arteritis?

Onset rare before the age of 50

Mean age of onset is 70

Females commonly more affected

Most common in Scandinavian populations

What is the most feared complication of giant cell arteritis?

Irreversible blindness

Cerebrovascular accident

What rheumatic condition is giant cell arteritis commonly associated with?

Polymyalgia rheumatica

Giant cell arteritis occurs in about 1/3 of polymyalgia rheumatica patients

What is polymyalgia rheumatica?

It is an inflammatory disorder that is typically characterized by pain and stiffness in the hip or shoulder area. It is typically worse in the morning and improves during the day.

What are some signs and symptoms of giant cell arteritis?

Unilateral burning headache

Worse at night

Accompanied with tender/pulseless temporal artery

Scalp tenderness

Jaw claudication (painful chewing)

Decreased visual acuity

What is an important diagnostic laboratory test to obtain in giant cell arteritis?

Erythrocyte sedimentation rate (ESR) (Between 50 and 100 mm/h)

Does a normal erythrocyte sedimentation rate rule-out giant cell arteritis?

No

What study confirms the diagnosis of giant cell arteritis?

Temporal artery biopsy (sensitivity will vary depending where the sample is obtained)

What are some critical actions in the management of giant cell arteritis?

Treatment must be started immediately if clinical suspicion is high and patient should be admitted for further evaluation

High-dose prednisone (use ranges from 60 to 120 mg/day)

Early involvement of neurology and/or ophthalmology

Subarachnoid Hemorrhage

What are some important facts to know about a subarachnoid hemorrhage?

Accounts for about 10% of cerebrovascular accidents

One of the most common causes of sudden death from stroke

What is the most common cause of a subarachnoid hemorrhage?

Ruptured saccular or berry aneurysms can account for up to 80% of all subarachnoid hemorrhages.

Name some genetic disorders associated with the development of a saccular aneurysm:

Marfan syndrome (mutated form of fibrillin protein of connective tissue)

Ehlers-Danlos syndrome (mutation of various genes involved in collagen formation)

Polycystic kidney disease (secondary to HTN, maybe also defective connective tissue)

What are other causes of a subarachnoid hemorrhage?

Arteriovenous malformation (AVM)

Illicit drug use (especially cocaine)

Intracranial arterial dissections

List some risk factors for the development of a subarachnoid hemorrhage:

Cigarette smoking

Moderate to heavy alcohol consumption

Hypertension

Family history of SAH

Antithrombotic therapy

Bleeding diathesis

What are some signs and symptoms of a subarachnoid hemorrhage?

Sudden, severe headache described as the "worst headache of my life"

Often described as a "thunderclap" headache

Seizure

Nausea

Vomiting

Meningismus (stiffness/rigidity of the neck)

What is a sentinel headache?

Also known as a "warning leak," it is a sudden and severe headache that often precedes a major subarachnoid hemorrhage by a few days to weeks.

What percentage of patients will manifest a sentinel headache prior to a subarachnoid hemorrhage?

Up to 50%

What is the diagnostic test of choice to obtain emergently?	Non-contrast CT of the brain
What is the sensitivity of the head CT with a subarachnoid hemorrhage?	While the sensitivity approaches greater than 90% in the first 24 hours, this drops off dramatically over time as the blood is reabsorbed.
Can you rule-out out a subarachnoid hemorrhage with a normal CT of the brain?	No! If your suspicion is high, a lumbar puncture is the next diagnostic test to obtain.
What is xanthochromia?	On a lumbar puncture, the pink or yellow tint of the CSF that represents hemoglobin degradation products, commonly seen 2 to 4 hours after a bleed but may take up to 12 hours.
What are the two most common reasons to miss a subarachnoid hemorrhage?	1. Failure to understand the limitations of head CT 2. Failure to obtain a lumbar puncture after a normal CT
What is the next diagnostic test to obtain once the diagnosis is established?	Angiography to evaluate the vascular anatomy Identify the source of hemorrhage Consider possible surgical intervention
What are some critical actions in the management of a subarachnoid hemorrhage?	Airway, breathing, circulation Urgent neurosurgical consultation Slowly lower blood pressure Treat for pain and emesis
What calcium channel blocker is often recommended due its ability to decrease vasospasm in the brain?	Nimodipine

CEREBRAL VENOUS SINUS THROMBOSIS

What is a cerebral venous thrombosis?	Thrombosis of the intracranial veins
List some factors associated with the development of a cerebral venous thrombosis:	Inflammatory systemic disorders Medications such as contraceptives Neurosurgical procedures Hypercoagulable disorders

What are some signs and symptoms of a cerebral venous thrombosis?

The clinical presentation is variable but can include headache, nausea, emesis, seizures, and may see papilledema on funduscopic examination.

What laboratory test may be useful to obtain?

D-dimer (not specific)

What imaging modality can be obtained to evaluate a patient with suspected cerebral venous thrombosis?

Non-contrast CT of the brain–while edema and infarct may be seen, the ideal test is to visualize the actual venous system (see below).

What is the ideal imaging test to visualize the venous system of the brain?

Often a combination of an MRI and MRV (magnetic resonance venography) is considered the gold standard by some neurologists.

POST-LUMBAR PUNCTURE HEADACHE

What is a post-lumbar puncture headache?

A post-lumbar puncture headache is thought to be due to a persistent CSF leak where the pain is worse in the upright position (traction on the pain fibers).

What is a useful maneuver to perform at the bedside which may help with the diagnosis?

Headache that is relieved on recumbency and worse in the upright position

List some factors that have been associated with the development of a post-lumbar puncture headache:

Orientation of the bevel during the procedure (bevel should by oriented superiorly/inferiorly)

Size of the spinal needle

Amount of fluid withdrawn

What are some signs and symptoms of a post-lumbar puncture headache?

A bilateral headache that tends to be throbbing with neck stiffness, nausea, and vomiting

Occurs following LP

What are some treatment options for a post-lumbar puncture headache?

Intravenous hydration

Mild analgesics

Methylxanthine (caffeine)

What is the treatment of choice for severe cases after failure of traditional treatment?

Epidural blood patch—autologous blood injected into the epidural space to aid in clotting off the leak (requires anesthesia consultation)

SEIZURES

What is the definition of a seizure?	Uncontrolled rhythmic electrical discharge within the brain that usually, but not always, results in characteristic abnormal movements of the body.
What is the general incidence of recurrent seizures?	1 to 2%
What is the cause of primary seizures (epilepsy)?	Commonly genetically determined, usually at an early age
What are some causes of secondary seizures?	Intracranial mass Vascular malformation Infections Endocrine (hypoglycemia) Electrolyte disturbances (sodium)
What are some elements in the history to obtain in a patient who presents with a seizure?	Whether the patient has a history of seizures The circumstances that led to the seizure Observed ictal behavior Identify potential triggers Loss of bladder/bowel function Current medication regimen
Define partial seizures:	Localized electrical discharge of the cerebral cortex; consciousness is often intact as it does not cross the midline of the brain.
Define the following types of partial seizures:	
Simple partial	No alteration of consciousness Symptoms based on cortex affected Visual changes if occipital area affected
Complex partial	Consciousness is impaired A simple partial with mentation affected Often due to discharge of temporal region
Partial seizure with secondary generalization	A seizure that starts localized and then spreads throughout the cerebrum Originally with localizing symptoms, then evolves into one of the types below

Define generalized seizures	Global discharge of both cerebral hemispheres that often results in loss of consciousness along with abnormal movements of the body.

Define the following types of complex seizures?

Absence (petit mal)	Typically very brief, lasting only a few seconds
	Loss of consciousness, but not postural tone
	Patient will often continue afterwards, unaware of event
	Classically affects school-aged children and may have hundreds of episodes in a day
Atonic	Less common type of seizure
	Sudden loss of postural tone
	May have brief loss of consciousness
Tonic	Less common type of seizure
	Prolonged contraction of the body
	Often will be pale and flush
Clonic	Less common type of seizure
	Repetitive clonic jerks without tonic element
Myoclonic	Less common type of seizure
	Brief and shock-like movement of extremity
	May affect entire body or just one limb
Tonic-clonic (grand mal)	Abrupt loss of consciousness
	Typically starts with tonic (rigid) phase
	Often clonic phase comes after tonic phase
	Loss of bladder/bowel function
	Consciousness returns slowly
What are important aspects of the physical exam?	Evaluation of fractures and injuries
	Particular attention to the head and spine
	Vitals as well as glucose is important
	A thorough neurological exam is crucial
What is Todd paralysis?	A focal neurological deficit that typically follows a simple-partial seizure that resolves within 48 hours

What are some other conditions that may mimic a seizure?

Syncope (may have myoclonic movements)

Neuromuscular disorders

Migraines

Narcolepsy

Pseudoseizure (underlying cause is psychiatric rather than medical)

What are four clinical features that help to distinguish seizures from other causes?

1. Inability to recall attack
2. Postictal confusion and lethargy
3. Abrupt onset
4. Purposeless movement

What are some diagnostic studies to consider in the evaluation of a seizure?

Glucose concentration

Anticonvulsant medication concentration

Chemistry panel

Complete blood count

Toxicology screen

Urinalysis

Non-contrast CT of the brain

What are some indications when to consider a non-contrast CT of the brain?

First-time seizure (absence of fever–simple febrile seizures do not require imaging which occur in the pediatric population)

Seizure pattern that is different

New focal deficits

Recent head trauma

Use of any anticoagulants

Any suspicion of meningitis

What is the role of electroencephalography (EEG) in the evaluation of seizures?

Not typically utilized in the emergency department

Typically done on outpatient basis

Can be used to classify seizure type

Important to obtain in a patient who is intubated for status epilepticus and receives a long-acting paralytic

What are some critical actions for an actively seizing patient?

Management is expectant most of the time

Most seizures self-terminate within minutes

Consider pharmacologic interventions for a prolonged seizure

Gentle firm restraint should be used

Turn to side to avoid aspiration

What is the most common reason for a seizure in a person with a seizure disorder?

Subtherapeutic anticonvulsant concentration

What is typically done for a patient with a seizure disorder who is therapeutic on anticonvulsant and still has a seizure?

If a single seizure, the focus is to identify precipitants that may have lowered the seizure threshold.

Name some commonly used anticonvulsants:

Carbamazepine

Phenytoin/Fosphenytoin

Valproic acid

What is the definition of status epilepticus?

Defined as a seizure that occurs non-stop for greater than 30 min or recurrent seizures without regaining consciousness for greater than 30 min.

What are some complications of status epilepticus?

Hypoxia

Hyperthermia

Rhabdomyolysis

Permanent neural damage

What are the three classes of medications used to treat status epilepticus?

1. Benzodiazepines
2. Phenytoin/Fosphenytoin (not efficacious for tox-related seizures)
3. Phenobarbital

What other medications should be considered in refractory cases of seizures?

Phenobarbital

Propofol

MENINGITIS

What is meningitis?

Inflammation of the leptomeninges typically from microorganisms such as bacteria and viruses but can also be from medication.

List important causes of meningitis:

Bacterial

Viral

Fungal

Tuberculosis

Table 2-1 Cerebrospinal Fluid (CSF)

	Normal	Viral	Bacterial	TB	Fungal
Protein (mg/dL)	<55	<200	>200	>200	>200
Glucose (mg/dL)	>40	>40	<40	<40	<40
WBCs (cells/μL)	<5	<1000	>1000	<1000	<500
Gram stain	negative	negative	positive	negative	negative
Opening pressure (mm CSF)	<170	~200	>300	~200	~300

WBC, white blood cell

What is important to know about meningitis?	One of the top 10 infectious causes of death
	Causes over 100,000 deaths worldwide
	80% of cases are caused by either *Streptococcus pneumoniae* or *Neisseria meningitides*
	Main cause was *H influenza*, prior to HIB vaccine
What is the mortality of a missed diagnosis of bacterial meningitis?	15 to 50%
What are the top three causes of meningitis:	Depends on the age group
In infants	*Streptococcous pneumoniae*
	Group B streptococcous infection
	E coli
	Listeria monocytogenes
In young adults	*S pneumoniae*
	N meningitidis
	H influenza (No longer common cause after introduction of HIB vaccine)
In people over 60	*S pneumoniae*
	Listeria monocytogenes
	N meningitidis/group B streptococcous infection
	H influenza

In nosocomial infections	*Pseudomonas aeruginosa* Other gram negatives *Staphylococcus aureus*
What are some risk factors for meningitis?	Colonization of the nasopharynx Bacteremia (endocarditis/UTI) Contiguous source (mastoid/sinus) Living in a dormitory or barracks
What are some host factors that can predispose to meningitis?	Asplenia HIV Complement deficiency Long-term steroid use
What is the classic triad of meningitis?	Fever Nuchal rigidity Mental status change
What are some other signs and symptoms of meningitis?	Headache Significant photophobia Nausea and vomiting Seizures and focal neurological deficits Rash (purpura of DIC secondary to *N meningitidis*, or viral exanthem)
What is Kernig sign?	Inability to extend patient's knee due to pain when leg is flexed with hip at 90°.
What is Brudzinski sign?	Passive flexion of the patient's neck causes flexion of both hips.
Name two important diagnostic tests to obtain when evaluating meningitis:	1. Lumbar puncture 2. Non-contrast CT of the brain
What is the reason a non-contrast CT of the brain is done prior to a lumbar puncture?	A lumbar puncture in the presence of increased intracranial pressure may be fatal if herniation occurs
What are some considerations in the management of meningitis?	Empirical treatment should not be withheld for diagnostic tests Always maintain a high index of suspicion Do not wait for CT→LP to start treatment (particular if testing will take over an hour)

What empiric treatment is commonly used?	Ceftriaxone (High dose such as 2 grams for blood brain penetration)
	Vancomycin
	Ampicillin
	Acyclovir
When is chemoprophylaxis indicated?	High-risk contacts of patients with *N meningitides* or *H influenzae* type B.
What is the drug of choice for chemoprophylaxis?	Rifampin
What role do steroids play in meningitis?	Should be given before or with the first dose of antibiotics, mostly beneficial in pneumococcal meningitis which may help to reduce neurologic sequelae.

CEREBROVASCULAR ACCIDENT

Name some important causes of a cerebrovascular accident and some examples:

Ischemic stroke	Embolic
	Emboli from the heart (ie, atrial fibrillation)
	Endocarditis
	Plaques from large vessels (ie, carotid)
Thrombotic	Atherosclerosis
	Sickle cell disease
	Mycotic aneurysms
	Hypercoagulable states
	Vasculitis
Hemorrhagic stroke	Trauma
	AV malformation
	Bleeding disorders
	Spontaneous rupture of berry aneurysm
	Transformation of an ischemic stroke

Table 2-2 NIH Stroke Scale

Category	Patient Response and Score
1. a. Level of consciousness:	0 Alert
	1 Not alert, but arousable with minimal stimulation
	2 Not alert, but requires repeated stimulation
	3 Coma
1. b. Ask patient the month and age:	0 Answers both questions correctly
	1 Answers one question correctly
	2 Both questions answered incorrectly
1. c. Ask patient to open and close eyes and fist:	0 Obeys both correctly
	1 Obeys one correctly
	2 Does not obey either commands
2. Best gaze:	0 Normal
	1 Partial gaze palsy
	2 Forced deviation
3. Vision field testing:	0 No visual field loss
	1 Partial hemianopia
	2 Complete hemianopia
	3 Bilateral hemianopia
4. Facial paresis:	0 Normal symmetrical movement
	1 Minor paralysis
	2 Partial paralysis
	3 Complete paralysis of one or both sides of the face
5. Motor function—arm: right arm_____ left arm_____	0 Normal
	1 Drift
	2 Some effort against gravity
	3 No effort against gravity
	4 No movement
6. Motor function—leg: right leg_____ left leg_____	0 Normal
	1 Drift
	2 Some effort against gravity
	3 No effort against gravity
	4 No movement

(Continued)

Table 2-2 NIH Stroke Scale (*Continued*)

Category	Patient Response and Score
7. Limb ataxia:	0 No ataxia
	1 Present in one limb
	2 Present in two limbs
8. Sensory:	0 Normal
	1 Mild to moderate decrease in sensations
	2 Severe to total loss of sensation
9. Best language: look at pictures and read words	0 No aphasia
	1 Mild to moderate aphasia
	2 Severe aphasia
	3 Mute
10. Dysarthria: read several words	0 Normal articulation
	1 Mild to moderate slurring of words
	2 Unintelligible or unable to speak
11. Extinction and inattention:	0 Normal
	1 Inattention/extinction to bilateral simultaneous stimulation
	2 Severe hemi-inattention to more than one modality

National Institute of Neurological Disorders and Stroke Health

What is the NIH stroke scale?

Objective way to rapidly assess and determine the extent of neurologic deficits of a stroke patient and helps to determine if thrombolytics are needed.

What are some important things to note about the posterior circulation?

Originates from the vertebrobasilar arteries

Supplies 20% of cerebral blood flow

The following structures are supplied:

Brainstem

Upper spinal cord

Medial portion of temporal lobe

Cerebellum

Thalamus

Occipital lobe

What are some important things to note about the anterior circulation?

Originates from the carotid arteries

Supplies 80% of cerebral blood flow

The following structures are supplied:

Anterior portion of temporal lobe

Frontoparietal lobes

Optic nerve and retina

What is the Circle of Willis?

Circle of arteries that supply the brain

Creates redundancies in the cerebral circulation so if one vessel is blocked, blood flow from other vessels can maintain perfusion

List some risk factors for a cerebrovascular accident:

Transient ischemic attack

Hypertension

Cardiac disease

Diabetes

Atherosclerosis

Erythrocytosis

Dyslipidemia

What are some other conditions that may mimic a stroke?

Migraines

Hypoglycemia

Hepatic encephalopathy

Seizures

What is the definition of a transient ischemic attack?

Blood supply to a part of the brain is briefly interrupted, resulting in a transient stroke that lasts only a few minutes, but may persist up to 24 hours.

What is the clinical significance of a transient ischemic attack?

"Red flag" of an impending stroke in evolution.

What are some signs and symptoms for the following stroke syndrome based on the occluded vessel:

Middle cerebral artery (MCA)

Contralateral hemiplegia/hemianesthesia

Upper extremity deficit more severe than lower extremity deficit

Gaze preference toward the affected side

Aphasia (dominant hemisphere affected)

Constructional apraxia/agnosia (non-dominant hemisphere affected)

Posterior cerebral artery (PCA)	Ipsilateral cranial nerve (CN) III nerve palsy
	Contralateral homonymous hemianopsia, hemisensory loss, and hemiparesis
Anterior cerebral artery (ACA)	Contralateral foot, leg, and arm paralysis
	Lower extremity deficit more severe than upper extremity deficit
	Frontal lobe disinhibition (ie, abulia)
Cerebellar infarct	Nausea, vomiting, ataxia, vertigo, lateralizing dysmetria, and nystagmus
Basilar artery	Quadriplegia: severe bilateral signs
	Coma: "Locked-in syndrome"—no motor function except upward gaze of eyes

What is an important consideration in a stroke patient with a depressed level of consciousness?

Airway management

Although hypertension is commonly associated with cerebrovascular accident, should it be treated in the emergency department?

Generally not—lowering the blood pressure aggressively may worsen the stroke

What is an important diagnostic test to obtain early in the evaluation of a stroke patient?

ECG

What is the initial diagnostic test of choice to obtain in an emergent stroke?

Non-contrast CT of the brain

What are some possible findings on a CT brain that may be seen in a stroke?

Hyperdense artery sign (acute thrombus in a vessel)

Loss of gray-white interface

Sulcal effacement

Acute hypodensity

What are the advantages in using an MRI to evaluate a stroke?

May identify infarcts earlier

Accurately evaluate acute posterior circulation strokes

What is diffusion-weighted imaging (DWI) and perfusion-weighted imaging (PWI)?

MRI techniques that allow differentiation between irreversible and reversible neuronal injury.

What therapeutic option is available for patients who present with an ischemic stroke within three hours?

Thrombolysis

List three thrombolytics available for use:

Alteplase (Activase)

Reteplase (Retavase)

Tenecteplase (TNKase)

What CT findings are associated with an increased risk of an intracranial hemorrhage from use of thrombolytics?

Mass effect

Acute hypodensity

What are some important guidelines in determining if a patient is a candidate for thrombolytic therapy?

If symptom onset is within 3 hours

Significant neurologic deficit (NIH >20 may be associated with increased risk of ICH)

Recommended blood pressure limits

No contraindications

List some contraindications regarding the use of thrombolytics in acute stroke:

History of structural CNS disease

Systolic pressure >180 mm Hg

Significant head trauma in <3 months

History of intracranial hemorrhage

Recent trauma >6 weeks

Recent GI/GU bleeding

VERTIGO

Table 2-3 Central Versus Peripheral Vertigo

	Central	Peripheral
Onset	Slow (can be sudden)	Sudden
Severity	Vague	Intense
Nystagmus	Vertical	Horizontal-rotatory
Auditory symptoms	No	Can have Sx
Pattern	Constant	Intermittent
CNS symptoms	Yes	No
Prognosis	Usually serious	Usually benign

What is the definition of vertigo?

Sensation of movement of oneself or the surrounding area most often described as a feeling of spinning.

What is the pathophysiology of peripheral vertigo?

Disorders of the ear or cranial nerve VIII

How much does peripheral vertigo account for all cases of vertigo?

85%

What are some signs and symptoms of peripheral vertigo?

Sudden onset of intense sensation of intermittent disequilibrium

Nausea and vomiting

Hearing loss/tinnitus common

Nystagmus

What are some important causes of peripheral vertigo?

Benign positional vertigo (BPV)

Ototoxic drugs

Otitis media

Menière disease

What is the Dix-Hallpike maneuver?

Used to diagnose and treat BPV

What are some key steps in the Dix-Hallpike maneuver?

Sit with patient's legs extended on the examination table; patient is brought rapidly from sitting to supine, head slightly extended below horizontal, and then head is rotated to right and left quickly

What are some treatment options for peripheral vertigo?

Antihistamine

Antiemetics

Anticholinergics

Benzodiazepines in severe cases

Despite intense symptoms of peripheral vertigo, do patients typically require admission?

No—usually can treat on outpatient basis with referral to ENT clinic.

What is the pathophysiology of central vertigo?

Commonly due to lesions of the cerebellum or brainstem.

What are some signs and symptoms of central vertigo?

Mild, but constant disequilibrium that may present acutely, nausea/vomiting, vertical nystagmus, and often will have associated CNS symptoms.

What are some CNS symptoms that can be associated with central vertigo?

Lateralizing dysmetria

Ataxia

Dysarthria

Scotomata

Blindness

What are some important causes of central vertigo?

Multiple sclerosis

Cerebellar tumors

Brainstem infarct

Vertebrobasilar insufficiency

What is the disposition of patients with central vertigo?

Often requires admission for further evaluation.

PERIPHERAL NEUROLOGIC LESIONS

Table 2-4 Muscles and Motor Function

Upper extremities	Deltoid	C5 C6	Hand extensors	C6 C7
	Biceps	C5 C6	Finger extensors	C7 C8
	Triceps	C6 C7 C8	Finger flexors	C7 C8 T1
Lower extremities	Quadriceps	L2 L3 L4	Dorsiflexors	L5
	Iliopsoas	L2 L3 L4	Big toe extensors	L4 L5 S1
	Gluteal	L5 S1	Plantar flexors	S1 S2
	Anterior tibial	L4 L5	Toe extensors	L5 S1
Reflexes	Supinator	C5 C6	Knee	L3 L4
	Biceps	C5 C6	Tibialis post	L5
	Triceps	C7 C8	Ankle	S1 S2

Myopathies and Myelopathies

What are some defining features of myopathies?

Proximal weakness (ie, standing up)

Deep tendon reflexes are typically intact

No alterations in sensation

Often have abnormal laboratory test results (ie, CPK, sedimentation rate, and elevated WBC)

What are some signs and symptoms for the following types of common myopathies:

Steroid myopathy

Long-term steroid use that is associated with muscle weakness and pain

Polymyositis	Acute inflammation often leads to proximal muscles weakness and pain
	Often have elevated CPK
	Patients can also have low-grade fever
Hypokalemic myopathy	Typically due to renal tubular acidosis
	Toluene abuse (glue sniffing)
	Fanconi syndrome

What are some clinical features for the following types of myelopathies:

Multiple sclerosis	Demyelinating disorder thought to be autoimmune in origin
	Often have spinal cord involvement that results in upper motor neurons (UMNs) signs and bladder/bowel dysfunction
	Corticosteroids often used for exacerbations
Syringomyelia	Cyst forms within the spinal cord and over time destroys the center of the spinal cord
	Sensory disruption, especially the bilateral upper extremities (cape like distribution)
	Can adversely affect sweating, sexual function, and bladder/bowel control
Epidural mass	Can be due to abscesses, metastatic tumor, and epidural hemorrhage
	Commonly severe pain and signs of cord compression (ie, sensory alterations)
Dorsal column disorders	Commonly due to B$_{12}$ deficiency or syphilis (tabes dorsalis)
	Loss of position sense, vibration, and light touch

Neuromuscular Junction

What is the most common disorder of the neuromuscular junction?	Myasthenia gravis
What is myasthenia gravis?	Auto-immune destruction of acetylcholine receptors leading to a chronic neuromuscular disease characterized by varying degrees of weakness of the skeletal muscles with no sensory involvement.

What is the hallmark of myasthenia gravis?

Weakness that is typically first evident in the eyelids and extraocular muscles followed by generalized weakness of the limbs.

What are some ways that myasthenia gravis can be diagnosed?

Electromyogram

Serology (used with clinical picture)

Edrophonium test (giving a short acting acetylcholine esterase inhibitor temporarily resolves symptoms—use with caution as it may precipitate a cholinergic crisis)

What are some treatment options in myasthenia gravis?

Pyridostigmine

Prednisone

IV gamma globulin

Thymectomy

What is the most important complication to consider in myasthenia gravis?

Respiratory failure requiring intubation.

What is myasthenic crisis?

Severe weakness from acquired myasthenia gravis that is severe enough to require intubation often due to dysfunctional deficiency of acetylcholine.

What is the treatment of choice for myasthenic crisis?

Intravenous immunoglobulin G

Plasmapheresis

What other crisis can also occur with myasthenia gravis?

Cholinergic crisis

How does cholinergic crisis commonly occur?

When too much acetylcholinesterase inhibitors are used that result in an excess of acetylcholine.

What are some signs and symptoms of a cholinergic crisis?

Often cholinergic with muscarinic effects such as excessive salivation and urination along with severe muscle weakness and possible respiratory failure.

What treatment is commonly used for a cholinergic crisis?

Atropine

What is Eaton-Lambert syndrome?

Pre-synaptic disorder of neuromuscular transmission defined by impaired release of acetylcholine (ACh) that causes proximal muscle weakness, depressed tendon reflexes, and autonomic changes.

What disease does Eaton-Lambert syndrome have a high association with?	Lung cancer
What are other important differentials to consider in patients with generalized weakness?	Tick paralysis Botulism Amyotrophic lateral sclerosis (ALS) Organophosphate poisoning

Neuropathies

What is the definition of a neuropathy?	Disorders of peripheral nerves
What are the three types of nerves that make up the peripheral nervous system (PNS)?	1. Motor nerves 2. Sensory nerves 3. Autonomic nerves
What are some signs and symptoms of peripheral neuropathies?	Mixed sensory/motor involvement typical Reflexes usually absent Impairment is typically symmetrical/distal
What disorders are commonly associated with peripheral neuropathies?	Diabetes Uremia Cancer Hypothyroidism Tick paralysis Guillain-Barré syndrome
What toxins are also commonly associated with peripheral neuropathies?	Organophosphates Tetanus Heavy metals (ie, lead) Ethanol

LOWER BACK PAIN

What are some important things to know about lower back pain?	Up to 80% of the population have experienced lower back pain Lower back pain is more prevalent between the ages of 20 and 40 years Lower back pain in elderly patients is more concerning

What are red flags in the history of a patient that presents with lower back pain?

Age >50 years

History of cancer

Constitutional symptoms: fever, weight loss, etc.

Intravenous drug abuse (IVDA)

Recent instrumentation

Incontinence

Focal neurologic deficits

What are some findings on physical exam that is more concerning for serious pathology?

Positive straight leg raise

Neurological deficit

Any midline vertebral point tenderness

What are some physical exam findings of the affected nerve roots:

L3/L4

Diminished or absent knee jerk

Weakness in the quadriceps

Anteromedial thigh and knee pain

L5

There is usually no reflex loss

Foot drop common

S1

Ankle jerk is often diminished or absent

There may be weakness of toe flexors

Leg pain is often worse than LBP

What is straight leg raising?

Stretching of impinged nerve roots that may cause radiating pain

What is the most common cause of back pain?

Strain of soft tissue elements in the back

What is sciatica?

Pain radiating from back down lower extremity in a dermatomal distribution typically from nerve root impingement.

What are some common causes of sciatica?

Herniated disc

Tumor

Infection

Hematoma compression

Spinal stenosis

How long does it typically take for non-specific lower back pain to resolve?

Within a month

What are some options in the management of non-specific lower back pain?

Appropriate analgesia

Activity as tolerated

Discourage bed rest

Muscle relaxants if needed

Is imaging always required to evaluate non-specific back pain?

No—unless there are concerning elements in the history or physical.

What are some imaging tests to consider in lower back pain?

Plain spinal films—concern of fracture

CT—superior for vertebral fractures

MRI—for emergent conditions

List some laboratory tests obtained for lower back pain that are possibly caused by an infection or tumor:

Complete blood count

ESR/C-reactive protein (CRP)

Urinalysis

What are some important features in each of the "can't miss" diagnosis?

   Metastasis

Often older than 50 with hx of cancer

Often >1 month of weight loss and LBP

Often requires a variety of imaging tests

   Spinal epidural abscess

Immunocompromised and IVDA at risk

Often have fever and local spine tenderness

Focal neurological deficit not uncommon

Broad-spectrum Abx/neurosurgery consult

   Disc herniation

Common in >30 years with progressive LBP; sciatica and L4-L5 involvement common; treat conservatively; neurosurgery consult if evidence of cord compression

   Vertebral fracture

Often history of trauma or mets; sudden onset of pain and neurologic logic deficits; imaging is important for further evaluation

   Cauda equina syndrome

Often in those with mets or hx of trauma; incontinence/saddle paresthesias common; MRI test of choice; neurological emergency

SYNCOPE

What is the definition of syncope?	Abrupt/transient loss of consciousness associated with absence of postural tone, followed by a rapid and usually complete recovery.

List important conditions that should be considered for each category:

Cardiovascular	Dysrhythmias; obstruction (ie, aortic stenosis); myocardial infarction
Neurologic	Seizure; subarachnoid hemorrhage; posterior circulation infarct
Medication	Diuretics; beta-blockers; nitrates
Miscellaneous	Vasovagal; carotid sinus hypersensitivity

What are important elements in the history to gather to help determine cause of syncope?	Events prior to the episode; any associated pain (HA/chest/abdominal pain); diaphoresis and emesis; exertion; dyspnea
What are some findings to look for on physical exam?	Carotid bruits; cardiac murmurs; evidence of bleeding (ie, GI bleed); pulsatile abdominal mass; adnexal tenderness (ie, ectopic)

What is an important diagnosis to consider in the following scenario of a patient who presents with syncope and the following associated symptom:

A 21-year-old healthy male presents to the ED after passing out during soccer practice. Family history is significant for an uncle who died from sudden death at 27	Hypertrophic cardiomyopathy
A 31-year-old female presents to the ED after a syncopal episode while taking care of her kids. Her physical exam is significant only for right adnexal tenderness	Ectopic pregnancy
A 17-year-old female with no past medical history presents to the ED after passing out while giving blood at Red Cross. Observers noted she seemed diaphoretic and nauseous prior to passing out	Vasovagal

A 65-year-old male with history of hypertension, dyslipidemia, and CAD presents after passing out. His physical exam is significant for abdominal tenderness and bruits	Abdominal aortic aneurysm
A 24-year-old female is brought in by emergency medical service (EMS) when she was observed to pass out at the mall soon followed by rhythmic movements of her extremities. Physical exam is significant for lateral tongue bites	Seizure
A 62-year-old male is brought from home by his wife after he passed out. His history is only significant for HTN and DM. She mentioned he seemed diaphoretic prior to the event and also missed breakfast	Hypoglycemia
What are some considerations in the evaluation of syncope?	To separate benign from serious causes; a careful history and physical is paramount; initial ECG is also the mainstay in evaluation
What is an important point to keep in mind about syncope?	Although most cases of syncope are benign, syncope may be an initial symptom of something life-threatening such as AAA or SAH.
What patients are often admitted for syncope?	Elderly patients with many comorbidities; syncope with worse HA, pelvic pain, etc.; risk for fall and injury (typically elderly)
Which patients are typically safe to discharge?	No evidence of structural heart defects Isolated episode of syncope

CLINICAL VIGNETTES—MAKE THE DIAGNOSIS

60-year-old man presents with loss of short-term memory, urinary incontinence, and dementia; PE: wide-based gait; CT brain: massively dilated ventricular space

Normal pressure hydrocephalus

51-year-old man with PMH of heart disease presents with a sudden onset of left-sided extremity weakness that has not resolved; PE: flaccidity of left arms and leg along with Babinski (+) on left; CT brain: normal

Cerebrovascular accident (Right MCA)

27-year-old woman with hx of gastroenteritis 1 week ago now presents with symmetric ascending weakness of her legs and paresthesias; PE: diminished reflexes; LP: above normal protein

Guillain-Barré syndrome

58-year-old woman with an hx of breast cancer presents with radicular pain of her legs, urinary retention, and lower back pain; PE: saddle anesthesia and absent ankle jerk reflexes

Cauda equine syndrome

18-year-old woman presents with slow onset of paresthesias, diplopia, numbness of left upper extremity; MRI: discrete areas of periventricular demyelination

Multiple sclerosis

21-year-old man with a long hx of headaches presents with a unilateral headache, nausea, vomiting, and photophobia that typically occurs during her menstrual period

Migraine headache—common

21-year-old woman presents with a headache, nausea, and vomiting soon after being struck in the side of the head during a bar fight but then losses consciousness while in the ED; CT brain: lens-shaped, left-sided hyperdense mass near the temporal bone

Epidural hematoma

61-year-old man with an hx of colon cancer presents with an insidious onset of disequilibrium and dizziness that has been present for months; PE: vertical nystagmus and ataxia

Central vertigo

41-year-old man with a long hx of alcohol abuse presents with confusion, ataxia, and difficulty seeing; MRI brain: mamillary body atrophy and diffuse cortical atrophy

Wernicke encephalopathy

21-year-old college student presents with a high-grade fever, headache, and neck stiffness; PE: Kernig sign and nuchal rigidity; LP: decreased glucose, increased protein, and high polymorphonuclear leukocytes

Bacterial meningitis

12-year-old boy is referred to the ED from school due to frequent brief lapses of consciousness with slight limb jerking; PE: during exam, patient again has his brief lapse of consciousness with rapid eye-blinking

Absence seizure (petit mal)

67-year-old woman presents with a gradual decline in memory and having increasing difficulties with normal day-to-day routine, often getting lost when she walks back home; CT brain: diffuse cortical atrophy

Alzheimer disease

25-year-old man presents with unilateral periorbital headache with periods of multiple headaches alternating with symptom-free intervals; PE: ipsilateral tearing and conjunctival injection

Cluster headache

CHAPTER 3

Ophthalmologic Emergencies

BASIC OPHTHALMOLOGY

What are the two chambers of the aqueous part of the eye called?
1. Anterior chamber
2. Posterior chamber

What is the jelly-like substance in the back part of the eyeball which provides shape and is relatively inert?
Vitreous humor

What are some components that make up the anterior segment of the eye?
Cornea; conjunctiva; anterior chamber; lens; iris; ciliary body

What components make up the fundus of the eye?
Macula; optic nerve; retina

Please define the following forms:

Anisocoria
Unequal pupil size under equal lighting

Hyphema
Red blood cells in the anterior chamber

Hypopyon
White blood cells in the anterior chamber

Limbus
Circumferential border of the cornea and white sclera

Tonopen
Pen-shaped device to measure intraocular pressure

What are some important elements in the history that should be obtained in any general eye exam?
History of diabetes or hypertension; use of contact lenses (ie, extended wear); past visual acuity; occupation; any prior ocular procedure

What are eight components of the eye exam that should be obtained with all eye complaints?	1. Visual acuity (most important!) 2. External eye 3. Pupils 4. Confrontation of visual fields 5. Extraocular movement 6. Fundus examination 7. Anterior segment 8. Intraocular pressure

TRAUMA OF THE EYE

Corneal Foreign Bodies

What is important to confirm during examination of the eye with regards to a foreign body?	Assess superficial penetration versus full-thickness injury
What is the best way to assess foreign body depth in the emergency department (ED)?	Slit-lamp exam
Can a superficial corneal foreign body be removed in the ED?	Yes—under best magnification available
What are some key steps in the removal of a superficial corneal foreign body?	Instill topical anesthetics in both eyes; use slit-lamp magnification; can use a 30-gauge needle to remove or a moistened cotton-tipped applicator; most superficial objects can be removed
What are some key steps in the removal of a full-thickness foreign body?	Do not remove in the ED—should be done by ophthalmology
What is an additional concern if a foreign body is metallic?	Metallic bodies can leave behind rust rings that are toxic to the cornea.
Should rust rings be removed in the ED?	Can be removed with an ophthalmic burr, but only the superficial layer.
A corneal abrasion will be present after foreign body removal, what are some treatments for it?	Antibiotic ointment; cycloplegia; referral to ophthalmology

Corneal Abrasions

What should always be done as part of an eye exam with corneal abrasions?	Check under the eyelids
What is usually done for conjunctival abrasions?	Erythromycin drops (ointment); ensure no other ocular injuries
What are some signs and symptoms of corneal abrasions?	Photophobia, tearing, and eye pain
What are two common causes of corneal abrasions?	1. Trauma 2. Use of contact lenses
What is typically a limiting factor to do a complete eye exam?	Patient is typically in extreme discomfort
What is an effective way to reduce pain?	Adequate cycloplegia, topical anesthetic
What is the optimal way to visualize corneal abrasions?	Fluorescein staining with cobalt-blue lighting
What is an effective long-acting cycloplegia for large or very painful abrasions?	Scopolamine
What are some considerations in the management of corneal abrasions?	Adequate pain control with cycloplegias; antibiotic drops; abrasion typically heal without problems
What is a particular concern of corneal abrasions from contacts?	*Pseudomonas* infections
What other antibiotic ointment should be added if concerned about *Pseudomonas* infection?	Tobramycin or fluoroquinolone drops
Should patients be sent home with topical anesthetics for pain control?	No—can cause corneal toxicity if improperly dosed and can also erode the cornea

Subconjunctival Hemorrhage

What is the mechanism by which a subconjunctival hemorrhage occurs?	Rupture of conjunctival vessels

What are some common causes of a subconjunctival hemorrhage?	Trauma; hypertension; sudden valsalva (ie, coughing)
What is the treatment of choice for a subconjunctival hemorrhage?	Nothing—will resolve in 1 to 2 weeks

Chemical Injuries

What is the most important point to remember about ocular chemical injuries?	True ocular emergency
What is considered a more devastating injury: acidic or alkali?	Alkali burns as they penetrate deeper
What are some common causes of alkali burns?	Ammonia; lye; industrial solvents
What is the immediate management of ocular chemical injuries?	Topical anesthetic; placement of Morgan lens; copious irrigation with 1 to 2 L of normal saline
When should the copious irrigation be stopped?	Once pH of the tears is near normal (7.5–8)—can use litmus paper before and after irrigation
What are some long-term complications of chemical burns?	Symblepharon; cataracts; scarring/ neovascularization of the cornea
When should patients be referred to ophthalmology?	Corneal clouding; epithelial defect
Assuming there are no corneal clouding or anterior chamber findings, what is the general disposition?	Erythromycin drops; cycloplegics for pain control; ophthalmologic follow-up within 2 days

Blunt Injuries

What is important to assess after blunt injury to the eye?	Vision and globe integrity
What is an important diagnosis to consider in any blunt trauma to the eye?	Ruptured globe

What are some signs and symptoms of a ruptured globe?	Obvious full-thickness laceration, blindness, flat anterior chamber, irregular pupil, and hyphema
What is important not to do during an eye exam if a ruptured globe is suspected?	Checking intraocular pressure (IOP)
What are some considerations in the management of a ruptured globe?	Avoid any pressure on the globe; place a metal eye shield; update tetanus status; consider antibiotic use depending on object; emergent consultation with ophthalmology
What is a hyphema?	Blood in the anterior chamber of the eye
What are some common causes of hyphema?	Trauma (blunt or penetrating); spontaneous (esp. sickle-cell disease)
What vessel is typically responsible for a hyphema?	Iris root vessel
What is also important to assess in a patient with a hyphema?	Any other associated trauma such as a ruptured globe
Why is it recommended to dilate the pupil?	To avoid pupillary movement which may increase bleeding from an iris root vessel
What is an important complication of hyphema?	Increased IOP
What is the general disposition of patients with hyphema?	Consultation with ophthalmology; elevate patient's head; administer dilating agent (ie, atropine); treat significant IOP increase; also protect eye from further trauma
How is increased IOP typically treated?	Topical beta-blocker; topical alpha-adrenergic agonists; intravenous mannitol
What is an important diagnosis to consider in a patient with blunt trauma and inability to gaze upward?	Orbital blowout fracture
What is the most frequent site of an orbital blowout fracture?	Inferior-medial wall

How is the diagnosis of an orbital blowout fracture made?	CT (axial and coronal scans)
What is the general disposition of an isolated orbital blowout fracture?	Referral for surgery within 3 to 9 days (if no ocular involvement)
What are other important injuries to examine for with orbital blowout fractures?	Hyphema; abrasions; traumatic iritis; retinal detachment

INFECTIONS OF THE EYE

Conjunctivitis

What is the common element in the history of a patient with viral conjunctivitis?	Preceding upper respiratory infection
What are some signs and symptoms of viral conjunctivitis?	May initially have one eye involvement with watery discharge, reddened conjunctiva, and often normal cornea
What is the primary reason the cornea should be stained?	Avoid missing a herpes dendritic keratitis
What are some considerations in the management of viral conjunctivitis?	Typically self-limiting (1–3 weeks); highly contagious; naphcon-A for congestion/itching; consider topical antibiotic in suspected bacterial conjunctivitis
What are some signs and symptoms of bacterial conjunctivitis?	Mucopurulent discharge, inflammation of eye, and often a history of exposure to someone with viral conjunctivitis
What should be done to avoid missing a corneal abrasion or ulcer?	Fluorescein staining
What is the treatment of choice for patients with bacterial conjunctivitis?	Broad-spectrum topical antibiotic
What is a special consideration for contact lens-wearing patients with bacterial conjunctivitis?	*Pseudomonas* infection
What topical antibiotic should be used for contact lens-wearers with bacterial conjunctivitis?	Topical aminoglycoside or fluoroquinolone

What parts of the eye can be affected by herpes simplex virus (HSV)?	Conjunctiva; cornea; lids
What does fluorescein staining typically show with HSV involvement of the eye?	Linear branching pattern with terminal bulbs
What is an important concern with HSV keratitis?	Corneal scarring
What should be avoided with HSV keratitis?	Topical steroids
How is HSV keratitis commonly treated?	Viroptic drops (ie, longer if cornea involved); erythromycin drops to avoid secondary bacterial involvement
What is herpes zoster ophthalmicus (HZO)?	Shingles of CNV with involvement of eye
What is Hutchinson sign?	Cutaneous lesions on the tip of the nose
What are some signs and symptoms of HZO?	Iritis with pain and photophobia with possible cutaneous lesions
How is HZO commonly treated?	Topical steroids for iritis; topical cycloplegic agents for pain; consider IV acyclovir; distinguish from primary HSV infection

Corneal Ulcer

What is a corneal ulcer?	Serious infection involving multiple layers of the cornea
What is the pathophysiology of a corneal ulcer?	Break in the epithelial layer that allows bacteria to invade the corneal stroma
What are some causes of corneal epithelial break?	Trauma; contact lenses; incomplete lid closure
What are some signs and symptoms of a corneal ulcer?	Eye pain, photophobia, tearing, and redness
What does a slit-lamp exam commonly reveal in a corneal ulcer?	Staining shows epithelial defect with underlying infiltrate as well as possible hypopyon

How corneal ulcers are commonly treated?	Topical aminoglycoside or fluoroquinolone; topical cycloplegic for pain; ophthalmology follow-up within 24 hours

Periorbital/Orbital Cellulitis

What is periorbital cellulitis?	Superficial cellulitis of the periorbital area
What are some signs and symptoms of periorbital cellulitis?	Surrounding area of the eye (ie, eyelid) is red, warm, and edematous with no involvement of the eye itself
What is the most common organism involved with periorbital cellulitis?	*Staphylococcus aureus*
What is the typical management for periorbital cellulitis without eye involvement?	Oral antibiotic is sufficient
What is a special concern of periorbital cellulitis in young children?	High risk of bacteremia and meningitis
What are some considerations in the management of young children with periorbital cellulitis?	Full evaluation with Abx and blood cultures (**Must differentiate** between pre-septal cellulitis vs orbital cellulitis)
What is orbital cellulitis?	Potentially life-threatening orbital infection that lies deep to the orbital septum
What are some common organisms to consider in orbital cellulitis?	*S aureus; H influenzae* (in children); mucormycosis (in immunocompromised patients)
What is the most common source of orbital cellulitis?	Paranasal sinus
What are some signs and symptoms of orbital cellulitis?	Fever, pain, extraocular muscle (EOM) impairment, proptosis, decreased visual acuity
What are some considerations in the management of orbital cellulitis?	Admission for full evaluation; CT scan of orbital/nasal area; IV antibiotics

Hordeolum

What is an external hordeolum (stye)?	Acute infection of an oil gland associated with an eyelash
What is the most common organism involved with a stye?	*S aureus*
What is the typical appearance of a stye?	A small pustule at the lash line
What is the treatment of a stye?	Warm compresses with erythromycin ointment
What is an internal hordeolum known as?	Chalazion
What is a chalazion?	Acute or chronic inflammation of the eyelid commonly due to blockage of an oil gland
What is the appearance of a chalazion?	Tender red lump at the lid, cystic mass can occur with recurrent chronic inflammation
What is the treatment of an acute chalazion?	Warm compresses with erythromycin ointment; consider doxycycline if chronic inflammation

ACUTE VISUAL LOSS

Central Retinal Artery Occlusion

What vessel provides blood supply to the inner retina?	Central retinal artery from the ophthalmic artery
What are some signs and symptoms of central retinal artery occlusion (CRAO)?	Sudden, **painless**, and profound monocular loss of vision
What is a possible warning symptom of a CRAO?	Amaurosis fugax
What is the definition of amaurosis fugax?	Loss of vision in one eye caused by a temporary lack of blood flow to the retina

What are some important causes of CRAO?

Giant cell arteritis; embolus; sickle-cell disease; thrombosis; trauma

What is the most common cause of CRAO?

Embolus (ie, atrial fibrillation)

How long does it take before irreversible damage to the retina can occur?

60 to 90 minutes

What is the main focus in treatment of CRAO?

Dislodging the embolus

What are some considerations in the management of CRAO?

Initiate treatment as rapidly as possible; ocular massage (attempt to dislodge the embolus); acetazolamide and topical beta-blockers; immediate ophthalmology consultation—newer treatment options include use of thrombolytics through interventional

Central Retinal Vein Occlusion

What is typically the mechanism of central retinal vein occlusion (CRVO)?

Thrombosis of the central retinal vein

Name some conditions that are associated with CRVO:

Glaucoma; hypertension; hypercoagulable disorders

What are some signs and symptoms of CRVO?

Acute, **painless**, and monocular involvement with variable vision loss

What is the typical funduscopic finding in CRVO?

Diffuse retinal hemorrhage in all quadrants; optic disc edema

What is the typical treatment option for CRVO?

Ophthalmology consultation; may consider giving aspirin

Narrow-Angle Glaucoma

Is a history of glaucoma common in patients who present with narrow-angle glaucoma?

No—patients will typically have an undiagnosed narrow anterior chamber angle

What is the mechanism by which aqueous humor is produced?	Aqueous humor is produced in the ciliary body from the posterior chamber which flows through the pupil and into the anterior chamber, where it is reabsorbed
What is the pathophysiology of narrow-angle glaucoma?	When the pupil becomes mid-dilated, the lens touches the iris leaflet, blocking the flow of aqueous humor and causing an increase in IOP, causing the cornea to become edematous and distorted
What are some signs and symptoms of narrow-angle glaucoma?	Headache, eye ache, cloudy vision, nausea/vomiting, and increased IOP
How high can the IOP be in narrow-angle glaucoma?	Higher then 50 mmHg
What is the typical finding on exam of the pupil?	Mid-dilated and non-reactive
What is the focus of treating narrow-angle glaucoma?	Quickly lowering IOP and decrease production of aqueous humor
What are some agents commonly used to suppress aqueous humor production?	Topical beta-blockers and alpha-agonists; acetazolamide
What is another agent to consider that is effective in lowering IOP?	Mannitol
What agent is commonly used to constrict the pupil once the IOP has been reduced?	Pilocarpine (will not typically work during an acute attack)
What is the definitive treatment for narrow-angle glaucoma?	Peripheral laser iridectomy

Optic Neuritis

What is optic neuritis?	Optic nerve dysfunction that is the most common cause of acute reduction of vision
What are some causes of optic neuritis?	Ischemia; embolus; nerve compression; multiple sclerosis (MS); lupus
What are some signs and symptoms of optic neuritis?	Rapid and painful reduction of visual acuity, but more commonly affects color vision and afferent pupillary defect

What test is useful to detect alteration in color vision?	Red desaturation test
How is the red desaturation test carried out?	Have the patient look at a red object with each eye individually, the affected eye will often see the red object as pink or lighter
What is a possible finding on funduscopic exam of a patient with optic neuritis?	Optic disc is swollen (anterior neuritis)
In what case will the optic disc be normal during a funduscopic exam?	Retrobulbar neuritis
What is the typical disposition of patients with optic neuritis?	Discuss with ophthalmology on the use of steroids and follow-up

CLINICAL VIGNETTES—MAKE THE DIAGNOSIS

21-year-old male steel worker presents to the ED with right eye pain and blurring vision; eye exam: small metallic flecks in the cornea

   Corneal foreign body

16-year-old woman with no PMH presents with a 1 week history of tearing, photophobia, and left eye pain. She does have a history of sleeping with her contacts on; eye exam: fluorescein staining with cobalt-blue lighting

   Corneal abrasions

21-year-old man with no PMH presents with a sudden onset of blood visible in the right eye, patient does not complain of any vision problems or pain, but is otherwise very concerned

   Subconjunctival hemorrhage

35-year-old female chemist presents to the ED with recent history of lye splashing in her eyes. What is the most crucial aspect in management?

   Immediate copious irrigation

28-year-old man presents to the ED soon after being hit directly in his right eye with a baseball during a game. He now complains of pain and blindness; eye exam: irregular pupil, hyphema, and flat anterior chamber

   Ruptured globe

3-year-old girl is brought in by her mother due to concerns of bilateral red eyes with watery discharge. Significant history includes day care three times a week

Viral conjunctivitis

19-year-old college student with eye history of contact lens use presents with inflammation of her eyes along with mucopurulent discharge; eye exam: unremarkable for fluorescein staining

Bacterial conjunctivitis

47-year-old man presents with inflammation of the eyes with watery discharge for about 3 days; eye exam: linear branching pattern with fluorescein staining

HSV keratitis

20-year-old man with recent eye injury presents to the ED with left eye pain, photophobia, redness, and tearing for 2 days; eye exam: hypopyon and staining that shows epithelial defects

Corneal ulcers

68-year-old diabetic man presents with surrounding area of redness and edema around his left eye that is warm to the touch; eye exam: normal

Periorbital cellulitis

21-year-old man presents to the ED due to concern of a small growth around his upper eyelash, but otherwise has no changes in vision; eye exam: remarkable for a small pustule at the lash line

Stye

61-year-old woman with an Hx of comorbid disease (CAD), DM, atrial fibrillation (afib), and cerebral vascular accident (CVA) presents with sudden and painless loss of vision in her left eye

CRAO

63-year-old woman with history of DM presents with a pounding headache, cloudy vision, nausea, and eye pain soon after coming out from the movies; eye exam: mid-dilated and non-reactive pupil with IOP >50 mm Hg

Acute angle-closure glaucoma

CHAPTER 4

ENT and Dental Emergencies

ACUTE OTITIS MEDIA

What are some important things to know about acute otitis media (AOM)?

Most frequent diagnosis in sick children; the highest incidence between 6 and 24 months of age; often occur during winter/spring after an upper respiratory infection (URI)

What are some risk factors associated with the development of AOM?

Age; day care; second-hand smoke; immunocompromised

What is the pathogenesis of AOM?

Obstruction of the eustachian tube that results in a sterile effusion with aspiration of nasopharyngeal secretions into the middle ear that can result in acute infection.

What are the three most common bacterial pathogens involved in AOM?

1. *Streptococcus pneumoniae*
2. *Haemophilus influenza*
3. *Moraxella catarrhalis*

What are some signs and symptoms of AOM?

Examination of the ear often shows distortion of the tympanic membrane (TM), erythema, decreased motility of TM on pneumatic otoscopy, and fever.

What are some complications of untreated AOM?

Hearing loss, TM perforation, mastoiditis, lateral sinus thrombosis, and meningitis.

What is the most reliable sign of AOM?

Decreased motility of the TM on pneumatic otoscopy

What is the first-line treatment for AOM?	Amoxicillin
What are two other drugs to consider in penicillin-allergic patients?	1. Erythromycin 2. Trimethoprim-sulfamethoxazole
What are some considerations in the management of AOM?	Local heat application for relief; antibiotic for treatment; return if AOM does not improve within 3 to 5 days or development of additional concerning symptoms
Which patients with AOM need ENT referral?	Recurrent otitis media (3 or more in 6 months or 4 in 1 year) **WITH** Failure on prophylactic Tx (2 infections in 6 months) or Failure to respond to at least 2 antibiotics Effusion persistent for >3 months Effusion 6 months or more out of 12 months
What is the definition of bullous myringitis?	Inflammation of the TM with bullae that are present on the TM (typically more painful).
What agents are often associated with bullous myringitis?	Mycoplasma or viral infection
What is the treatment for bullous myringitis?	Macrolide antibiotics; topical Auralgan for intact TM; ENT follow-up as needed

OTITIS EXTERNA (SWIMMER'S EAR)

What is the definition of otitis externa?	Inflammation of the external auditory canal or auricle typically due to infection, allergic reaction, or dermal disease.
What are some inherent defenses that contribute to protection against infection?	Hair follicles; tragus and conchal cartilage; cerumen
What are the two most common organisms associated with otitis externa?	1. *Pseudomonas aeruginosa* 2. *Staphylococcus aureus*
What are some risk factors that contribute to the development of otitis externa?	Warm, moist environment (ie, swimming); excessive cleaning; devices that occlude the auditory canal

What are some signs and symptoms of otitis externa?	Pain, itching, fullness of ear, redness or swelling of external ear, and cheesy or purulent green discharge.
What are some features of severe cases of otitis externa?	Complete obstruction of canal due to edema, auricular erythema, adenopathy, and fever.
What are some considerations in the management of otitis externa?	Clean the canal thoroughly; control pain; topical agents in mild cases (ie, cortisporin); antibiotic in more severe cases
Most common organism associated with necrotizing otitis externa?	*Pseudomonas aeruginosa*
What is the definition of necrotizing otitis externa?	Serious complication of acute bacterial otitis externa where infection spreads from the skin to the soft tissue, cartilage, and bone of the temporal region and skull base.
Which population is more commonly affected by necrotizing otitis externa?	Elderly; diabetic; immunocompromised
What is the mortality rate of necrotizing otitis externa if left untreated?	Approaches up to 50%
What are some signs and symptoms of necrotizing otitis externa?	Otorrhea, pain that is out of proportion to the exam, granulation tissue at the bony cartilaginous junction of the ear canal floor, and cranial nerve palsies.
What are some considerations in the management of necrotizing otitis externa?	Intravenous (IV) antibiotics; ENT consult; possible surgical debridement; MRI/CT diagnostic test of choice to visualize complications if needed

ACUTE HEARING LOSS

What are the three components of the ear?	1. Outer ear: auricle and ear canal 2. Middle ear: TM and ossicles 3. Inner ear: cochlea and semicircular canals
How is hearing loss classified?	Conductive; sensorineural; mixed

What areas of the ear often result in conductive hearing loss if damaged?

External auditory canal; tympanic membrane; middle ear components (ie, ossicles)

What are some important causes of conductive hearing loss?

Middle ear effusion; TM perforation; otitis externa; foreign body impaction

What areas of the ear often result in sensorineural hearing loss if damaged?

Cochlea; auditory nerve; inner ear

What are some important causes of sensorineural hearing loss?

Acoustic neuroma; viral neuritis; temporal bone fracture; presbycusis

What are some common causes of bilateral sensorineural hearing loss?

Exposure to loud noise; antibiotics (ie, aminoglycosides); non-steroidal anti-inflammatory drugs (NSAIDs); loop diuretics

What are important elements in the exam to evaluate acute hearing loss?

History of vertigo and tinnitus; cranial nerve examination; thorough otoscopic exam; CT if any suspicion of tumor

What two tests are useful to distinguish sensorineural from conductive hearing loss?

1. Weber test
2. Rinne test

What is the Weber test?

Tuning fork is struck and placed on the patient's forehead. The patient is asked to report in which ear the sound is heard loudest.

In a patient with unilateral conductive hearing loss, in which ear would the sound be loudest in a Weber test?

A patient would hear the tuning fork loudest in the affected ear.

In a patient with unilateral sensorineural hearing loss, in which ear would the sound be loudest in a Weber test?

A patient would hear the tuning fork loudest in the unaffected ear.

How is a Rinne test done?

This is achieved by placing a vibrating tuning fork (512 Hz) initially on the mastoid, then next to the ear and asking which sound is loudest.

What are some possibilities with the Rinne test?

In a normal ear, air conduction (AC) is better than bone conduction (BC); in conductive hearing loss, BC is better than AC; in sensorineural hearing loss, BC and AC are both equally depreciated, maintaining the relative difference of AC > BC

What are some considerations in the management of acute hearing loss?	Primarily depends on the cause; foreign body should be removed; offending medication should be discontinued; tumors require admission/consultation

NASAL

Nasal Trauma

What is a common diagnosis in any nasal trauma?	Nasal fracture
What are some signs and symptoms of nasal fractures?	Deformity, nasal swelling, ecchymosis, tenderness, or crepitance
What role does x-ray play in the evaluation of uncomplicated nasal fractures?	Not commonly used-clinical diagnosis
What are some considerations in the management of uncomplicated nasal fractures?	Early reduction if swelling is not severe; delay reduction (2-3 days) if severe swelling; reevaluation after edema has resolved
What are some examples of complicated nasal fractures?	Other facial fractures (ie, orbital floor); nasoethmoid fracture
What is the test of choice to further evaluate complicated nasal fractures?	CT scan
What are some possible indications for the use of prophylactic antibiotics?	Use of nasal packing if epistaxis; laceration of nasal mucosa; immunocompromised
What is another major complication of nasal trauma?	Septal hematoma
What are some signs and symptoms of a septal hematoma?	Bluish-purple swelling of the nasal septum
What are some considerations in the management of a septal hematoma?	Vertical incision of the hematoma; pack the anterior nasal cavity; antibiotic coverage (Staph coverage); ENT follow-up
What is the consequence of failure to drain a septal hematoma?	Avascular necrosis; septal abscess

What is the common deformity that occurs due to avascular necrosis of the nasal septum?	Saddle-nose deformity
What can occur if the cribriform plate is fractured?	Cerebrospinal fluid (CSF) rhinorrhea
What is the timeline for when this can occur?	CSF rhinorrhea may not occur until weeks after the cribriform fracture
What is a common clinical scenario when this can occur?	Typically occurs in the setting of a facial trauma followed by clear nasal discharge that can be associated with anosmia and headache.
What diagnostic test can be used to detect cribriform plate fracture?	CT scan
What are some things to do if one suspects CSF rhinorrhea?	Keep the patient upright; avoid coughing/ sneezing; consult a neurosurgeon
What is the major concern of CSF rhinorrhea in regard to infections?	Meningitis
What role do antibiotics play in regard to CSF rhinorrhea?	Controversial—use in consultation with neurosurgery

Nasal Foreign Bodies

What age group do nasal foreign bodies occur in?	Children 2 to 4 years of age
What is the common clinical presentation of a child with a nasal foreign body?	Unilateral foul-smelling nasal discharge or persistent epistaxis
In many cases, can a history of an object being inserted into the nares be recalled?	No
How is the diagnosis of a nasal foreign body commonly made?	Inspection of nares with nasal speculum or otoscope
What are some commonly used methods to remove a nasal foreign body?	Forceps, wire loops, or right angle probes; suction catheter; positive pressure (ie, blow via nose)
What is typically done if the foreign object cannot be removed?	ENT follow-up within 24 hours (most can be done as outpatient)

What are some indications for admission for immediate nasal foreign body removal?

Associated infections (ie, facial cellulites); sharp objects; button batteries

Epistaxis

What is more common: anterior nosebleeds or posterior nosebleeds?

Anterior nosebleeds (90% of cases)

What is the most common source of anterior nosebleeds?

Kiesselbach plexus

What age group is commonly affected with anterior nosebleeds?

Children and young adults

What are some important causes of anterior nosebleeds to consider?

Foreign body; trauma; nose picking (digital trauma); blood dyscrasias; infections

What are some important elements in the history to consider with respect to anterior nosebleeds?

Recurrent; onset; duration; medication; illicit drug; underlying medical problems

What are some important elements in the physical to focus on?

Vitals (ie, orthostatics); evidence of coagulopathy (ie, bruising); location (anterior versus posterior)

What simple thing can be done prior to further evaluation of nosebleeds?

Apply a topical vasoconstrictor/ anesthetic; pinch nose firmly and keep head forward

What are some commonly used methods to gain hemostatic control of anterior nosebleeds?

Silver nitrate sticks (cautery); anterior nose packing; piece of hemostatic material (ie, gelfoam)

What is the most common source of posterior nosebleeds?

Sphenopalatine artery (arterial source); Woodruff plexus (venous source)

What age group is commonly affected with posterior nosebleeds?

Elderly

What are some important causes of posterior nosebleeds to consider?

Cancer; coagulopathy

What are some considerations in the management of posterior nosebleeds?

Particular importance on airway; posterior packing with premade posterior nasal-packing balloon; admit with ENT consultation

How is posterior packing commonly done?	Use gauze pack with an intranasal balloon device or Foley catheter
What are some important complications of epistaxis?	Severe bleeding; airway obstruction from bleeding; sinusitis; AOM

ENT INFECTIONS

Pharyngitis

What is the definition of pharyngitis?	Inflammation of the mucous membrane of the oropharynx with potential for airway compromise.
What are some important causes of pharyngitis?	Infections; trauma (ie, caustic ingestions); irritant inhalant
What is the most common cause of pharyngitis?	Viral infections
What are some viruses that are commonly implicated in pharyngitis?	Epstein-Barr virus; influenza virus; parainfluenza virus; adenovirus
What are some signs and symptoms of infectious pharyngitis?	Fever, sore throat, dysphagia, and cervical adenopathy
What are some signs and symptoms of herpes simplex virus (HSV) pharyngitis?	May present with features of infectious pharyngitis with grouped vesicles in the oropharynx that erode to form ulcers
What is the treatment for HSV pharyngitis?	Acyclovir for immunocompromised patients, may benefit other patients (ie, healthy)
What is the cause of infectious mononucleosis?	Epstein-Barr virus
What age group is commonly affected by infectious mononucleosis?	Young adults (10 to 26 years of age)
What are some signs and symptoms of infectious mononucleosis?	Fever, sore throat, malaise, fatigue, and cervical adenopathy (especially, posterior) with exudative pharyngitis and hepatosplenomegaly
What is an important complication of infectious mononucleosis?	Splenic rupture

What is a common finding on a peripheral blood smear?	Lymphocytosis
What diagnostic test can be used to support the diagnosis of infectious mononucleosis?	Monospot test
What are some considerations in the management of infectious mononucleosis?	Treatment is primarily supportive; avoid contact sports for a month or so
List some indications for steroid use in infectious mononucleosis:	Neurologic complications (ie, encephalitis); airway compromise; severe hemolytic anemia
What infectious organisms should be considered in a patient with infectious pharyngitis and a history of orogenital sex?	Gonorrhea
What is the significance of pharyngitis caused by gonorrhea in children?	Sexual abuse
What are some commonly used antibiotics for the treatment of pharyngitis caused by gonorrhea?	Ceftriaxone + Chlamydia coverage (macrolide)
What other organisms should be considered in pharyngitis caused by gonorrhea?	Chlamydia
What are two antibiotics commonly used to treat chlamydia?	1. Macrolides 2. Doxycycline
Is diphtheria a common cause of pharyngitis?	No—not with DPT immunizations, but can still occur for patients who did not receive DPT immunization
Who are at risk for diphtheria?	Really young or old patients; DPT immunization not up-to-date; developing countries
What is the organism responsible for diphtheria?	*Corynebacterium diphtheriae*
What is the pathophysiology of diphtheria?	Invasive infection that primarily affects the throat and nose causing tissue necrosis often producing the characteristic pseudomembrane in the posterior pharynx

What are some signs and symptoms of diphtheria?

Typically toxic-appearing with acute onset of fever, malaise, sore throat, and hoarse voice. PE: exudative pharyngitis with adherent pseudomembrane in the posterior pharynx and cervical adenopathy

What are the systemic complications of diphtheria primarily due to?

Powerful exotoxin that primarily affects the cardiovascular system and central nervous system

What are some important complications of diphtheria?

Airway obstruction; neuritis; atrioventricular (AV) block; myocarditis/endocarditis

What are some common laboratory findings of diphtheria?

Positive culture on the Loeffler media; gram (+) rods with clubbing on swab; complete blood count (CBC) showing thrombocytopenia

What are some considerations in the management of diphtheria?

Airway, breathing, circulation (ABC) (especially airway); respiratory isolation; treatment aimed at bacteria and toxin; consider tetanus and diptheria (Td) booster in close contacts

What is the typical medical treatment for a patient with diphtheria?

Diphtheria antitoxin; penicillin or macrolide

What is the most common cause of bacterial pharyngitis?

Group A *beta-hemolytic Streptococcus*

Who are more commonly affected with Group A streptococcus?

Young adults during winter

What is the Centor criteria?

Used to predict group A streptococcal (GAS) pharyngitis in adults, therefore help to guide use of Abx

What are the four clinical features of the Centor criteria?

1. Fever
2. Absence of cough
3. Cervical lymphadenopathy
4. Tonsillar exudates

How is the Centor criteria used?

Used in conjunction with a rapid Streptococcus screen whether to treat for Group B streptococcus

What are some commonly used antibiotics to treat GAS?

Penicillin; azithromycin (for recurrent infections); first- and second-generation cephalosporin

What role does the use of intramuscular (IM) dexamethasone play?	Often used for severe symptoms; decreases severity of symptoms; provides pain relief
What are some important complications of GAS?	Rheumatic fever; glomerulonephritis; pharyngeal space infections
Is the timely treatment of GAS enough to prevent the three mentioned complications?	All but glomerulonephritis
What is rheumatic fever?	Non-suppurative complication of GAS, it is a serious inflammatory condition that can affect the heart, joints, nervous system, and skin. It most frequently occurs in children between the ages 6 and 16 years.
What is the Jones criteria?	Used to help diagnose rheumatic fever in conjugation with laboratory findings **Major.** Carditis; polyarthritis; subcutaneous nodules; erythema marginatum; chorea **Minor.** History of rheumatic fever or heart disease; fever; arthralgias
What is the treatment of choice for rheumatic fever?	Penicillin; steroids for carditis; NSAIDs for arthritis
What common organisms can produce pharyngitis in immunocompromised patients?	Fungi (cryptococcus; histoplasma; candida)
What does the physical exam commonly reveal for candida pharyngitis?	White/removable plaques on an erythematous base
What are two medications that can be used to treat candida pharyngitis?	1. Nystatin swish and swallow 2. Systemic fluconazole

Oral and Facial Infections

What is the biggest concern of any abscess within the oral cavity?	Airway compromise
What is the Ludwig angina?	Progressive cellulitis of the floor of the mouth involving sublingual and submandibular space.

What is a common cause of the Ludwig angina?	Trauma or abscess to the posterior mandibular molars.
Name the three potential spaces that the infection can tract to:	1. Sublingual space 2. Submandibular space 3. Submaxillary space
Name some commonly involved organisms in Ludwig's angina:	Streptococcus; staphylococcus; anaerobic organisms (ie, bacteroides)
What are some signs and symptoms of Ludwig's angina?	Often appear toxic with odynophagia, dysphonia, dysphagia, drooling, trismus, massive swelling of the floor of the mouth, and an elevated tongue
What are some considerations in the management of patients with Ludwig's angina?	Airway management should be top priority; immediate ENT consultation; avoid putting the patient in a supine position; IV antibiotics (ie, ampicillin-sulbactam); admit to ICU
What are some organisms involved with a masticator space abscess?	Anaerobes; streptococcus
What is the pathophysiology of how a masticator space abscess occurs?	Infection secondary to infection around third molar or extension from anterior space such as buccal space
What are some signs and symptoms of a masticator space abscess?	Fever, trismus, and face swelling
What are some considerations in the management of a masticator space abscess?	Careful attention to airway; Immediate ENT consultation; IV antibiotics
Name four potential spaces that can become infected in pharyngeal space infections:	1. Retropharyngeal space 2. Peritonsillar space 3. Peripharyngeal space 4. Prevertebral space
Where do retropharyngeal abscesses occur?	In the space posterior to the pharynx and anterior to the prevertebral fascia.
In what age groups do retropharyngeal abscesses occur?	Most common in children <3 years of age
List the most common pathogens involved in retropharyngeal abscesses:	Anaerobes; *Group A Streptococcus; S aureus*

What are some signs and symptoms of retropharyngeal abscesses?	Often appears toxic with fever, dysphagia, sore throat, swelling of neck, unilateral bulge of posterior pharynx wall, and stridor.
What is the initial diagnostic test of choice for retropharyngeal abscesses?	Soft-tissue lateral film of neck
What are some findings of the lateral neck film that points to a retropharyngeal abscess?	Widening of the retropharyngeal space; displacement of the larynx; presence of air-fluid level in the space
What are some significant complications to keep in mind?	Airway obstruction; invasion to adjacent structures; sepsis; aspiration
What are some considerations in the management of retropharyngeal abscesses?	Careful attention to airway; immediate ENT consultation for incision and drainage (I&D); IV antibiotics (ie, ampicillin/sulbactam)
Where do prevertebral abscesses occur?	In the space anterior to the cervical spine and posterior to the prevertebral fascia
What are some signs and symptoms of prevertebral abscesses?	Due to the very close proximity of the prevertebral space and retropharyngeal space, the clinical features are very similar to a retropharyngeal abscess
What distinguishing factor can help to distinguish one from the other?	Age (prevertebral abscesses more likely in older patients)
What is a common cause of prevertebral abscesses?	Cervical osteomyelitis
What is the initial diagnostic test of choice for prevertebral abscesses?	Lateral neck film
What are some findings of the lateral neck film that point to prevertebral abscesses?	Widening of the retropharyngeal space; displacement of the larynx; evidence of osteomyelitis of cervical spine
What three possible diagnostic tests can be used to confirm prevertebral abscesses?	1. CT 2. MRI 3. Cervical myelogram (not commonly used)
What are some considerations in the management of prevertebral abscesses?	IV antibiotics; neurosurgical consultation; patient requires admission

Where do peritonsillar abscesses occur?

Between the superior constrictor muscle and tonsillar capsule.

What are peritonsillar abscesses commonly due to?

Untreated tonsillitis

What age group are peritonsillar abscesses common in?

Young adults

What are some organisms involved with peritonsillar abscesses?

Usually polymicrobial

What are some signs and symptoms of peritonsillar abscesses?

Typically a history of sore throat and fever that becomes progressively worse and unilateral, can also have trismus, dysphagia, ear pain, tender cervical adenopathy, and deviated uvula to opposite side.

What are some diagnostic studies that can help confirm the diagnosis of peritonsillar abscesses?

CT; ultrasound

What are some considerations in the management of peritonsillar abscesses?

ABC—ensure airway and hydration; IV antibiotics; ENT consultation for I&D; culture for pathogen; if uncomplicated can discharge with 24 hour follow-up

Where do peripharyngeal abscesses occur?

Occur in the space lateral to the pharynx and medial to the masticator space

What are some common causes of peripharyngeal abscesses?

Tonsillar infections; dental infections

What are some signs and symptoms of peripharyngeal abscess?

Unilateral neck swelling, fever, neck pain, dysphagia, drooling, cervical adenopathy, and sore throat.

What are some complication of peripharyngeal abscesses?

Airway obstruction; cranial nerve involvement; erosion into carotids or jugular veins

What are some considerations in the management of peripharyngeal abscesses?

ABC—ensure intact airway; admission for further care; ENT consultation; IV antibiotics

Facial Infections

What is the definition of sinusitis?	Infection of the paranasal sinuses typically from a preceding URI.
Name four paranasal sinuses:	1. Maxillary 2. Ethmoid 3. Frontal 4. Sphenoid
What is the most commonly involved sinus in sinusitis?	Maxillary
What is the pathophysiology of sinusitis?	Occlusion of the sinus ostia which is usually precipitated by a URI or allergic rhinitis that results in a culture medium ideal for bacterial growth and infection.
Name some pathogens typically involved in sinusitis:	*S pneumoniae;* non-typeable *H influenza; S aureus; M catarrhalis*
What are some signs and symptoms of sinusitis?	Nasal congestion, fever, purulent yellow-green discharge, headache, nasal congestion, tenderness over the affected sinus, and opacification of the sinus on transillumination.
What are some diagnostic tests to consider in sinusitis?	Diagnosis can typically be made on history and physical, but a CT of the sinuses can be done
What are some considerations in the management of sinusitis?	Decongestants; mucolytics; analgesics; antibiotics for severe cases or complications
What are some complications of sinusitis?	CNS involvement (ie, meningitis, brain abscesses, etc.), cavernous sinus thrombosis, periorbital/orbital sinus, and surrounding abscess formation.
What is the definition of mastoiditis?	Infection of the mastoid air cells most commonly from AOM.
Name some pathogens typically involved in mastoiditis:	*S pneumoniae;* non-typeable *H influenza; S aureus*
What are some signs and symptoms of mastoiditis?	Posterior auricular tenderness, headache, hearing loss, otorrhea, and abnormal TM, pinna displaced outward and down

What are some commonly used diagnostic studies to evaluate mastoiditis?	MRI; CT of temporal bone
What are some complications of untreated mastoiditis?	CNS involvement (ie, meningitis, brain abscesses, etc.), CN VII involvement, and labyrinthitis
What are some considerations in the management of mastoiditis?	ENT consultation for possible debridement; IV antibiotics; adequate pain control; admission for further care

DENTAL EMERGENCIES

What cranial nerve (CN) provides primary sensation to the face?	Trigeminal nerve (CNV) Ophthalmic branch; maxillary branch; mandibular branch
What are branching nerves of the ophthalmic branch and the area they innervate:	
Nasociliary nerve	Dorsal nose and cornea
Supraorbital nerve	Forehead and scalp
What are branching nerves of the maxillary branch and the area they innervate:	
Superior alveolar nerves	
Posterior	Maxillary molar
Middle	First and second bicuspid
Anterior	Maxillary central, lateral, and cuspid teeth
Nasopalatine and greater palatine nerves	Hard palate (along with gingiva)
Infraorbital nerve (with part of the superior alveolar nerve)	Midface, maxillary incisors, side of nose, upper lip, and lower eyelids
What are two commonly used local anesthetics to achieve oral anesthesia?	1. Lidocaine 2. Marcaine (longer acting)

Name four nerves that are commonly blocked to achieve anesthesia:	1. Inferior alveolar nerve 2. Posterior superior alveolar nerve 3. Infraorbital nerve 4. Supraorbital nerve
What type of infiltration is commonly used to achieve individual tooth anesthesia?	Supraperiosteal infiltrations
What are some important complications of performing nerve blocks in patients?	Vascular injury; facial nerve damage (motor paralysis); neural injury
What are the major portions of a tooth?	Root; crown
What key structure keeps the tooth anchored into the alveolar bone?	Periodontal ligament
What are some considerations in the initial management of an avulsed permanent tooth?	Hold tooth by crown and gently wash root (normal saline); place tooth back into socket; do not brush root of the tooth; immediate dental consultation
What is the key determinant of the viability of an avulsed tooth?	Time outside the socket (>60 min: poor outcome)
What is the reason why the root should not be brushed or wiped?	Preserving the periodontal ligament is vital
What are two other management points to consider?	1. Prophylactic antibiotics if indicated 2. Tetanus status
Are deciduous (primary) teeth typically placed back into the socket?	No—alveolar ankylosis may result
How are alveolar fractures typically noticed?	Panorex film or evident on exam
What are other possible dental injuries from alveolar fractures?	Avulsion or subluxation of tooth; dental fractures
What is typically done for alveolar fractures?	Immediate dental consultation; reduction and fixation (via wire); antibiotics and tetanus when indicated

What are some important points and management for the following classification of tooth fractures:

Ellis I

Isolated enamel fracture; no pain; elective treatment

Ellis II

Fracture of enamel; dentin exposed; sensitive to temperature changes of hot/cold; calcium hydroxide paste over dentin if <14 years of age; dressing over tooth if >14 years of age; dental follow-up in timely manner

Ellis III

Fracture of tooth with pulp exposure; pink tinge may be seen on exam; this is a true dental emergency; immediately consult a dentist and place wet cotton with dental or aluminum foil wrapped if there is a delay

What is typically done for dental caries?

Proper pain control and dentist referral

What is a complication of dental caries to consider?

Periapical abscess

What are some clinical features of a periapical abscess?

A fluctuant swelling, sharp/severe pain when tooth is percussed, and temperature sensitivity.

What are some considerations in the management of a periapical abscess?

I&D of the abscess; antibiotic coverage (may or may not help); dental referral

CLINICAL VIGNETTES—MAKE THE DIAGNOSIS

18-year-old man with a recent URI presents with fever, fatigue, and right ear pain, but is otherwise healthy; PE: right TM shows bullae and is erythematous in appearance

Bullous myringitis

24-year-old woman with no past medical history (PMH) presents after being involved in a bar fight and complains of a bruise on her leg and some facial pain; PE: ecchymosis of left thigh and nasal swelling with tenderness and crepitence

Nasal fracture

17-year-old woman presents with a 1-week history of sore throat with low-grade fevers and fatigue. Patient mentions her sore throat is getting progressively worse; PE: exudative pharyngitis with posterior cervical adenopathy along with left upper quadrant (LUQ) tenderness

Mononucleosis with splenomegaly

3-year-old infant presents with low-grade fever, decreased appetite and mother mentions that he is tugging at his ear; PE: decreased mobility of TM on pneumatic otoscopy

Acute otitis media

51-year-old woman who just recently finished her antibiotics for a UTI presents with bilateral hearing loss, but is otherwise healthy; PE: decreased hearing acuity and normal Rinne and Weber test

Sensorineural hearing loss secondary to antibiotic use

3-year-old boy was brought in by mother due to purulent drainage from left nasal passage, but swears that the child did not place any objects in the nose; PE: general exam was unremarkable

Nasal foreign bodies (often occurs unwitnessed)

6-year-old boy is brought in by mother for persistent nosebleeds, but is otherwise healthy with immunizations up-to-date; PE: child was actively picking his nose during the exam

Anterior nosebleed

13-year-old girl with a sore throat 1 month ago now presents with fevers, joint pain, and what the mom notes as "weird movements"; PE: pain of joints with movement and subcutaneous nodules

Rheumatic fever

19-year-old man presents with severe left ear pain and complains of decreased hearing with occasional purulent discharge; PE: TM could not be visualized due to the purulent discharge in the external canal

Otitis externa

9-year-old girl presents with a 3-day history of low-grade fevers, sore throat, and fatigue but otherwise healthy; PE: cervical adenopathy with exudative pharyngitis

Streptococcal pharyngitis

2-year-old boy is brought in by mom for high fevers, sore throat, and some swelling of her neck; PE: sick-appearing child with unilateral bulge of posterior pharynx wall and stridor

Retropharyngeal abscesses

61-year-old woman present with epistaxis that began 2-hours earlier and has not stopped bleeding from conventional means; PE: epistaxis that is refractory to all methods that are used for anterior nosebleeds

Posterior nosebleed

31-year-old man with a recent history of AOM that was not treated presents otorrhea, pain around the ear, and a moderate headache; PE: tender posterior auricular area and distorted TM

Mastoiditis

24-year-old woman presents with a history of nasal congestion, fever, purulent yellow-green discharge, and headache; PE: yellowish discharge from nose and tender maxillary sinus

Sinusitis

CHAPTER 5

Pulmonary Emergencies

ASTHMA

What is the definition of asthma?

It is a chronic condition characterized by *reversible* airway constriction typically initiated by a variety of stimuli.

What are some important things to know about asthma?

More common in children and adolescents; prevalence is increasing; asthma-related morbidity is also increasing

Name some common triggers of an asthma exacerbation:

Allergens; exercise; medications; cold exposure

What are some risk factors for death from asthma?

>2 hospitalization or > 3 ED visits for asthma exacerbation in a year; recent use of corticosteroids; prior ICU admission or intubation; going through >2 inhalers in a month

What are some signs and symptoms of an asthma exacerbation?

Dyspnea, cough, and wheezing are considered the triad. There may be a lack of wheezing if airway diameter is decreased enough to impede air flow.

What are some important physical exam findings that may indicate impending respiratory failure?

Altered mental status; pulsus paradoxus; cyanosis (not common); tachycardia greater than 130 beats/min

What are some important diagnostic tests to consider in asthma?

Pulmonary function tests (ie, PEFR); ABG (if impending respiratory failure); CXR (more to rule out other conditions); ECG (if you suspect ischemia)

What are some considerations in the management of asthma?

Ensure adequate oxygenation; optimize lung function (ie, medication); identify the cause of exacerbation

What are the three classes of drugs that are the mainstay for the treatment of asthma exacerbation?

1. Beta-adrenergic (albuterol)
2. Anticholinergic (ipratropium)
3. Corticosteroids (prednisone)

When should intravenous adrenergic agonists be considered?

Should be used in severe cases as they have more adverse drug reactions with intravenous use; IM epinephrine should be strongly considered

Are there any advantages of intravenous administration of corticosteroids over oral?

Many studies have clearly demonstrated that oral corticosteroids are as beneficial as intravenous corticosteroids.

Do methylxanthines or leukotriene modifiers play a role in the acute management of asthma?

No—often used as maintenance therapy

What role does non-invasive positive pressure ventilation (NPPV) play?

Impending respiratory failure where the patient is able to cooperate; should not be considered a substitute for intubation for a deteriorating patient

What is the definition of status asthmaticus?

Severe exacerbation that does not respond to aggressive interventions within 30 min.

What procedure should be considered in the setting of impending respiratory failure?

Intubation

What is considered the induction agent of choice when intubating an asthmatic?

Ketamine due to ability to dilate bronchioles.

What are some critical issues to consider in the intubated asthmatic?

Minimizing high airway pressure to avoid barotrauma; permissive hypercapnia (ie, using lower vent settings despite increased pCO_2)

What should be a strong consideration in any intubated patient who suddenly deteriorates?

Pneumothorax

What are some other agents that can be considered when the mainstay treatment of asthma shows little improvement?

Magnesium sulfate; heliox (helium to improve airflow); terbutaline

What are some important elements to consider when deciding to admit a patient with an asthma exacerbation?	Social supports; recent hospitalizations and past intubations; compliance with medication; severity of the exacerbation

CHRONIC OBSTRUCTIVE PULMONARY DISEASE

What are the disease entities that make up chronic obstructive pulmonary disease (COPD)?	Emphysema; asthma; chronic bronchitis

What are some important features for each of the following elements:

Emphysema	Irreversible airway destruction
Chronic bronchitis	Cough/sputum production for at least 3 months for two consecutive years
Asthma	Hyperactive airway and inflammation that is reversible

What are some important risk factors for the development of COPD?	Tobacco use (most common cause); environmental pollution; $alpha_1$–antitrypsin deficiency; cystic fibrosis
What are some signs and symptoms of a COPD exacerbation?	Dyspnea, cough, chest tightness, occasional hemoptysis; increased sputum production
What are some common causes of a COPD exacerbation?	Infections; pulmonary embolism (PE); congestive heart failure (CHF) exacerbation; tobacco use; non-compliance with medication

What are some of the common signs and symptoms of the following COPD variant (more of a classic description):

Chronic bronchitis (blue bloaters)	Tend to be heavy set; normal chest diameter; productive wet cough
Emphysema (pink puffer)	Tend to be thin; increased AP chest diameter

What are some common findings on CXR?	Increased AP diameter; overinflation; presence of bullae
What are some other diagnostic tests to consider in COPD?	ABG; ECG (for ischemia or dysrhythmias)

Does a culture of sputum or gram stain have any role in the management of a COPD exacerbation?

No—while it may be useful to guide antibiotic management when patient is admitted.

What two dysrhythmias are common in COPD?

1. Multifocal atrial tachycardia
2. Atrial fibrillation

What are some considerations in the management of a COPD exacerbation?

Oxygenation is the cornerstone; beta-adrenergic agonist; anticholinergics; corticosteroids use; Abx if signs of infection—purulent sputum

Name three common organisms associated with a COPD exacerbation:

Moraxella catarrhalis

Streptococcus pneumonia

Haemophilus influenza

List some common antibiotics commonly used in a COPD exacerbation:

Macrolides, third-generation cephalosporin, and fluoroquinolones

PNEUMONIA

What are some facts about bacterial pneumonia?

It accounts for about 10 to 15% of admissions; *Streptococcus pneumoniae* is the most common agent in community acquired pneumonia; most common mechanism is aspiration

Name some other important bacterial agents in bacterial pneumonia:

Pseudomonas aeruginosa; Hemophilus influenza; Staphylococcus aureus; E coli

List some predisposing factors that increases susceptibility to bacterial pneumonia:

Impaired immunity; impaired gag reflex/mucociliary transport; iatrogenic (ie, endotracheal tube); chest wall dysfunction

What are some signs and symptoms of bacterial pneumonia?

Fever, chills, productive cough, purulent sputum, and pleuritic chest pain.

What are some common physical findings in a patient with pneumonia?

Crackles, wheezes, dullness to percussion, egophony, and tactile fremitus

Name the most likely organism for
each of the following scenarios:

Alcoholic who presents with fever, chills, and productive cough. Chest x-ray (CXR) shows lobar pneumonia	*Klebsiella pneumoniae*
45-year-old man who has been in the ICU for 2 weeks on vent support develops fever and chills with productive green sputum on suction	*P aeruginosa*
63-year-old man with a history of COPD, DM, and debilitation presents with shortness of breath, fever, and a CXR that shows patchy infiltrates	*H influenza*
35-year-old woman bird-breeder presents with a 3-day history of high fever, hacking cough, and severe headache which she feels is like the flu	*Chlamydia psittaci*
21-year-old male farmer presents with a sudden onset of high fever, myalgias, and hacking cough. He mentions he often cleans at one of the slaughterhouses	*Coxiella burnetii*
40-year-old man presents with SOB and productive cough recalls onset of symptoms after returning from a spa	*Legionella pneumophila*
31-year-old woman who typically skins rabbits presents with high fever, SOB, and hemoptysis	*Francisella tularensis*
19-year-old patient with AIDS and a cell count of <200 cells/mm^3 presents with fever, non-productive cough, and dyspnea	*Pneumocystis jirovecii* (formerly called *Pneumocystis carinii*)

What are some diagnostic tests to consider in addition to the CXR?	Arterial blood gas; sputum culture (often low yield unless done under bronchoscopy); blood culture prior to administration of antibiotics
What are some complications of bacterial pneumonia?	Abscess formation (especially *S aureus*); sepsis; empyema

Name some of the most common agents in the following age group:

Neonates

Group B streptococci, *E coli*, and *Chlamydophila pneumoniae*

Children (5 weeks to 18 years)

Respiratory syncytial virus (RSV), *Mycoplasma pneumoniae*, *C pneumoniae*, and *S pneumoniae*

Adults (18-40 years)

M pneumoniae, *C pneumoniae*, and *S pneumoniae*

Adults (45 years and older)

S pneumoniae, *H influenzae*, anaerobes, and gram-negatives

What are some commonly used antibiotics in uncomplicated pneumonia?

Penicillin, macrolides, and doxycycline

Name three common causes of atypical pneumonia:

1. *M pneumoniae*
2. *C pneumoniae*
3. *L pneumophilia*

What are some signs and symptoms of atypical pneumonia?

Headache, fever, non-productive cough, and myalgias (often described as a "walking pneumonia")

What are some facts to know about mycoplasma pneumonia?

Most common cause of atypical pneumonia with 1 to 3 weeks incubation; most common in ages 4 to 40 years; CXR often show a reticulonodular pattern

What are some complications of mycoplasma pneumonia?

Splenomegaly; aseptic meningitis; encephalitis; respiratory failure

What is the preferred antibiotic of choice for atypical pneumonia?

Erythromycin; tetracycline or doxycycline are alternatives

Name the most likely organism for each of the following scenarios involving viral pneumonia and the preferred treatment:

34-year-old with a history of a kidney transplant presents with fever, cough, and a CXR showing interstitial infiltrates

Cytomegalovirus; treatment (Tx): ganciclovir or foscarnet

3-year-old child presents with a 4-day history of fever, chills, and coryza with a CXR that shows patchy infiltrates

RSV; Tx: primarily supportive

| 20-year-old man presents with a 2-week history of fever, chills, and non-productive cough during winter | Influenza virus; Tx Amantadine |
| 34-year-old woman presents with fever, headache, and myalgia. She primarily works with rodents and is from Arizona | Hantavirus; Tx: supportive/ribavirin |

HEMOPTYSIS

What is the definition of hemoptysis?	Coughing up of blood that originates from the tracheobronchial tree or pulmonary parenchyma.
What are some characteristics of hemoptysis that help to distinguish it from hematemesis?	Bright red and foamy; usually preceded by a vigorous cough; lack of food particles
What is the definition of massive hemoptysis?	Coughing up of blood that typically exceeds 50 mL in a single expectoration or 500 mL in a 24 hour period.
What are some important causes of hemoptysis?	Infection and inflammation (most common); trauma; CA—especially bronchogenic; iatrogenic; pulmonary embolism
What are some important causes of massive hemoptysis?	Lung abscess; bronchiectasis; tuberculosis
What are some considerations in the management of hemoptysis?	Focus should be on underlying cause; low threshold to secure the airway; patient will often require a bronchoscopy

PLEURAL EFFUSION AND EMPYEMA

| What is the definition of a pleural effusion? | An abnormal accumulation of fluid in the pleural space. |

What are some of the characteristics of the following types of pleural effusion:

Transudate

Increase in hydrostatic pressure; decreased oncotic pressure; CHF is the most common cause; low protein infiltrate

Exudate

Lymphatic blockage; typically due to malignancy or infection; high protein infiltrate

What are some signs and symptoms of pleural effusion?

Pleuritic chest pain, cough, and SOB; PE: dullness to percussion and pleurisy

Which CXR view is more sensitive for detecting a pleural effusion?

Lateral decubitus (as little as 5 mL can be seen)

What procedure is commonly used to analyze pleural effusions?

Thoracentesis

What are some laboratory tests to consider when analyzing pleural fluid?

Gram stain and cultures; pleural fluid lactate dehydrogenase (LDH) and protein; serum LDH, protein, and glucose

List some of the criteria that may indicate an exudative pleural effusion:

Pleural fluid LDH >200 IU/mL; pleural fluid cholesterol >60 mg/dL; pleural fluid protein/serum protein >0.5

Name some important causes of transudative pleural effusion:

CHF; low protein states (ie, cirrhosis); peritoneal dialysis

Name some important causes of an exudative pleural effusion:

Bacterial pneumonia; TB; malignancy; connective tissue disorder (ie, systemic lupus erythematosus)

What is the definition of an empyema?

Collection of pus in the pleural space.

What are some common causes of an empyema?

Infections (ie, gram negatives)
Iatrogenic (ie, chest tube)

What are some signs and symptoms of an empyema?

Fever, chills, pleuritic chest pain, SOB, fatigue, and weight loss

What are some diagnostic tests used to diagnose an empyema?

CXR; thoracentesis

What are some complications of empyema?

Loss of lung tissue; bronchopleural fistula; pleural adhesions secondary to a loculation

What are some important management issues of an empyema?	Pleural drainage via chest tube; broad spectrum Abx; video-assisted thoracoscopic surgery (VATS) may be required for loculations

LUNG ABSCESS

What is the definition of a lung abscess?	It is a cavitation of the lung parenchyma due to central necrosis.
What is the most common cause of a lung abscess?	Aspiration
What class of bacteria are typically involved in a lung abscess?	Typically mixed anaerobic and gram (–) bacteria
What are some signs and symptoms of a lung abscess?	Weakness, fever, SOB, pleuritic chest pain, putrid sputum, and hemoptysis.
What are some important diagnostic tests to consider in a lung abscess?	Complete blood count (CBC); CXR (shows cavitation); sputum stain; a chest CT will often show abscesses
What are some complications of a lung abscess?	Empyema; bronchopleural abscess; chronic lung abscess
What are some considerations in management of a lung abscess?	Abx therapy (clindamycin preferred); surgical intervention if cause is a tumor or fistula

TUBERCULOSIS

What are some important points to know about tuberculosis (TB)?	The incidence of TB is rising (especially in AIDS patients); top cause of infectious death worldwide; transmission is primarily respiratory
What is the pathophysiology of infection from *M tuberculosis*?	Obligate aerobic rod (acid-fast staining) that is phagocytized by macrophages, but not killed and allowed to grow (albeit slowly).
What is the primary determinant of whether the infection is contained or likely to spread?	Immune status (lifetime risk of activation is still 10% in the general population)

What are some factors that are associated with an increase in reactivation?

DM; immunocompromised (ie, AIDS, transplant recipient); malignant disease

What are some of the signs and symptoms for each of the following TB states:

Primary

Asymptomatic in most patients; positive purified protein derivative (PPD) test primary way to detect; sometimes Ghon complex seen on CXR

Secondary (reactivation)

Constitutional symptoms (ie, weight loss); productive cough; hemoptysis; up to 20% have extrapulmonary features

Name the four most common sites of extrapulmonary involvement:

1. CNS (TB meningitis)
2. Vertebral bodies (the Pott disease)
3. Liver
4. Psoas muscle

What are some important diagnostic tests to consider in TB?

CXR; sputum (acid-fast bacilli); PPD test

What are the criteria for a positive PPD test?

Less than 5 mm indurations for immunocompromised patients (ie, AIDS); less than 10 mm indurations for high-risk individuals (IV drug abusers and immigrants from high-risk areas); less than 15 mm indurations in healthy individuals

What are two common causes of a false negative PPD test?

Anergy; infection with a mycobacterium species such as *M avium*

What are some considerations in the management of TB?

Respiratory isolation once TB is suspected; multidrug therapy for more than 6 months; baseline liver/kidney test and visual acuity

Describe the main side effects for each of the drug used to treat TB (RIPE):

Rifampin

Orange-colored urine, tears, and saliva; increase P450 activity

Isoniazid (INH)

Hepatitis; neuropathy (prevented with supplemental vitamin B_6)

Pyrazinamide (PZA)

Hepatitis; hyperuricemia; arthralgias

Ethambutol

Optic neuritis; rash

SPONTANEOUS PNEUMOTHORAX

What is the definition of a spontaneous pneumothorax?

It is collection of air in the pleural space (assuming that no trauma is involved).

List some important facts for the following:

Primary spontaneous pneumothorax

Typically occurs in healthy individuals; most have a history of smoking; results from rupture of a bleb

Secondary spontaneous pneumothorax

Typically will have underlying lung disease; COPD and asthma most common cause; usually patients are older than 45 years

What are some signs and symptoms of a spontaneous pneumothorax?

Sudden onset of dyspnea and pleuritic chest pain. PE: decreased breath sounds and hyperresonance on the affected side.

What is the diagnostic test of choice?

Chest radiograph

What are critical management issues for a spontaneous pneumothorax?

All patients should receive oxygen; observation and serial CXR if small; a large (often greater than 20% or expending) pneumothorax is an indication for a tube thoracostomy

What is a feared complication of a spontaneous pneumothorax?

Tension pneumothorax

What are some signs and symptoms of tension pneumothorax?

Hypotension, absent breath sounds on the affected side, jugular venous distension (JVD), and trachea deviation to the opposite side.

What is a critical action in the management of a tension pneumothorax?

Immediate chest decompression (14 gauge) followed with a chest tube.

What are some specifics of chest decompression in a tension pneumothorax?

If any evidence of tension pneumothorax, immediate needle decompression should be done with a needle placed into the second and third intercostal space at the anterior axillary line followed by a chest tube in the fifth intercostal space in the mid-axillary line.

CLINICAL VIGNETTES—MAKE THE DIAGNOSIS

8-year-old child with history of multiple allergies presents with acute respiratory distress; PE: tachypnea, intercostal retractions, and audible wheezing; CXR: hyperinflation of lung

Bronchial asthma

41-year-old man with recent "flu" presents with a 2-day history of fever, chill, productive cough, and pleuritic chest pain; PE: ill-appearing patient, crackles, wheezes, and dullness to percussion of the left lung

Community-acquired pneumonia

32-year-old man with a long history of ethanol use presents to the ED with fever, hemoptysis, SOB, and purulent sputum; PE: lung fields relatively clear; CXR: central cavitation

Lung abscess

65-year-old woman with a long history of smoking presents in acute respiratory distress with a recent illness; PE: hyperresonant chest, decreased breath sounds bilateral; CXR: hyperinflation of lung and small infiltrate of right lower lobe

COPD exacerbation

67-year-old man with a long history of smoking presents with a 2-week history of worsening hemoptysis and a 20-lb weight loss in a month period; CXR: a spiculated mass is seen on the left side

Bronchogenic cancer

41-year-old man with an PMH of CHF presents with SOB and wet cough, but otherwise has been doing well; PE: dullness to percussion and pleurisy; lateral decubitus CXR: dependant fluid collection

Pleural effusion

23-year-old slender man with a smoking history presents with sudden onset of dyspnea and pleuritic chest pain, but is otherwise healthy; PE: an area of hyperresonance on the left side

Spontaneous pneumothorax

31-year-old man with PMH of HIV presents with hemoptysis and recent weight loss along with a CD4+ count of <200; PE: cachectic appearance, is actively coughing

Tuberculosis

CHAPTER 6

Cardiovascular and Vascular Emergencies

DYSRHYTHMIAS

What is the normal range of sinus rhythm?

60 to 100 beats/min

What is sinus tachycardia?

Appears like sinus rhythm except that the rate is >100 beats/min.

What are some causes of sinus tachycardia to consider?

1. Fever
2. Drug-induced
3. Hypovolemia
4. Hyperthyroid
5. Anxiety

What is the treatment for sinus tachycardia?

The objective is to search for the underlying cause and avoid using medications such as a beta-blocker to mask the vital signs unless directed for treatment.

What is sinus bradycardia?

Appears like sinus rhythm except that the rate is <60 beats/min.

What are some causes of sinus bradycardia to consider?

Sick sinus syndrome

Hypothermia

Drug effect

Inferior wall MI

Increased vagal tone (valsalva maneuver)

What are some indications for the treatment of sinus bradycardia?

Based on symptoms: hypotension, altered mental status, shortness of breath, and chest pain (treatment should not be based on a number)

What are some considerations for the management of sinus bradycardia?

Atropine, transcutaneous pacing, transvenous pacing

What does the term SVT refer to?

Generic term that refers to all dysrhythmias above the bifurcation of the bundle of His which can include MAT or PSVT.

What is the typical atrial rate for paroxysmal supraventricular tachycardia (PSVT)?

120 to 200 beats/min

What are some other characteristic findings of PSVT on ECG?

Rhythm is regular; QRS complex is typically narrow unless there is aberrant conduction through a bypass tract; p-waves are visible

What is atrial fibrillation?

Irregularly irregular rhythm due to uncoordinated atrial activity with randomly conducted ventricular depolarization.

What are some other characteristic findings of atrial fibrillation on ECG?

P waves are typically absent with no PR interval; rhythm is irregular; QRS complex is typically normal unless aberrant conduction

What are some features of paroxysmal versus permanent atrial fibrillation?

Paroxysmal tends to last less than 24 hours in many cases and often terminate spontaneously, whereas permanent often greater for one year and difficult to terminate.

What is the primary concern for untreated atrial fibrillation?

Thromboembolic events such as stroke

What are some considerations in the management of atrial fibrillation?

Duration of the episode
Search for underlying cause/trigger
Presence of an accessory pathway
Patient's stability

What is an important distinction to make with any patient who presents with atrial fibrillation?

If the patient is hemodynamically stable

What is the immediate action required in any unstable patient due to uncontrolled atrial fibrillation?

Electrical cardioversion

For the stable patient with uncontrolled atrial fibrillation, should the focus be on conversion or rate-control?

Generally speaking, ventricular rate control should be the mainstay of treatment.

What are some pharmacologic interventions to consider with ventricular control of atrial fibrillation?

Cardioactive calcium channel blocker such as diltiazem

Beta-blocker

Cardioactive steroids (digoxin)

What is an important contraindication to consider in the treatment of atrial fibrillation with the above agents?

Undiagnosed Wolff–Parkinson–White (WPW) syndrome which may lead to conduction solely down the accessory pathway: life-threatening in which case amiodarone or Class IA/IC can be considered, but again if unstable cardioversion is indicated.

What is atrial flutter?

A very rapid rhythm with a slower ventricular response due to nodal delay. They typically occur with some type of AV block such as 2:1 or 3:1.

What are some other characteristic findings of atrial flutter on ECG?

P waves have a characteristic sawtooth appearance; PR interval is normal as well as QRS complex; the ventricular rate is normally 100 to 150

What are some considerations in the management of atrial flutter?

Similar to atrial fibrillation: if unstable consider electrocardioversion and may consider vagal maneuvers or rate-controlling agents such as beta-blockers

What is multifocal atrial tachycardia (MAT)?

It is an irregular rhythm that is mistaken for atrial fibrillation, but often is characterized by P waves of varying morphology.

What is the most common cause of MAT?

COPD decompensation

What is premature atrial contractions?

They are extra beats that originate from an ectopic origin in the atrium outside the sinus node.

What are premature ventricular contraction (PVC)?

Abnormal QRS complex that originates from an ectopic site on the ventricle

What are some other characteristic findings of a PVC on ECG?

Preceding P wave is missing; QRS complex is wide and occur earlier than the next expected QRS complex; generally followed by a compensatory pause

What is ventricular tachycardia?

Typically consecutive PVCs at a rate >100 beats/min.

What are some other characteristic findings of ventricular tachycardia on ECG?

P waves are absent; wide QRS complex is a defining feature; fusion beats may be present; deflection of the ST segment and T waves is generally opposite to that of the QRS complex

What is a fusion beat?

Intermediate between a normal QRS and a PVC.

What is the most common cause of ventricular tachycardia?

Ischemic heart disease

What is the immediate action required in any unstable patient with ventricular tachycardia?

Electrical cardioversion starting at 100 joules

What is another rhythm sometimes mistaken for ventricular tachycardia?

SVT with aberrancy (assume all patients have ventricular tachycardia until proven otherwise!)

What are some pharmacologic agents for stable patients with ventricular tachycardia?

Amiodarone, procainamide, and lidocaine are good options

What is torsades de pointes ("twisting of the pointes")?

Sine wave in appearance, it is also known as polymorphic ventricular tachycardia

What are some treatment options for the treatment of torsades?

Magnesium sulfate (primarily for prevention and not termination)

Overdrive pacing

What is ventricular fibrillation?

Uncoordinated contraction of the cardiac muscle of the ventricles in the heart which does not allow for effective contractions.

What are some other characteristic findings of ventricular fibrillation on ECG?

Commonly appear as a fine or course zigzag pattern without any discernible P waves, QRS complexes, or T waves

What is pulseless electrical activity (PEA)?

It is some type of non-perfusing rhythm that is not v-tach or v-fib; they are often associated with a specific clinical scenario such as hypoxia or overdose.

What are the five Hs and Ts to consider for causes of PEA and Vfib?	Hypoxemia
	Hypovolemia
	Hydrogen ions (acidemia)
	Hyperkalemia
	Hypothermia
	Trauma
	Toxic overdose
	Tension pneumothorax
	Thrombosis (MI)
	Thrombosis (PE)
What is the treatment for PEA/Vfib arrest?	Search and treat any underlying cause
	IMMEDIATE defibrillation
	ACLS protocol (ie, epi)
What is a bundle branch block?	They are abnormal conduction in which the ventricles depolarize in sequence as opposed to simultaneously.
What is a right bundle branch block (RBBB)?	It is a unifascicular block where the ventricular activation occurs by the left bundle branch with activation of the left ventricle before the right ventricle (the opposite occurs with a left bundle branch block).
What are some other characteristic findings of an RBBB on ECG?	Wide QRS (>0.12 seconds); wide S waves in Leads I, V_5, and V_6; T wave has a deflection opposite the terminal half of the QRS complex
What are some other characteristic findings of a left bundle branch block (LBBB) on ECG?	Wide QRS (>0.12 seconds); large wide R waves in Leads I, aVL, V_5, and V_6; T wave has a deflection opposite to that of the terminal half of the QRS complex
What is an atrioventricular (AV) block?	Occurs due to abnormal conduction between the atria and ventricles at the AV node in many cases.
What are some other characteristic findings of an AV block on ECG?	Will depend on the following:
First-degree AV block:	AV conduction is slightly prolonged; 1:1 relationship between the P wave and QRS complex; PR interval is >0.20 seconds; block is most often at the level of the AV node

Second-degree AV block- Mobitz I (Wenckebach):	The defining feature is the progressive prolongation of the PR interval with each beat until a beat is dropped; P wave and QRS complex are normal; block is typically within the AV node
Second-degree AV block- Mobitz II:	PR interval is usually similar as opposed to Type I, but they are dropped beats; P waves are normal; QRS complex are usually normal but may be wide due to a associated BBB; block is typically below the AV node
Third-degree AV block:	No atrial pulses are conducted; the block may occur either at the node or anywhere below; NO relationship between the P waves or QRS complex
Name two common pre-excitation syndromes:	1. Wolff-Parkinson-White (WPW) 2. Lown-Ganong-Levine (LGL)
What is the basic pathophysiology of these syndromes?	Abnormal conduction pathway (accessory pathway) between the atrium and ventricle. Impulses may bypass the normal conduction pathway.
What are some other characteristic findings of WPW on ECG?	Short PR interval (<0.12 seconds); wide QRS with a delta wave (slurred upstroke to the QRS)
What are some other characteristic findings of WPW on ECG?	Also a short PR interval as in WPW but no delta wave with normal QRS interval
What pharmacologic agents are contraindicated?	Any nodal blockers such as beta-blockers
What is the treatment of choice in any unstable patient with WPW?	Electrical cardioversion
What pharmacologic agents should be considered in the treatment of WPW?	Procainamide (normal ejection fraction) or amiodarone (good if patient have impaired cardiac function)

CARDIAC DEVICES

What are some indications for the placement of a permanent pacemaker?	1. Symptomatic sinus bradycardia 2. Symptomatic heart block 3. Atrial fibrillation with a symptomatic bradycardia

What are two primary function of a pacemaker?

1. Sense the intrinsic cardiac activity
2. Stimulate the heart

What are some indications for the placement of a cardioverter-defibrillator?

1. Spontaneous sustained VT
2. Cardiac arrest from VT or VF

Name three components that make up a pacemaker:

1. Battery
2. Electronic circuitry
3. Lead system

What is the most common battery type used?

Lithium-ion (4-10 year life)

What are two possible lead configurations used?

Bipolar:

Have both the negative and the positive electrodes within the heart

Unipolar:

Positive pole is the metallic casing of the pulse generator and negative electrode in contact with the heart

What is a pacer spike?

It is a narrow deflection on ECG that usually appears prior to a depolarization. Appearance will depend on whether the pacemaker uses a bipolar or unipolar lead system.

Is a right bundle branch pattern normal with a pacemaker?

No—a left bundle branch pattern should be seen, a right bundle pattern suggests a lead displacement.

What are some important complications of a pacemaker to consider?

1. Infection
2. Thrombophlebitis
3. Malfunction

Name some examples of pacemaker malfunction:

Undersensing—ie, the device fails to recognize the electrical activity of beats that are present

Oversensing—ie, the device falsely interprets signals as beats that are not actually present

Failure to capture

Inappropriate rate

What is failure to capture?

It may range from a lack of stimulus-induced complex after a spike or lack of a spike at all.

Does placing a magnet externally over the pulse generator turn the pacemaker off?

No—it converts the pacemaker to an asynchronous/fixed-rate pacing mode.

What is the most common cause for failure to capture?

Lead displacement (typically first month after placement)

What is the initial diagnostic test of choice to obtain in the emergency department when evaluating a pacemaker problem?

Chest radiograph (evaluate for lead fracture or displacement) and ECG

What are some signs and symptoms of a patient with a pacemaker malfunction?

Dizziness, syncope, palpitations, and dyspnea

What is Twiddler syndrome?

Permanent malfunction of a pacemaker due to the patient's manipulation of the pulse generator. This may result in stimulation of the ipsilateral phrenic nerve resulting in diaphragmatic pacing and the sensation of abdominal pulsations.

Can electrical defibrillation be applied to a patient with a pacemaker who has cardiac arrest?

Yes

What are the components of an implantable cardioverter-defibrillator (ICD)?

Similar to a pacemaker

What is the most common complaint of patients with an ICD?

When the ICD discharges to terminate a malignant rhythm (often described as being kicked in the chest by a horse)

What are some potential causes of an increase in shock frequency?

1. Non-sustained VT
2. Inappropriately sensing supraventricular tachyarrhythmia as a VT
3. T waves are sensed as a QRS complex and interpreted as an increased heart rate

Will the use of a magnet deactivate an ICD?

Yes

What is a left ventricular assist device (LVAD)?

A mechanical device that supports the function of the left ventricle, often a bridge to cardiac transplantation.

What are some signs and symptoms of an LVAD failure?

Often severe congestive heart failure

What are some important considerations in the management of a patient with an LVAD failure?

Should be managed as severe congestive heart failure with use of dobutamine and pressors; will often require transfer to a cardiac transplantation center

PERIPHERAL ARTERIOVASCULAR DISEASE

Name the three categories of arteries:

1. Large or elastic arteries
2. Medium or muscular arteries
3. Small arteries

Define the three primary layers of an artery:

1. Intima
2. Media
3. Adventitia

Please define the following terms:

Arterial Thrombosis:

In situ formation of a blood clot typically from endothelial damage or abnormal flow causing shear stress

Aneurysms:

Abnormal dilatation of the arterial wall, a true aneurysm involves all three layers of the arterial wall

Atherosclerosis:

A disease of medium-to-large arteries. An atheroma develops which is a fatty plaque that can damage arterial walls or impede blood flow

Vasospasm:

Abnormal vasomotor response in small arteries

What are some signs and symptoms of patients who present with peripheral artery disease?

Clinical presentation will depend primarily on the location of the diseased artery as well as onset of occlusion but can include pain, pallor, and dysfunction.

What are the 6 Ps of an acute arterial occlusion?

Pulselessness

Paralysis

Pain

Pallor

Paresthesias

Poikilothermia

What are two common causes of acute arterial occlusion?

Embolism

In situ thrombosis

Is it important to determine the cause of suspected arterial occlusion?

In the setting of limb-threatening ischemia, it is more important to surgically intervene. Cause is important when there is time, as this will determine intervention.

What are some signs and symptoms of chronic arterial insufficiency?

One can have intermittent claudication and ischemic pain at rest with the latter signifying progression of the disease. Often will sleep with leg dangling over the edge to improve perfusion pressure.

Match the corresponding area of arterial occlusion with the following claudication pain pattern:

Calf claudication:

Femoral and popliteal occlusion

Hip and buttock claudication:

Aortoiliac occlusion

What is the hallmark of an arterial embolism?

Sudden loss of pulse

What is a diagnostic test to consider when pulses are difficult to palpate?

Doppler

What are some important points to consider in the following diagnostic tests used to evaluate arterial occlusion?

Contrast angiography:

It is considered the gold standard to define abnormal peripheral artery anatomy; invasive with risk of contrast reaction; catheter-related complications

Computed tomography angiography:

Readily available at most institutions; less invasive; can also visualize abdominal aorta; substantial radiation exposure; possible contrast reaction

Magnetic resonance imaging:

Expensive; not available at many instructions; accurate visualization of anatomy by various section cuts

What is the treatment of choice in limb-threatening ischemia?

Fogarty catheter embolectomy for an embolism, bypass can be used for thrombosis

What are some non-invasive treatment options that should be considered?	Heparin is an important treatment Low-dose arterial fibrinolytic therapy is finding increasing use

ACUTE CORONARY SYNDROME

What is acute coronary syndrome (ACS)?	It is a continuum of coronary artery disease where the symptoms are due to myocardial ischemia. The underlying cause of ACS is an imbalance between demand and supply of myocardial oxygen.
What are three clinical presentations that cover the ACS spectrum?	1. Unstable angina 2. Non–ST-elevation MI (NSTEMI) 3. ST-elevation MI (STEMI)
What are three non-modifiable risk factors associated with development of ACS?	1. Gender 2. Age 3. Family history
What are four modifiable risk factors associated with the development of ACS?	1. Cholesterol 2. Hypertension 3. Diabetes 4. Smoking
What are some signs and symptoms of the following presentations of coronary artery disease:	
Stable angina	Episodic pain that is transient and predictable, typically reproducible on exertion and improves with rest or use of nitroglycerin
Unstable angina	New-onset angina that can be exertional or at rest, different from previous stable angina, increased frequency of attack or increased resistance to relief such as nitroglycerin
Acute myocardial infarction (AMI)	Substernal chest discomfort that lasts longer than 20 minutes, typically associated with nausea, vomiting, dyspnea, diaphoresis, and radiation to arms/jaw/back with evidence of myocardial damage such as ECG changes suggestive of ischemia or elevated cardiac markers

| What are some signs and symptoms of atypical AMI? | Vague chest discomfort/pressure, nausea and vomiting, short of breath, confusion, dizziness, abdominal pain, weakness, or syncope. |

| What population group can frequently present with atypical symptoms? | Diabetics; women; elderly; patients with a neurological dysfunction with altered perception of pain |

| What are three important elements in the patient's presentation to consider in an AMI? | 1. History and physical
2. Cardiac enzymes
3. ECG |

| What is the single most important diagnostic test to obtain in a patient with suspected AMI? | ECG (within 10 minutes of arrival) |

| What are other uses of the initial ECG aside from screening for cardiac ischemia? | Evaluating for other disease processes such as pulmonary embolism and pericarditis |

Table 6-1 ECG Infarct Region

I: lateral	aVR:	V1: septal	V4: anterior
II: inferior	aVL: lateral	V2: septal	V5: lateral
III: inferior	aVF: inferior	V3: anterior	V6: lateral

| What are some caveats to note about the use of an ECG? | Initial ECG is diagnostic 50% of the time; serial ECGs are more useful for evolving MI; comparison with a previous ECG for any changes is also crucial |

| What are some ECG findings in a patient who presents with a STEMI? | Inverted T-waves; Q-waves; ST segment elevation >1 mm in two or more contiguous leads; new left bundle branch block |

What are some common complications for the following infarct location?	
Inferior	Increased vagal tone; bradyarrhythmias are more common; high association with right ventricular wall infarct
Lateral	Greater risk of left ventricular (LV) dysfunction

| Anterior | Greater risk of LV dysfunction (CHF); conduction abnormalities |
| | |

Right ventricular — Hypotension (preload dependent); cardiogenic shock

What are limitations concerning the role of biomarkers used in the diagnosis of an AMI? — Initial level cannot be used to exclude an AMI; serial levels are more useful; detection requires enough time/tissue death. Troponin will stay elevated for prolonged periods, limiting their usefulness in assessing re-infarction.

Table 6-2 Cardiac Biomarkers

Cardiac Enzymes	Initial Elevation	Peak	Return to Baseline
Troponin	2-6 h	12-16 h	5-14 days
CK-MB	4-6 h	12-24 h	2-3 days
Myoglobin	2 h	6-8 h	3-4 days

What is MONA? — It is the initial treatment for all patients with suspected ACS

Morphine

Oxygen

Nitro

Aspirin

What treatment within MONA is clearly shown to improve morbidity and mortality of ACS and should *always* be given (assuming no contraindications)? — Aspirin

What else should be done for all patients with suspected ACS? — Intravenous access

Oxygen supplementation

Placed on a monitor

What are some important points for the following treatments used in ACS:

Aspirin (ASA) — Antiplatelet medication; should be given within 4 hours of chest pain onset; clearly shown to improve outcome; often 4 baby aspirins (81 mg) are given to chew

Glycoprotein IIb/IIIa inhibitors — Abciximab, tirofiban, and eptifibatide; platelet inhibitors; used prior to percutaneous coronary intervention; also indicated in some cases of NSTEMI

ADP-receptor inhibitors	Clopidogrel and ticlopidine (increased risk of thrombotic thrombocytopenic purpura (TTP) and neutropenia); also prevents platelets aggregation; second-line if ASA cannot be used: reduce risk of recurrence in patients with recent MI or stroke
Heparin	Potentiates the action of antithrombin III; patients with ACS (UA/NSTEMI/STEMI); decrease re-infarction, deep vein thrombosis (DVT), LV thrombus; adverse drug reactions include bleeding complications and heparin-induced thrombocytopenia
Beta-blockers	Improved outcome in acute MI; prior recommendations were that they were to be given in the ED, now can be given within 24 hours so can withhold in the ED; contraindications include high-degree heart block, bradycardia, severe CHF
Nitroglycerin	Decreases preload/dilates coronary arteries; should be given in ischemic chest pain; avoid if hypotensive or if on sildenafil
Morphine	Decreases anxiety, preload, and afterload; should be given if pain persists after nitros; can cause hypotension/decrease respiratory drive; use with caution in inferior/posterior AMI as they may drop BP
What is the treatment of choice for STEMI?	Reperfusion therapy 1. Percutaneous coronary intervention (PCI) 2. Thrombolytics "Door to balloon time" of 90 min
What are some commonly used thrombolytics in AMI?	Streptokinase (not commonly used); tissue plasminogen activator such as alteplase
What is the most serious complication of thrombolytics?	Intracranial hemorrhage (ICH)
Which is the preferred reperfusion modality?	PCI is associated with slightly better outcomes, lower incidence of reinfarction, and death

Should thrombolytics be withheld if PCI is anticipated?	They should not be withheld if transfer to a cath lab will be greater than 90 min despite better outcomes with PCI.
What are other complications to consider in AMI?	Arrhythmias (especially ventricular fibrillation); cardiac rupture; congestive heart failure; septal rupture

CONGESTIVE HEART DISEASE AND PULMONARY EDEMA

What is the definition of congestive heart failure (CHF)?	A pathophysiologic state in which, at normal filling pressures, the heart is incapable of pumping a sufficient supply of blood to meet the metabolic demands of the body.
What are four classifications commonly used in CHF:	
Class I	Not limited with normal physical activity by symptoms
Class II	Ordinary physical activity results in fatigue, dyspnea, or other symptoms
Class III	Marked limitation in normal physical activity
Class IV	Symptomatic at rest or with any physical activity
How is congestive heart failure classified?	While many classification methods exist (high output vs. low; systolic vs. diastolic), a useful clinical construct is the distinction of left versus right heart failure.
What are other signs and symptoms of left ventricular failure?	Nocturnal angina, paroxysmal nocturnal dyspnea, orthopnea, fatigue, diaphoretic, and anxious. Physical Exam: rales/wheezes, S3 or S4 gallop, tachycardia and tachypnea, and pulsus alternans.
What are some causes of left ventricular failure?	Ischemic heart disease (no. 1 cause); HTN; valvular heart disease; dilated cardiomyopathy

What is cardiogenic pulmonary edema?

Acute presentation of left heart failure resulting from an imbalance in pulmonary vascular hydrostatic and oncotic forces, leading to transudation of fluid into the pulmonary interstitium.

What is the most common cause of right heart failure?

Left heart failure

What are some other common causes of right heart failure?

Pulmonary hypertension; pulmonary embolism; chronic obstructive pulmonary disease; right ventricular infarct

What are some physical exam findings of right ventricular failure?

Neck vein distension, ascites, dependent edema, and hepatojugular reflux.

What are important elements in the history for patient who present with acute CHF?

Prior history of heart failure, prior catheterization, presence of chest pain, and medication list.

Define orthopnea:

Common in patients with CHF, it is a type of dyspnea worse in the supine position due to increased venous return with an increase in diastolic pressure which is improved upon sitting.

What are some precipitating factors of acute pulmonary edema?

Myocardial ischemia; high sodium diet; non-compliance with medications; dysrhythmias; COPD (chronic cor pulmonale)

How is hypertension a precipitating cause of acute CHF?

A sudden increase in blood pressure or afterload can cause acute CHF

Name some common radiographic findings on a CXR in acute pulmonary edema:

Generally an enlarged cardiac silhouette (may be normal is acute), pleural effusions, cephalization (vascular redistribution to upper lung fields), and bilateral perihilar infiltrates

Does a normal CXR exclude acute pulmonary edema?

No—CXR findings may be delayed up to 12 hours after symptom onset

What is β-type natriuretic peptide (BNP)?

Cardiac myocytes secrete BNP in response to the high atrial and ventricular filling pressures.

How is BNP used clinically?	Increasingly used as a serum marker for CHF; levels of <100 pg/mL reliably exclude acute CHF; high negative predictive value with low BNP; BNP levels above 500 pg/mL were highly associated with HF; often not needed in acute management as it is a clinical diagnosis
What is the single most important agent for the treatment of acute CHF?	Oxygen
Patients with decompensated left heart failure frequently require assistance in maintaining adequate oxygenation/ventilation. What are some treatment options?	
High-flow via non-rebreather mask	Optimal option to deliver 100% oxygen; used to maintain adequate oxygen saturation; commonly used to avoid hypoxia
Non-invasive positive pressure ventilation	Continuous positive airway pressure (CPAP) and bilevel positive airway pressure (BiPAP) commonly used; improves oxygenation and dyspnea; early use helps avoid intubation
Endotracheal intubation	Final pathway if other methods fail; typically used for the following conditions: cannot maintain PaO_2 above 60 mm Hg; obtunded; progressive increase in CO_2 resulting in worsening respiratory acidosis
What should be the initial approach for all patients who present with acute CHF?	1. Identify the underlying cardiac disease 2. Identify the precipating cause such as AMI or poor compliance with diet or medications 3. Initiate treatment
What is the focus of treatment for acute CHF?	1. Reducing the cardiac workload by decreasing both the afterload and preload 2. Improve heart function 3. Control excessive salt and water
What are some options to decrease preload?	Nitrites and morphine

What are some important considerations for the following treatment options?

Nitrites

At low doses they are primarily venodilators while they will cause arteriolar dilation at high doses; prolonged nitrate use leads to tachyphylaxis; can be given sublingual or intravenously; titratable agent with rapid onset and offset of action; may cause hypotension in excessive amounts

Morphine

Peripheral vasodilation is from histamine release; has a central sympatholytic effect; decreases heart rate/blood pressure and myocardial oxygen consumption; given in repetitive 2- to 4-mg intravenous doses titrated to effect; may cause respiratory depression in excessive amounts

Loop diuretics

Furosemide is commonly administrated intravenously; inhibit sodium resorption from the renal filtrate with significant increase in excretion of salt and water

Phosphodiesterase type III inhibitors

Amrinone is commonly used; results in increased levels of cyclic adenosine monophosphate in the myocardium and peripheral smooth muscle; increase cardiac output and reduce left ventricular pressures; prodysrhythmic; should be used with invasive hemodynamic monitoring

Vasoactive pressors

Norepinephrine should be considered in hypotensive patients in acute CHF to increase blood pressure and coronary perfusion pressure, but will also increase afterload (worsening heart failure); these patients are complex and often require more definitive treatment such as angioplasty; dobutamine will increase cardiac output but can decrease blood pressure; isoproterenol should be avoided as it causes tachycardia and hypotension

THROMBOEMBOLIC DISEASE

What is Virchow triad?

Factors predisposing to vascular thrombosis with risk of pulmonary embolism: hypercoagulability; vessel wall injury; venostasis

List some other important risk factors for the development of a deep vein thrombosis (DVT):

Cancer; pregnancy and postpartum; recent trauma and surgery; estrogen therapy; obesity; protein C and S deficiency

What determines the clinical presentation of a DVT?

Degree of occlusion; location of occlusion; extent of collaterals

What are some signs and symptoms of a DVT?

Unilateral leg swelling, tenderness, edema, discoloration, palpable cord, and Homans sign

What is the most reliable finding on physical exam for a DVT?

Unilateral leg swelling with more than 3 cm difference from the other leg

Can a DVT be diagnosed by physical exam alone?

Due to variability of presentation, it cannot be used to exclude or make the diagnosis

What are some considerations of commonly used ancillary testing for the diagnosis of a DVT:

    D-dimer assay

Fibrin degradation product found with a DVT/PE; other conditions such as cancer or recent surgery can cause an elevation in d-dimer; more sensitive for proximal clots; it is not specific and a positive test often mandates further diagnostic evaluation

    Duplex ultrasonography

Initial diagnostic test in many cases; ideal for patients who are pregnant, diabetic, or have a contrast allergy; non-invasive; highly sensitive/specific for proximal DVT; less sensitive for deep vein, pelvic, and IVC thrombosis

    MRI

MRI rarely used in the ED; highly sensitive/specific for a DVT; non-invasive but expensive; can detect pelvic, renal, and calf thrombi; useful for second/third trimester pregnancy

    Contrast venography

Once the gold standard diagnostic test; invasive/painful and requires contrast; very high sensitivity/specificity

What are the primary goals for the treatment of a DVT?

Primarily to prevent the development of a pulmonary embolism (PE); prevent post-phlebitic syndrome, which is the result of prolonged venous insufficiency.

What are some pharmacologic agents to consider in the management of a DVT?

Heparin

Low-molecular-weight heparin (LMWH)

Warfarin

What are some advantages with the use of LMWH?

Patients can be discharged home; does not require monitoring such as heparin or warfarin; dalteparin and enoxaparin commonly used

What are some indications for the use of an inferior vena cava filter?

Contraindication to anticoagulation; urgent surgery (cannot anticoagulate prior); anticoagulation has failed (still clotting)

What are the general indications for admission for patients with a DVT?

Limited cardiopulmonary reserve and high risk for embolization; IV heparin use (contraindications to LMWH); poor compliance with medications

What is the epidemiology of a pulmonary embolism?

Third most common cause of death in the United States; most common preventable death in the hospital setting; up to 1/3 of all PEs are undiagnosed

What is a major source of a PE?

Venous thrombi from lower extremities and pelvis

What are some other possible sources of a PE?

Renal and ovarian veins; paradoxical left-to-right shunts from emboli originating in the left atrium; right side of heart

What are some risk factors for the development of a PE?

Similar to those for a DVT

What is the most common symptom of a PE?

Dyspnea

What are some signs and symptoms of a PE?

Pleuritic chest pain, hemoptysis, cough, tachycardia, sweating, elevated temperature, and syncope/hypotension in the setting of a massive PE.

What is the classic triad of a PE?

Pleuritic chest pain

Dyspnea

Hemoptysis

What are some commonly used screening tests used to evaluate a possible PE?

ABG (often will have an A-a gradient)

Chest radiograph

Electrocardiogram

D-dimer

What are some consideration with the use of these screening tests?

May help to exclude other disease processes; may support the diagnosis of a PE; a majority of these test often are poor at excluding a PE

What are some common findings in an arterial blood gas for a patient with PE?

PO_2 <80 mm Hg; mild respiratory alkalosis; elevated alveolar-arterial (A-a) gradient

Does a normal A-a gradient, normal PO_2, and normal vital signs exclude a PE?

No

What is the most common CXR finding in a patient with suspected PE?

Normal CXR

What are some radiographic abnormalities that can be seen on CXR in a PE?

Elevated hemidiaphragm; atelectasis; small pleural effusion

What is Hampton's hump?

The chest x-ray finding of a triangular density with a rounded apex that points toward the hilum representing pulmonary infarction.

What is Westermark sign?

The chest x-ray finding of regional oligemia.

How common are Hampton's hump and Westermark sign?

Rare—if present highly suggestive of PE in the correct clinical context

What are some common findings on ECG of a patient with a PE?

Sinus tachycardia (most common finding); evidence of right heart strain (S1, Q3, T3); transient non-specific ST-T wave changes

What are some characteristics of the following diagnostic tests:

    Computed tomography of the chest with intravenous contrast

Extensively used diagnostic test; rapidly performed; exclude other disease processes; disadvantage include contrast allergy, significant radiation exposure, and risk of acute renal failure

Ventilation-Perfusion (V/Q) scan	Commonly used as a screening test; normal V/Q scan virtually excludes PE; must also look at clinical probability; typically either read as normal, indeterminate, or high probability; if indeterminate it implies further testing (ie, CTA) may be required
Pulmonary angiography	Considered the gold standard for the diagnosis of a PE; it is invasive, not available everywhere, and carries a small mortality risk; complications more common in elderly patients; rarely used as diagnostic testing supplanted by CT
What are the treatment goals for a PE?	Prevent recurrent PEs with the use of anticoagulation as the cornerstone of management
What are some commonly used anticoagulants for PE?	Heparin Low-molecular-weight heparin (LMWH) Warfarin
What are two complications of heparin and LMWH?	1. Thrombocytopenia 2. Hemorrhage (risk is substantial in the setting of renal failure with LMWH)
What are two commonly used thrombolytics for PE?	1. Streptokinase (often not used) 2. Tissue plasminogen activator (TPA) such as alteplase
What is an important indication for the use of thrombolytics in the setting of a PE?	Hemodynamic instability Cardiac arrest where a PE is a consideration

CARDIOMYOPATHIES

What is a cardiomyopathy?	Disease of the myocardium associated with cardiac dysfunction.
What are some classifications of cardiomyopathies?	Dilated cardiomyopathy Hypertrophic cardiomyopathy Restrictive cardiomyopathy

What diagnostic test is commonly used to evaluate cardiomyopathies?

Echocardiographic evaluation

What is the definition of a dilated cardiomyopathy?

Dilatation and impaired contraction of one or both ventricles, affected patients have impaired systolic function and may or may not develop overt heart failure.

What is commonly associated with dilated cardiomyopathy?

Viral myocarditis

What are some other important causes of dilated cardiomyopathy?

Idiopathic; toxins (especially ethanol/cocaine/lithium); peripartum; nutritional deficiencies (thiamine deficiency)

What are some signs and symptoms of dilated cardiomyopathy?

Signs and symptoms of right and left-sided heart failure such as exertional fatigue, dyspnea, JVD, orthopnea, and ascites.

What are some common findings in the following diagnostic tests used for diluted cardiomyopathy:

ECG

Poor R-wave progression; atrial or ventricular enlargement; AV block; atrial fibrillation most common dysrhythmia

CXR

Cardiomegaly; pulmonary venous congestion

Echocardiogram

Decreased ejection fraction; enlarged heart chambers; mural thrombi; abnormal ventricle contraction

What are some considerations in the management of dilated cardiomyopathy?

Alleviation of symptoms; consider anticoagulation if there is a mural thrombi or in atrial fibrillation

What are commonly used agents in alleviating symptoms of dilated cardiomyopathy?

Diuretics, vasodilators, and cardioactive steroids

What is the definition of restrictive cardiomyopathy?

Non-dilated ventricles with impaired ventricular filling due to diastolic restriction usually from infiltration of the myocardium causing stiffening.

What are some important causes of restrictive cardiomyopathy?

Amyloidosis; endomyocardial fibrosis; hemochromatosis; type II glycogen storage disease

What are some signs and symptoms of restrictive cardiomyopathy?

Similar to constrictive pericarditis: often will have symptoms of right-sided heat failure with exercise intolerance being very common. Physical Exam: abnormal heart sounds (S3/S4 gallop), dependent edema, and rales/wheezes

What are some common findings in the following diagnostic tests in restrictive cardiomyopathy:

ECG

Commonly show atrial fibrillation (afib); non-specific ST-T wave changes; low voltage

CXR

Cardiomegaly can be seen; may initially show a normal heart

Echocardiogram

Normal systolic function; thickened wall; atria size is greater than ventricle size

What are some points in the management of restrictive cardiomyopathy?

Diuretics often used for relief; vasodilators may decrease afterload; diagnosis is confirmed with biopsy

What is the definition of hypertrophic cardiomyopathy?

Left ventricular hypertrophy without dilation that often results in impaired diastolic relaxation and can result in decreased cardiac output.

What is the most common cause of hypertrophic cardiomyopathy?

50% is autosomal dominant inherited

What is the most common presenting symptom of hypertrophic cardiomyopathy?

Dyspnea on exertion

What are some other signs and symptoms of hypertrophic cardiomyopathy?

Syncope, dysrhythmias (afib most common), ischemic chest pain, and sudden death (especially from ventricular fibrillation. Physical Exam: systolic ejection murmur especially with valsalva, rapid biphasic carotid pulse, and prominent A wave of neck veins.

What are some common findings in the following diagnostic tests:

ECG

Afib and PVCs are common; changes in anterior, inferior, or lateral leads; left ventricular hypertrophy

CXR	Typically normal
Echocardiogram	LVH especially with septal hypertrophy; small left ventricular chamber

What are some components in the management of hypertrophic cardiomyopathy?

Beta-blockers are the mainstay for symptom relief; calcium (channel blocker in select patients); amiodarone for ventricular dysrhythmias; avoid inotropic agents; consider anticoagulation for afib

What treatment is reserved for severely symptomatic patients who fail medication?

Septal myomectomy

ENDOCARDITIS

What is the definition of endocarditis?

Localized infection of the endocardium that is typically characterized by vegetations.

What is the pathophysiology of endocarditis?

Any injury to the endocardium can result in platelet-fibrin complex that can be colonized by organisms such as bacteria or fungus.

What are some risk factors of endocarditis?

Prosthetic valves; intravenous drug abuse (IVDA); any acquired or congenital valvular lesions; indwelling lines (ie, shunts or catheters); hemodialysis or peritoneal dialysis

Name two sites that commonly allow entry of bacteria in endocarditis:

1. Oral cavity
2. Genitourinary tract

What are some classes of organisms involved in endocarditis?

Bacteria (most common); fungi; viruses; rickettsiae

What are the top three causes of endocarditis in the following:

    Intravenous drug use or immunocompromised

Streptococcus species; *S aureus*; gram-negative bacteria

    Normal valves

Streptococcus viridans; S aureus; Enterococci

    Prosthetic valves

Staphylococcus (coagulase negative); *Streptococcus viridans; S aureus*

What are some important things to know about right-sided endocarditis?

Commonly involves the tricuspid valve; typically an acute presentation; very common in intravenous drug use; *S aureus* most common agent

What are some important things to know about left-sided endocarditis?

Commonly involves the mitral valve; more common in valvular defects; *S viridans* and *S aureus* common organisms involved

What are some signs and symptoms of endocarditis?

Typically non-specific such as fever, fatigue, weight loss, neurologic complaints, and chest pain. Physical Exam: heart murmur, seeding to other sites such as lung, cutaneous signs (ie, petechiae), and eye findings (ie, conjunctival hemorrhages)

What are Janeway lesions?

Non-tender and small erythematous/hemorrhagic nodules in the palms or soles, which are pathognomonic of infective endocarditis. The pathology is due to a type III hypersensitivity reaction.

What are Osler nodes?

Painful, red, raised lesions on the finger pulps that are indicative of subacute bacterial endocarditis (can be seen elsewhere such as systemic lupus erythematosus).

What are some important diagnostic tests to consider in evaluating endocarditis?

Blood culture: positive in most cases; CBC; CXR; ESR/C-protein: often elevated; echocardiography: often show vegetations

What is the ideal method to draw blood cultures?

Three sets of blood culture should be drawn from three separate sites with at least 1 hour between the first and last blood culture.

How often do blood cultures return positive?

90 to 95% unless antibiotics have been administered in which case it may be lower

What is Duke Criteria for the diagnosis of infective endocarditis?

Any of the following:

Two major criteria

One major and three minor criteria

Five minor criteria

What are the major criteria used in Duke criteria?

Positive blood culture from at least two separate sets of culture

Evidence of endocarditis demonstrated by echo (ie, vegetations)

What are some minor criteria used in Duke criteria?

Physical findings such as Osler nodes, Janeway lesions, Splinter hemorrhages, etc.

Fever

Risk factors such as intravenous drug use or structural problem

What is the ideal antibiotic regiment to initiate in patients with suspected infective endocarditis?

Depends on if the valve is native, intravenous drug use, or mechanical heart valve:

If native heart valve consider penicillin or vancomycin AND gentamycin

If intravenous drug use: vancomycin

If prosthetic valve: vancomycin and gentamycin

What are some conditions that require the use of prophylaxis for endocarditis?

Prosthetic heart valves; any acquired or congenital valvular lesions; any congenital malformation; hypertrophic cardiomyopathy

MYOCARDITIS

What is the definition of myocarditis?

Inflammation of the muscles of the heart, often due to infection that is also often associated with acute pericarditis.

Name some examples for the following causes of myocarditis:

Viruses (most common cause)

Coxsackie A and B; poliovirus; CMV

Bacteria

N meningitidis; Beta-hemolytic streptococcus; C diphtheriae

Parasites

Chagas disease; trichinosis; toxoplasmosis

Drugs/Toxins

Cocaine; inhalants; methyldopa

Systemic diseases

Lupus; Kawasaki syndrome; sarcoidosis

What are some signs and symptoms of myocarditis?

Highly variable depending on degree of cardiac involvement that can range from chest pain, signs of heart failure, to dysrhythmias and tachycardia. Physical exam: S3/S4 gallop, pericardial friction rub (if pericarditis present), and various murmurs

What history is common to those who present with myocarditis?	Preceding viral illness in many cases
What are some common findings for the following diagnostic studies that may be used to evaluate myocarditis:	
ECG	Any type of dysrhythmias may be present; low-voltage QRS; non-specific ST-T wave changes
Echocardiography	Dilated chambers; focal wall motion abnormalities
CXR	Typically normal; may show cardiomegaly; may also show pulmonary edema
Cardiac enzymes	Unlike AMI, they will rise and fall slowly; elevations of cardiac troponin I or T more common than CK-MB
In what case should one suspect myocarditis?	A young healthy male who presents with unexplained cardiac abnormalities, especially if recent history of viral infections.
How is myocarditis confirmed in combination with clinical history?	Endomyocardial biopsy
What are some components in the management of myocarditis?	Primarily supportive; Abx if bacterial cause is suspected; avoid steroids/ NSAIDs in early course; IVIG may be useful in pediatric patients, especially with Kawasaki syndrome; intensive care unit in severe cases

PERICARDIAL DISEASE

What is the primary presentation of pericardial disease?	The principal manifestations of pericardial disease are pericarditis and pericardial effusion.
What are the two most common causes of pericardial disease?	1. Infections (ie, Coxsackie viruses A and B) 2. Idiopathic
List some other important causes of pericardial disease:	Rheumatologic disease (ie, lupus); cancer (ie, metastatic); radiation; cardiac injury (ie, post MI); medication (ie, hydralazine)

What are some signs and symptoms of pericarditis?	Sharp inspirational chest pain that is relieved when leaning forward, low-grade fever, and dyspnea.
What physical finding is pathognomonic for pericarditis?	Pericardial friction rub
What is the best way to elicit a pericardial friction rub?	Sitting and leaning forward
What is the most common ECG finding?	Sinus tachycardia (dysrhythmias are rare)

What are some common findings for the following diagnostic studies that may be used to evaluate pericarditis:

CBC	Often show an elevated white count
ESR/CRP	Typically elevated due to inflammation, but it is non-specific
Cardiac enzymes	May be mildly elevated; often increase in setting of myocarditis
ECG	Diffuse ST-segment elevation; reciprocal ST segment depression in aVR and V1; PR segment depression; diffuse T wave inversion—late finding
CXR	Typically normal; may show enlarged silhouette if pericardial effusion >200 mL
Echocardiography	Test of choice to evaluate effusion; echo can also assess cardiac function; can detect as little as 15 mL of effusion

What are some considerations in the management of pericarditis?	Treat the underlying cause Pain control with NSAIDs commonly used Important to consider tamponade as a complication
What are some guidelines to admit patients with pericarditis?	Serious underlying cause (ie, MI); severe pain refractory to medication; most can be managed on a outpatient basis
What is the most serious complication of pericardial disease?	Cardiac tamponade
What is Beck triad?	Jugular venous distension (JVD); hypotension; muffled heart sounds—rare to have all three

What are some other common clinical features of cardiac tamponade?	Dyspnea, narrow pulse pressure, pulse paradoxus, and tachycardia
What are some possible ECG findings in cardiac tamponade?	Low QRS voltage; total electrical alternans (beat-to-beat alternating pattern)—not always present
What are some important differentials to consider in patients with JVD and hypotension?	Cardiac tamponade; tension pneumothorax; massive pulmonary embolism
What is the gold standard to diagnose cardiac tamponade?	Echocardiography
What are some considerations in the management of cardiac tamponade?	Immediate pericardiocentesis if unstable with suspected tamponade Aggressive fluid resuscitation Inotropic agents (ie, dopamine)

VALVULAR DISEASE

Tricuspid Stenosis

What are some causes of tricuspid stenosis?	Endocarditis secondary to IVDA; rheumatic fever; congenital tricuspid atresia; carcinoid syndrome
What is important to note about tricuspid stenosis?	Tricuspid stenosis often coexist with other valvular disease (ie, mitral stenosis)
What are some common clinical features of tricuspid stenosis?	Systemic venous congestion, fatigue, and dyspnea in some cases. Physical Exam: diastolic murmur, ascites, and JVD
What is the most common dysrhythmia associated with tricuspid stenosis?	Atrial fibrillation
What are some common findings for the following diagnostic studies that may be used to evaluate tricuspid stenosis:	
CXR	May show an enlarged right atrium
ECG	Tall and pointed P-waves; Afib if present

What are some considerations in the management of tricuspid stenosis?	Treat for afib (rate control/anticoagulate); antibiotic prophylaxis when indicated

Tricuspid Regurgitation

What are some causes of tricuspid regurgitation?	Rheumatic fever; RV dilation due to pulmonary HTN; infective endocarditis; trauma
What are some signs and symptoms of tricuspid regurgitation?	Dyspnea on exertion, fatigue, anorexia, peripheral edema, and JVD. Physical Exam: holosystolic murmur and palpable left ventricular heave
What are some common findings for the following diagnostic studies that may be used to evaluate tricuspid regurgitation:	
CXR	May show an enlarged right atrium/ ventricle; pulmonary vasculature often normal
ECG	Right atrial and ventricular hypertrophy; incomplete right RBBB; Afib if present
What are some considerations in the management of tricuspid regurgitation?	Treat for afib (rate control/ anticoagulate); adequate control of fluid overload and failure symptoms; surgical intervention for structural deformity

Mitral Stenosis

What are some causes of mitral stenosis?	Rheumatic fever (>90% of cases); left atrial myxoma; congenital
What are some signs and symptoms of mitral stenosis?	Dyspnea on exertion, hemoptysis, fatigue, orthopnea, and palpitations. Physical Exam: early diastolic opening snap, palpable diastolic thrill, and loud S1

What are some common findings for the following diagnostic studies that may be used to evaluate mitral stenosis:	
CXR	Pulmonary congestion; left atrial enlargement
ECG	P mitrale (left atrial enlargement); Afib if present
What are some considerations in the management of mitral stenosis?	Treat for afib (rate control/anticoagulate); diuretics for pulmonary congestion; Abx prophylaxis when indicated

Chronic Mitral Regurgitation

What are some causes of chronic mitral regurgitation?	Rheumatic fever; connective tissue disorder; mitral valve prolapse; infective endocarditis
What are some signs and symptoms of chronic mitral regurgitation?	Dyspnea on exertion and orthopnea, but even with severe MR, most are asymptomatic unless LV failure, pulmonary HTN, or afib. Physical Exam: S1 is diminished, S3/S4 gallop, and left parasternal heave
What are some common findings for the following diagnostic studies that may be used to evaluate chronic mitral regurgitation:	
CXR	May show an enlarged left atrium/ventricle; pulmonary vasculature often congested
ECG	Left ventricular hypertrophy; left atrial enlargement; Afib if present
What are some considerations in the management of mitral regurgitation?	Treat for afib (rate control/anticoagulate); adequate control of fluid overload and failure symptoms; Abx prophylaxis when indicated

Acute Mitral Regurgitation

What are some causes of acute mitral regurgitation?	Myocardial infarction; trauma; infective endocarditis

What structures associated with the mitral valve can be damaged?	Papillary muscle; valve leaflet; chordae tendineae
What are some signs and symptoms of acute mitral regurgitation?	Dyspnea on exertion and orthopnea, but will often present as fulminant CHF and symptoms of the cause of the rupture (ie, MI). Physical Exam: S1 is diminished, S3/S4 gallop, and left parasternal heave
What are some common findings for the following diagnostic studies that may be used to evaluate acute mitral regurgitation:	
CXR	Often have a normal cardiac silhouette; evidence of severe pulmonary edema
ECG	Often show sinus tachycardia; may also show evidence of myocardial infarction if that is the underlying etiology
What are some considerations in the management of mitral regurgitation?	Oxygen and afterload reduction; adequate control of fluid overload and failure symptoms; emergent consult with CT surgery

Mitral Valve Prolapse

What are some important things to know about mitral valve prolapse?	Most common valvular heart disease; more common in young females; present in up to 10% of the population
What are some causes of mitral valve prolapse?	Idiopathic; associated with tissue connective disorder; autosomal dominant congenital disorder
What are some signs and symptoms of mitral valve prolapse?	Palpitations, syncope, chest pain, or can be asymptomatic. Physical Exam: high-pitched late systolic murmur or late systolic click
What are some complications to consider for mitral valve prolapse?	Sudden death (very rare); CHF (due to severe regurgitation); embolization

What are some common findings for the following diagnostic studies that may be used to evaluate aortic stenosis:	
CXR	Typically normal unless severe regurgitation
ECG	Typically normal; may show T-wave changes in inferior lead; may show QT prolongation
What are some considerations in the management of mitral valve prolapse?	Abx prophylaxis when indicated (usually if with injury); beta-blockers for chest pain/dysrhythmias; anticoagulation for suspected embolization

Aortic Stenosis

What are some causes of aortic stenosis?	Congenital bicuspid valve; rheumatic heart disease; calcific aortic disease
When do patients generally become symptomatic with aortic stenosis?	Most are asymptomatic until very late in the disease—valve opening decreases <1 cm
What are some signs and symptoms of aortic stenosis?	Syncope, chest pain, dyspnea on exertion, sudden death, and symptoms of heart failure. Physical Exam: harsh systolic murmur (crescendo-decrescendo), narrow pulse pressure, and diminished carotid upstroke
What are some common findings for the following diagnostic studies that may be used to evaluate aortic stenosis:	
CXR	Aortic calcification; left ventricular enlargement; poststenotic dilatation of the aorta
ECG	Left ventricular hypertrophy; left or right BBB
What are some considerations in the management of aortic stenosis?	Symptomatic patients referred for either valve replacement or valvuloplasty; admit patients in CHF; Abx prophylaxis when indicated

Chronic Aortic Regurgitation

What are some causes of chronic aortic regurgitation?	Rheumatic heart disease; connective tissue disorder; bicuspid valve; infective endocarditis; tertiary syphilis
What are some signs and symptoms of chronic aortic regurgitation?	Dyspnea on exertion, orthopnea, fatigue and palpitations. Physical Exam: S1 is diminished, wide pulse pressure, high-pitched decrescendo blowing murmur, and displaced PMI

What are some common findings for the following diagnostic studies that may be used to evaluate chronic aortic regurgitation:

CXR	Often have cardiomegaly; pulmonary root congestion; aortic root dilation
ECG	Left ventricular hypertrophy; sometimes an LBBB can be seen
What are some considerations in the management of chronic aortic regurgitation?	Adequate control of fluid overload and failure symptoms (treat as CHF); Abx prophylaxis when indicated

Acute Aortic Regurgitation

What are some causes of acute aortic regurgitation?	Aortic dissection; trauma; infective endocarditis
What are some signs and symptoms of acute aortic regurgitation?	Severe dyspnea on exertion, signs of heart failure, and chest pain. Physical Exam: low blood pressure, tachycardia, normal pulse pressure, midsystolic flow murmur, and low CO

What are some common findings for the following diagnostic studies that may be used to evaluate acute aortic regurgitation:

CXR	Often have a normal cardiac silhouette; evidence of pulmonary edema
ECG	Often show sinus tachycardia; left ventricle strain; non-specific ST-T wave change

What are some considerations in the management of acute aortic regurgitation?	Determine cause and treat; adequate control of fluid overload and failure symptoms; emergent consult with CT surgery for valve replacement

Prosthetic Valves

What are two types of prosthetic valves commonly used?	1. Mechanical valves 2. Bioprosthetic valves (porcine or bovine)
What are some important points regarding mechanical valves?	Typically made from carbon alloys; most mechanical valves last 20 to 30 years and a metallic noise can be heard; life-long anticoagulation required; greater hemolysis than tissue valves
What are some important points regarding bioprosthetic valves?	Can be human, bovine, or porcine tissue; typically lasts <10 years; closure noise similar to native valves; anticoagulation required in some situations; less hemolysis then mechanical valves
What is the most serious complication of prosthetic valves?	Thromboembolic events
What are some other complications of prosthetic valves?	Structural failure leading to sudden heart failure; bleeding; embolization; hemolytic anemia; valvular obstruction (from thrombus)

THORACIC AORTIC DISSECTION

What is the epidemiology of thoracic aortic dissection (TAD)?	Males are affected more than females; most patients affected are over 50 years; TAD are more common than AAA
What is the pathophysiology of TAD?	Degeneration of the aortic media, or cystic medial necrosis that leads to a tear in the aortic intima. Propagation of the dissection to various areas (ie, coronary artery is the feared concern).
What are two factors that determine the rate of dissection propagation?	1. Blood pressure 2. Rate of ventricular contraction

What is the biggest risk factor for the development of TAD?	Uncontrolled blood pressure
What are some other important risk factors of TAD?	Connective tissue disorders—Marfan; congenital heart disease; Turner syndrome; infections (ie, syphilis); drugs that raise BP (ie, cocaine); trauma
What are the two major classification systems used to classify TAD based on location of dissection?	1. Stanford 2. DeBakey

What is the Stanford classification:

Type A	Ascending aorta
Type B	Descending aorta

What is the DeBakey classification:

Type I	Ascending aorta and part distal aorta
Type II	Ascending aorta only
Type III	Descending aorta only
Subtype IIIA	Dissection above the diaphragm
Subtype IIIB	Dissection below the diaphragm

What is the mortality rate for untreated TAD once the dissection begins:

1 day	33%
2 days	50%
2 weeks	75%
1 month	Approaches 90%

What is the character of chest pain in TAD?	Chest pain that is abrupt and maximal at onset, migrates as the dissection progresses that is typically described as tearing with radiation to jaw/arm/back.
What are some other signs and symptoms of TAD based on the location of the dissection?	Abdominal pain (mesenteric ischemia); flank pain/GU symptoms (< renal flow); cerebrovascular accident (dissection of carotid artery); myocardial infarction (dissection of coronary artery); CHF; syncope; spinal cord deficits
What are some important physical findings that help to establish the diagnosis of TAD?	Focal neurological deficits, a 20 mmHg extremity BP difference, and unequal or absent pulses between extremities.

What are some important points for the following initial tests that should be undertaken:

CXR

Should be done immediately and upright; CXR will almost be abnormal in TAD; mediastinal widening (>8 cm) common; other common findings include loss of aortic knob, deviation of trachea, effusion, etc. Important to realize non-specific findings

ECG

Will be abnormal in most cases; ischemic changes can be seen; LV hypertrophy is common as well; inferior wall MI most common pattern

Name four studies that are commonly used to confirm the diagnosis of TAD:

1. MRI
2. Aortography
3. Transesophageal echocardiography
4. CT aortography

Is a transthoracic echocardiography (TTE) a sensitive test?

No—it does not image the arch and the images are also dependent on the habitus of the person. A transesophageal echocardiography is a very sensitive test but may be difficult to obtain at some institutions

What is the test of choice at most institutions as it is non-invasive, inexpensive, and fast?

CT aortography

What are some findings on CT that may suggest a TAD?

Demonstration of both the false and true lumina

Identification of an intimal flap

Dilatation of the aorta

What is important initial management for any patient with suspected TAD?

Control of BP (ie, nitroprusside); control HR (ie, beta-blocker); avoid anticoagulants/lytics; also administer proper analgesia, opioids are ideal as they also decrease sympathetic outflow

Name some common pharmacologic agents used to manage TAD as well as important points for each:

Esmolol:

Very short acting; easy to titrate; should be used to decrease heart rate

Nitroprusside:

Often used in conjunction with a beta-blocker; often will cause reflex tachycardia if not used with beat-blocker

Nifedipine:

Not recommended as well as other dihydropyridines as they are poorly cardioselective and may cause reflex tachycardia

What is the disposition of patient with a type A dissection?

All type A dissections require surgical interventions

Do type B dissections require surgical intervention?

This patient population have worse surgical complications that so often are managed with medications to control hypertension.

What is another possible treatment option for type B dissections?

Placement of a stent by interventional radiology

ABDOMINAL AORTIC ANEURYSMS

What are some important things to know about abdominal aortic aneurysms (AAA)?

Involve all layers of the aorta; most AAA occur below the renal arteries; a ruptured AAA is surgical emergency

What is the diameter of the aorta that is considered pathologic?

Diameter >3.0 cm is generally considered aneurysmal

What is the pathophysiology of AAA?

Aortic aneurysms are caused by a progressive weakening of the aortic wall which results in a dilatation. The aneurysm will grow progressively larger and eventually rupture if it is not diagnosed and treated.

What are some risk factors for the development of AAA?

Age (most occur in >70 years); male gender; history of smoking; hypertension; family history in first degree relatives; history of CAD or PVD

What are some signs and symptoms of AAA rupture?

Classic presentation is sudden onset of severe abdominal, back, or flank pain that may be associated with syncope. Pain can radiate to the testicles/labia as well.

What is the most common misdiagnosis of AAA rupture?

Kidney stone

What are some important physical findings that help to establish the diagnosis of AAA rupture?

A ruptured AAA will often have a tender pulsatile mass in the epigastric area, bruits, and signs of distal extremity ischemia.

What are some considerations for the following diagnostic tests commonly utilized for AAA:

Plain abdominal film

Not very accurate for AAA; may show aneurysmal calcification; does not confirm/exclude diagnosis

Ultrasonography

Can be utilized on unstable patients; inexpensive, fast, sensitive; can only detect aneurysm, not leaks; limited by adipose tissue and gas

CT contrast

Very accurate and sensitive; can also detect other abnormalities; negative: IV contrast and long study test; not to be used on unstable patients

What are the critical actions in the management of a ruptured aneurysm?

Fluid resuscitation

Potential blood transfusion—6 to 8 units of blood should be made available

A hemodynamically unstable patient requires immediate operative intervention

What is another treatment option aside from open repair of a ruptured AAA?

Endovascular repair

What are some late complications of a AAA repair?

Pseudoaneurysm

Graft infection

What is an important consideration in a patient with a history of a AAA repair who now presents with GI bleeding?

Aortoenteric fistula

What is the diagnostic test of choice in a suspected aortoenteric fistula?

Can vary from an upper endoscopy or CT scan

CLINICAL VIGNETTES—MAKE THE DIAGNOSIS

65-year-old woman with no cardiac history presents as a transfer from an outside hospital for chest pain. She mentions that her CP started about 3 hours ago and describes it is substernal associated with diaphoresis and nausea; PE: unremarkable; ECG reveals 3-mm ST-elevations in V1-V4

Anterior STEMI

19-year-old woman with currently on birth control medication presents with unilateral left leg swelling soon after a trip to Mexico, but otherwise has been well; PE: unilateral swelling of left calf with a (+) Homans' sign

Deep vein thrombosis

23-year-old man with Hx of IVDA presents with fever, fatigue, and weight loss for the past 2 weeks; PE: heart murmur, petechiae, and conjunctival hemorrhages

Infective endocarditis

18-year-old man with no PMH presents with a sudden syncopal episode during soccer practice, but otherwise is now feeling fine in the ED; PE: rapid biphasic carotid pulse and systolic ejection murmur; ECG: left ventricular hypertrophy

Hypertrophic cardiomyopathy

65-year-old man with Hx of DM and HTN presents with CP. Patient mentions that he previously had CP only when he did any moderate activity and which was relieved by rest and his nitro, but now he gets CP when he is at rest, but it still does not last more than 5 minutes or so

Unstable angina

70-year-old man with Hx of DM and HTN presents with "chest pressure" for about 2 hours associated with dyspnea, diaphoresis, nausea, and radiation of pain to jaw; PE: unremarkable exam except patient is anxious; labs: elevated cardiac enzymes; ECG: ST-depression in inferior leads (II, III, and aVL)

NSTEMI

51-year-old woman with history of DM, HTN, and smoking presents with a sudden onset of abdomen pain with radiation to the left flank as well as her inner thigh; PE: pulsatile mass in the epigastric area as well as abdominal bruits

Aortic abdominal aneurysm

50-year-old woman with Hx of breast cancer presents with pleuritic chest pain and dyspnea on exertion for 3 days, but is otherwise stable; PE: tachycardia, but otherwise unremarkable exam; CXR: clear fields except for regional oligemia

Pulmonary embolism

80-year-old woman with Hx of HTN presents with syncope whenever she exerts herself, but otherwise no other complaints; PE: harsh systolic murmur (crescendo-decrescendo), narrow pulse pressure, and diminished carotid upstroke

Aortic stenosis

48-year-old man with Hx of uncontrolled hypertension presents with tearing chest pain with radiation to the back that has been refractory to nitro; PE: 20 mmHg extremity BP difference, and unequal or absent pulses between extremities

Thoracic aortic dissection

21-year-old woman presents with CP that she describes as sharp and more painful on deep inspiration, but relieved when she leans forward; PE: friction heard on cardiac exam; ECG: depressed PR interval and diffuse ST segment elevation

Pericarditis

29-year-old woman who recently arrived from South America presents with chest pain and recalls that it started about a week after her cold; PE: S3/S4 gallop with a pericardial friction rub; ECG: low-voltage complex

Myocarditis

CHAPTER 7

Gastrointestinal Emergencies

ESOPHAGUS

Anatomy

What are some important anatomic points to know about the esophagus?	It is 25 cm in length; upper third is striated muscle (under voluntary control); lower two-thirds is smooth muscle (involuntary)
What are the major nerves of the extrinsic nervous system that innervate the esophagus?	Vagus nerve; sympathetic fibers; spinal accessory nerve
What are the two major plexuses that are found within the esophagus?	1. Meissner's plexus 2. Auerbach's plexus
What are the three layers of the esophagus?	1. Inner mucosa 2. Submucosa 3. Muscle layer
What is the clinical significance for the lack of serosa?	Any compromise of the submucosa will lead to diffuse rapid mediastinitis.
Name the three anatomical constrictions within the esophagus that may represent points of obstruction:	1. Upper esophagus sphincter (UES) 2. Lower esophagus sphincter (LES) 3. Level of the aortic arch

Dysphagia/Odynophagia

What is the definition of dysphagia?	It is a subjective experience that ranges from the inability to swallow to the sensation of food "stuck" in the esophagus—not painful.

What is the definition of odynophagia?	The sensation of pain when swallowing.
What are some important elements in the history to obtain in dysphagia?	Whether it is acute versus chronic; dysphagia to food or liquids (or both); intermittent versus progressive

What are some important points for the two categories of dysphagia:

Transport dysphagia	Problem typically lies at the esophagus; often patient will complain of a sticking sensation; commonly due to anatomical problems
Transfer dysphagia	Problem typically is at the oropharynx; difficulty in transfer of food bolus to esophagus; commonly due to neuromuscular problems
List some common anatomical problems that may result in dysphagia:	Strictures (ie, radiation injury); malignancy; webs; diverticula
List some common neuromuscular problems that may result in dysphagia:	Achalasia; spasms; neurological insults (ie, stroke)
What are some considerations in the management of dysphagia?	Ensure the patient is stable; a careful history is paramount. Further workup likely will require a swallow study or esophagogastroduodenoscopy (EGD).
What is a common cause of odynophagia?	Esophagitis
What are some signs and symptoms of odynophagia?	Pain on swallowing and chest pain
What are two main causes of odynophagia?	1. Infectious 2. Inflammatory
List some examples of infectious esophagitis:	Candida; herpes simplex virus (HSV); cytomegalovirus (CMV); aphthous ulceration
List some examples that may cause inflammatory esophagitis:	Medication (ie, non-steroidal anti-inflammatory drugs [NSAIDs] and antibiotics); GERD
What are some considerations in the management of esophagitis?	If chest pain, distinguish from cardiac origin; monitor for bleed, perforation, and obstruction; typically managed on a outpatient basis

Gastroesophageal Reflux Disease

What is the definition of gastroesophageal reflux disease (GERD)?	Reflux of stomach acid typically from transient relaxation of LES or a weak LES.
What are some complications of GERD?	Esophageal erosions; esophageal strictures; Barrett esophagus; esophageal cancer
Name some major causes of GERD:	Decrease in esophageal motility (achalasia); prolonged gastric emptying (obstruction); transient decrease in LES tone (diet)
What are some signs and symptoms of GERD?	Dysphagia, odynophagia, heartburn, and presentation that may be similar to pain related to cardiac ischemia (ie, "squeezing pain,") pain that radiates to arms and jaw, and nausea/vomiting.
What are some factors that may exacerbate GERD?	Heavy meals; medication; supine position
What is an important pitfall to remember when dealing with GERD?	Not considering ACS as a possible cause of symptoms
What are some considerations in the management of GERD?	H_2-blockers, proton-pump inhibitors (PPI); avoid triggers (ie, eating before bed or laying completely flat); consider outpatient referral with GI

Esophageal Perforation

What are some causes of esophageal perforation?	Chest trauma; iatrogenic (endoscopy); swallowing (object); sudden increase in intra-abdominal pressure such as emesis
What is the most common cause of esophageal perforation?	Iatrogenic
What is Mallory-Weiss syndrome?	A partial-thickness tear of the esophagus.
What are some signs and symptoms of Mallory-Weiss syndrome?	Mild self-limiting upper GI bleeding, dysphagia, and odynophagia

What are some risk factors for Mallory-Weiss syndrome?	Hiatal hernia; EtOH abuse; esophagitis, vomiting
What is Boerhaave syndrome?	A full-thickness perforation of the esophagus.
What are some of the signs and symptoms of Boerhaave syndrome?	Severe tearing chest pain that often radiates to the back/neck, mediastinal crunch, and epigastric tenderness.
What are complications of Boerhaave syndrome?	Mediastinitis (high mortality); sepsis
What are some diagnostic tests used in Boerhaave syndrome and some possible findings:	
Chest x-ray	Widened mediastinum, left pneumothorax, left pleural effusion, and mediastinal emphysema
Esophagram (water-soluble contrast)	Leakage of content into the mediastinal area—avoid barium as it is irritating
What are some considerations in the management of esophageal rupture?	Aggressive fluids; broad spectrum intravenous (IV) antibiotics; surgical consult

Swallowed Foreign Body

What are some important things to know about a swallowed foreign body?	80% of complaints are in the pediatric population; most ingestions pass through the GI tract without intervention or problems
What types of foreign bodies are most commonly swallowed by children?	True foreign objects such as coins
What types of foreign bodies are most commonly swallowed by adults?	Food impactions
What portion of the esophagus do most objects get lodged in children?	Cricopharyngeal area
What portion of the esophagus do most objects get lodged in adults?	Distal portion of the esophagus
What are some signs and symptoms of a swallowed foreign body?	Dysphagia, foreign body sensation, gagging, emesis, drooling, and possible respiratory distress

What is the diagnostic test of choice in a swallowed foreign body?	Plain films with at least two views; endoscopy (diagnostic and therapeutic); esophagram (if perforation is suspected)
What are three complications of foreign body impaction?	1. Obstruction 2. Esophageal perforation 3. Esophageal strictures
What is the probability that a foreign body will pass completely once past the gastroesophageal junction?	90%
What is typically done for proximal impactions of the esophagus?	Removal of object via endoscopy
What are some commonly used medications to help with passage of distal esophagus impaction?	Nifedipine; sublingual nitroglycerin; glucagon
About what percentage of foreign bodies that are lodged and cannot be removed require surgical intervention?	1%
What are some considerations in the management of swallowed foreign bodies?	Most can be managed expectantly; lodged sharp objects and button batteries (if lodged in esophagus) mandate removal; most foreign bodies are cleared in 2 to 3 days

GASTROINTESTINAL BLEEDING

What are some important epidemiologic facts about GI bleeding?	Potentially life-threatening; upper GI bleeding is more common in elderly males; mortality rises with age
What are some factors that are associated with high mortality in GI bleeding?	Advanced age; co-existing organ disease; hemodynamic instability; repeated hematemesis/hematochezia
What defines upper GI bleeding?	Bleeding that is proximal to the ligament of Treitz.
What are some important points about each of the important causes of upper GI bleeding:	
Gastric and esophageal varices	Commonly from portal hypertension; very high rebleeding and mortality rate; comprise small number of upper GI bleeds

Peptic ulcer disease	Includes gastric, and duodenal ulcers; most common cause of upper GI bleed; gastric ulcers have higher rebleed rate than duodenal ulcers
Mallory-Weiss syndrome	Longitudinal tear of esophagus; classically, hematemesis following retching
What are some other less common causes of upper GI bleeding?	Arteriovenous malformation; malignancy; aortoenteric fistula
What is the most common cause of apparent lower GI bleeding?	Upper GI bleeding
What is the most common cause of actual lower GI bleeding?	Hemorrhoids
What are other some common causes of lower GI bleeding?	Inflammatory (ie, inflammatory bowel disease)
	Neoplasm (ie, colon cancer)
	Other (ie, hemorrhoids)
	Vascular (ie, arteriovenous malformation [AVM])
	Anatomical (ie, diverticulosis)
What are some important elements to obtain in a patient who presents with GI bleeding?	Characterize the bleeding; changes in bowel habits and weight loss; retching and vomiting; medications (ie, NSAIDs); alcohol use; ingestion of bismuth or iron
What are some elements on the physical exam to consider?	Vitals (ie, decreased pulse pressure); stigmata of liver disease (ie, jaundice); abdominal and rectal exam
What are some laboratory data to consider in GI bleeding?	Type and cross-match blood; complete blood count (CBC); coagulation studies; liver panel; Chem-7 (ie, BUN can be elevated)
What are some diagnostic studies to consider in GI bleeding?	CXR and abdominal films (low yield); endoscopy (EGD) and colonoscopy; scintigraphy
What is the most accurate test to perform in upper GI bleeding?	Endoscopy (EGD)
Why is EGD evaluation useful in upper GI bleeding?	Diagnostic and therapeutic such as band ligation of esophageal varices.

| What are some important management points with patients who present with GI bleeding? | GI bleeding is potentially life-threatening; immediate resuscitation (fluids and blood); nasogastric (NG) tube placement is controversial |

| What role does somatostatin or octreotide play in GI bleeding? | Effective in reducing bleeding from all splanchnic circulation, especially esophageal varices and peptic ulcers. |

| What role do proton pump inhibitors play in management of upper GI bleed? | Omeprazole has been shown to reduce rates of rebleeding, transfusion requirement, and surgery. |

| What role does balloon tamponade play in GI bleeding? | Sengstaken-Blakemore tube can limit unstable variceal hemorrhage |

PEPTIC ULCER DISEASE

| What is the definition of peptic ulcer disease (PUD)? | PUD is a chronic disease that is typically caused by defects in the mucosal barrier most commonly along the lesser curvature of the stomach and duodenum. |

| What are the two most common causes of PUD? | 1. NSAIDs
2. *Helicobacter pylori* |

| List some other predisposing factors for the development of ulcers: | Zollinger-Ellison syndrome; cigarette smoking; long-term steroid use; stress |

What are some important things to know about the following types of ulcers:

| Gastric ulcers | Damage is from mucosal breakdown; *H pylori* is found in over 75% of cases; pain is typically shortly after eating |

| Duodenal ulcers | Damage is usually from acid hypersecretion; *H pylori* is found in over 90% of cases; pain is typically 2 to 3 hours after meals |

| Stress ulcers | Commonly due to acute trauma/CNS tumors; usually located on fundus/body of stomach; very common cause of gastric bleeding |

| What conditions are *H pylori* usually implicated in? | PUD; lymphoid hypertrophy; adenocarcinoma of stomach; gastric lymphoma |

What are some common diagnostic methods used to identify *H pylori*?

Serology; endoscopy (ie, rapid urea); urease breath test

What are some signs and symptoms of PUD?

Epigastric pain that is vague and described as "burning" often relieved by food

What are some important diagnostic tests to consider in PUD?

Endoscopy; barium-contrast x-ray

What are some considerations in the management of uncomplicated PUD?

Avoid exacerbating factors (ie, NSAIDs); antacids—symptomatic relief; H2-blockers (cimetidine); proton pump inhibitors (omeprazole); eradication of *H pylori*

What is the importance in the eradication of *H pylori*?

Reduces the recurrence of PUD; reduces need for suppressive therapy

What are the three drugs commonly used as triple therapy in the eradication of *H pylori*?

1. Macrolide (clarithromycin)
2. Tetracycline
3. Omeprazole

What are some complications of PUD?

Bleeding; perforation; outlet obstruction

What are some considerations in the management of the following complications of PUD:

Upper GI bleeding

Volume replacement and transfuse if needed; administer PPI or H2-blocker; consider nasogastric (NG) tube; GI or surgery consult in severe cases

Perforation

Monitor for peritoneal signs; X-ray evidence of free air; IV fluids; broad-spectrum antibiotics; surgical consultation

Gastric outlet obstruction

Healed ulcer scar that blocks pyloric outlet; endoscopy; upright abdominal plain film; IV fluids/NG tube suction and admit

APPENDICITIS

What is the definition of appendicitis?

It is inflammation of the appendix due to obstruction of the outlet.

What are some important facts about appendicitis?

Most common cause of emergent surgery; highest incidence in males 10 to 30 years of age

What is the pathophysiology of appendicitis?

Obstruction of the lumen that leads to intraluminal distension, venous congestion, and eventually ischemia followed by perforation (bacterial invasion common).

What are some common causes of appendiceal obstruction?

Fecalith—most common; enlarged lymphoid follicles; tumors (carcinoid); adhesions

What are the most common symptoms of appendicitis?

Abdominal pain (periumbilical then right lower quadrant); anorexia; N/V (should occur after pain); fever and chills

What are some common signs of appendicitis?

Abdominal tenderness with/without rebound; Rovsing sign (RLQ pain when pressing left lower quadrant [LLQ]); Psoas sign (passive extension of right hip that causes RLQ pain); Obturator sign (passive internal rotation of flexed hip causes RLQ pain); cervical motion tenderness (also seen in pelvic inflammatory disease)

How common is the classic migratory pain with associated symptoms in appendicitis?

Found in up to 2/3 of patients with appendicitis

What is the concern in a patient with suspected appendicitis who has a sudden decrease in pain followed by a dramatic increase in pain?

Perforation

What other conditions can mimic appendicitis?

Nephrolithiasis; pelvic inflammatory disease; right upper quadrant pain in pregnant women; ectopic pregnancy

What are some important diagnostic tests to consider in appendicitis?

Pregnancy test—consider ectopic pregnancy; complete blood count (CBC)—elevated WBC is typical but not diagnostic; plain abdominal films—may show fecalith; CT with IV and rectal/oral contrast—first choice; ultrasound (U/S)—useful for children/pregnant women

| What are some considerations in the management of appendicitis? | NPO and IV fluids; pain control; early surgical consult if suspicion is high; if surgery—prophylactic antibiotics |

GALLBLADDER DISEASE

What is the definition of cholecystitis?	Acute inflammation of the gallbladder that is commonly caused by obstruction at the neck of the gallbladder or cystic duct.
What are some important points about cholecystitis?	It is more common in females; most cases (>90%) due to cystic stones; one of the most common indications for surgery
What are some risk factors for the development of cholelithiasis (hence cholecystitis)?	Obesity; female; previous pregnancy; rapid weight loss; advanced age; cystic fibrosis; long-term TPN use

What are some important points for each of the following types of gallbladder disease:

Calculous cholecystitis	It is the most frequent variant; most common cause of pancreatitis
Acalculous cholecystitis	It makes up about 5 to 10% of cases; more common in elderly, DM, and sepsis; perforation and gangrene are more common
Ascending cholangitis	Extending infection into the liver; Charcot triad: fever/jaundice/RUQ pain; Reynold pentad: Charcot triad plus shock/ΔMS; requires rapid surgical intervention
Gallstone ileus	Very rare cause of bowel obstruction; gallstone erodes through the gallbladder and impacts in bowel near the cecum; more common in elderly females
Emphysematous cholecystitis	Rare infection of the gallbladder; agents usually include anaerobes/gram (–)

| What are some signs and symptoms of cholecystitis? | RUQ pain, fatty food intolerance, gallstone risk factors, N/V, fever, and tachycardia |

What is Murphy's sign?

It is increase in pain and temporary cessation of breathing when direct pressure is applied to RUQ when the patient takes a deep breath

What are some important diagnostic studies to consider in cholecystitis?

CBC—elevated WBC is typical; liver function test (LFT)—enzymes and alkaline phosphate may be elevated; amylase/lipase—increased if pancreatitis; abdominal plain films: typically normal

What are the typical findings in the following imaging modalities in the assessment of cholecystitis:

    Ultrasound

The study of choice where common findings include presence of gall stones, gallbladder wall thickening (>5 mm), pericholecystic fluid, and dilated common ducts

    Hepatobiliary Imino-Diacetic Acid scan (HIDA)

Typically used if U/S results are indeterminate and clinical suspicion is high; positive results typically show lack of isotopes in the gallbladder

    CT

It is not any more sensitive or specific when compared to U/S and exposes patient to significant amount of radiation

What are some considerations in the management of cholecystitis?

NPO/IV fluids; broad-spectrum Abx; surgical consult; pain control

What are some general criteria for admission?

Fever, significant abdominal pain, elevated WBC; complications (ie, ascending cholangitis); cholecystectomy (usually within 72 h)

PANCREATITIS

What is the definition of pancreatitis?

It is acute inflammation of the pancreas.

What are the two most common causes of acute pancreatitis?

1. Bile duct disease (gallstones)
2. Alcohol abuse

What are some other causes of acute pancreatitis?

Surgery; complications of ERCP; hyperlipidemia; hypercalcemia

What are some signs and symptoms of acute pancreatitis?	Epigastric pain typically after ingestion of EtOH or a fatty meal, N/V, low-grade fever, and tachycardia
What is Grey Turner sign?	Bluish discoloration of the flank.
What is Cullen sign?	Bluish discoloration near the umbilicus.
What do these two signs point to?	Although not common, they indicate the presence of hemorrhagic pancreatitis.
What is chronic pancreatitis?	Progressive, irreversible structural pancreatic changes due to repeated bouts of acute pancreatitis.

Give some important features of the following diagnostic tests:

Amylase	Amylase is also found in other organs; 1.5 above upper limit points to pancreatitis
Lipase	More specific and as sensitive as amylase; lipase is found primarily in the pancreas; it is reliable and inexpensive
CBC	Low hematocrit points to hemorrhagic pancreatitis; high WBC is common

What is Ranson's Criteria?	It is a set of prognostic factors that correlate with mortality based on the number of prognostic signs that are met.
On admission	Age >55 years; hyperglycemia >200 mg/dL; leukocytosis >16,000 per mm^3; LDH >350 IU/L; AST >250
After 48 hours	PO_2 <60 mm Hg; calcium <8 mg/dL; Hct >10% drop; base deficit >4 mEq/L; sequestration >4 L of fluid; BUN >5 mg/dL
What are some complications of acute pancreatitis?	Abscess; hemorrhagic; fluid sequestration; acute respiratory distress syndrome (ARDS)

COLITIS AND ILEITIS

Crohn Disease

What is the definition of Crohn disease (CD)?	A chronic, recurrent inflammatory disease of the intestinal tract (primarily the ileum and colon).

What is the epidemiology of CD?	Greater incidence in whites between the age of 16 and 40, more common in Jewish ancestry; positive family history in up to 20%
What are some signs and symptoms of CD?	Recurrent abdominal pain, fever, and diarrhea with weight loss. RLQ pain that mimics appendicitis is also not uncommon
What are some extraintestinal manifestations of the following organ systems in CD?	**Dermatology.** Pyoderma gangrenosum; erythema nodosum **Ophthalmic.** Iritis; conjunctivitis; uveitis **Rheumatology.** Ankylosing spondylitis; arthritis **Vascular.** Arteritis; thromboembolic disease; vasculitis **Hepatobiliary.** Gallstones; pericholangitis
What are some complications of CD?	Strictures; perforation; perianal complications; abscess; fistulas
What is the diagnostic test of choice for CD?	Colonoscopy with histological sample
What are some considerations in the management of CD?	IV fluids and NG tube; steroids to reduce inflammation; azathioprine— steroid sparing; metronidazole for perianal complications; infliximab may help in severe cases
What are some indications for admission for CD?	Acute complications; unable to keep PO; intractable pain

Ulcerative Colitis

What is the definition of ulcerative colitis (UC)?	Chronic inflammatory disease of the colon that always has rectal involvement.
What is the pathophysiology of UC?	Mucosa/submucosa inflammation with sparing of the serosa with continuous involvement unlike Crohn disease.
What is the epidemiology of UC?	Greater incidence in whites and females between the age of 16 and 40, bimodal peak around age 60 as with Crohn, more common in Jewish ancestry.

What are some signs and symptoms of the following degrees of UC:

Mild disease

No systemic symptoms; less than 4 bowel movements per day; few extra-intestinal symptoms

Severe disease

Systemic response (F/C, weight loss, etc); greater than 4 bowel movements per day; extraintestinal symptoms

What is the diagnostic test of choice for UC?

Colonoscopy

What are some complications of UC?

Toxic megacolon (more common in UC); perforation; obstruction; perianal abscess and fistulas; colon carcinoma; hemorrhage

What are some considerations in the management of mild/moderate attack of UC?

Sulfasalazine—mainstay therapy; mesalamine/olsalazine—second line; corticosteroid—supplement; avoid antidiarrheal agents; azathioprine/cyclosporine—if steroids fail

What are some considerations in the management of severe UC?

IV fluids and NG tube; broad-spectrum Abx; monitor for hemorrhage/toxic megacolon; surgical consult

Pseudomembranous Enterocolitis

What is the definition of pseudomembranous enterocolitis?

Inflammatory bowel disease characterized by yellow exudative pseudomembranous plaque over necrotic colon.

What is the pathogenic species responsible for pseudomembranous enterocolitis?

Clostridium difficile

What antibiotics are commonly associated with the proliferation of *C difficile*?

Clindamycin; ampicillin; cephalosporins

What is the pathophysiology of *C difficile* associated pseudomembranous enterocolitis in relation to Abx use?

Abx use alters normal gut flora and allows *C difficile* to propagate

What are some common signs and symptoms of pseudomembranous enterocolitis?

Profuse watery diarrhea with crampy abdominal pain, stool may have blood, and fever.

What is the general time frame for the development of pseudomembranous enterocolitis after Abx use?

Generally 7 to 10 days after Abx use, but can occur weeks after discontinuation.

What is the diagnostic study of choice?

C difficile toxin in stool

What are some considerations in the management of pseudomembranous enterocolitis?

IV fluids and electrolyte balance; discontinue the offending agent; oral metronidazole is first-line; oral vancomycin if metronidazole does not work

What role do antidiarrheal drugs play in management?

None—they can worsen symptoms and increase likelihood of toxic megacolon

MESENTERIC ISCHEMIA

What is the pathophysiology of mesenteric ischemia?

Mesenteric arteries that do not deliver enough blood to the small or large intestine, typically due to sudden occlusion or decreased cardiac output (CO).

What are some important things to know about mesenteric ischemia?

Commonly affects elderly with vascular disease; mortality rate 50% once infarction occurs

What are some considerations in the following causes of mesenteric ischemia:

Non-occlusive

Typically due to reduction in CO (ie, CHF); account for up to 25% of all cases; commonly affects critically sick/elderly; presentation is more subtle and insidious

Acute occlusion

Typically due to embolization (ie, afib); accounts for the majority of cases; common in severe atherosclerotic patients; presentation is acute, sudden, and dramatic

Venous thrombosis

Typically due to hypercoagulable state; often have history of deep vein thrombosis/pulmonary embolism (DVT/PE)

What are some causes for the following causes of mesenteric ischemia:

Non-occlusive

Hypotension (ie, sepsis); CHF; hypovolemia

Acute occlusion

Recent MI; atherosclerotic heart disease; dysrhythmias (especially afib)

Venous thrombosis

History of DVT/PE; hypercoagulable

What are some signs and symptoms of mesenteric ischemia?

Vague abdominal pain that is out of proportion early in the course, sudden severe pain if cause is acute, guaiac positive stool, N/V, and peritoneal signs late in the course if infarction occurs.

What are some commonly used diagnostic tests?

CBC—often elevated white count; arterial blood gas (ABG)—metabolic acidosis is common; plain films—often normal; CT/US—not the first line choice; lactate level

What is the diagnostic test of choice in suspected mesenteric ischemia?

Angiography

What are the general considerations in the management of mesenteric ischemia?

IV fluids; broad-spectrum Abx; look for underlying cause and correct them; use of papaverine for diagnostic study; early surgical consult

What are the indications for surgical intervention in mesenteric ischemia?

Necrotic bowel requiring resection; revascularization; evidence of perforation (peritoneal signs)

DIVERTICULAR DISEASE

What is the definition of diverticula?

Sac-like herniations of the mucosa in the colon typically due to an increase in intra-luminal pressure often from lack of fiber.

What are some important things to know about diverticular disease?

Direct correlation with incidence and age; high in patients who consume low fiber; common cause of painless lower GI bleed

What are the two main manifestations of diverticular disease?

1. Diverticulosis
2. Diverticulitis

What are some signs and symptoms of diverticulosis?

Hallmark is self-limiting painless rectal bleeding that is typically bright red or maroon, although a small percentage have massive lower GI bleed.

What are some considerations in the management of diverticulosis?

Ensure that there is no massive GI bleeding; bleeding is typically self-limited; diagnosis requires colonoscopy; increase in fiber may reduce future attacks; avoidance of seeds—not really proven

What is the definition of diverticulitis?

Microperforation of diverticula that result in an inflammatory response that is typically walled off by pericolic fat.

What are some signs and symptoms of diverticulitis?

LLQ pain present for a few days is the hallmark, N/V, diarrhea, and changes in urinary symptoms.

What are some complications of diverticulitis?

Abscess formation; fistula; obstruction; perforation

How commonly do patients with diverticulitis present with RLQ pain?

Less than 5%—more common in Asians

What other differential should be considered in those who present with RLQ pain?

Appendicitis

What are some commonly used diagnostic tests in diverticulitis?

CBC—leukocytosis; Ab plain film—examine for complications; CT—test of choice to evaluate extent of disease

What are some considerations in the management of diverticulitis?

IV fluids and NPO; NG tube if suspected obstruction; broad-spectrum Abx; surgical consult if suspected complications

HERNIA

What is the definition of a hernia?

It is the protrusion of any body part out of its natural cavity primarily due to inherent weaknesses (congenital) or acquired (surgery).

Define the following possibilities for a hernia:

Reducible

The contents can be returned to its cavity

Irreducible/Incarcerated

Unable to reduce—no vascular compromise

Strangulated

Vascular compromise of herniation

What are some important points for the following types of hernia:

Femoral hernia

Protrudes below the inguinal ring; more common in females; high frequency of incarceration

Direct inguinal hernia

Directly via the floor of Hesselbach triangle; incidence increases with age; rarely incarcerates

Indirect inguinal hernia

Protrudes via the internal inguinal ring; more common in men; more common in younger population; high frequency of incarceration

Umbilical hernia

Represents a congenital defect in newborns; most will close by 3 years of age; rarely incarcerates

What are some signs and symptoms of a hernia?

Palpable bulge that often can be detected on exam and can be sore when pressed, but rarely painful unless incarcerated.

What are some considerations in the management of a hernia?

If hernia is recent, can try to reduce; if suspected necrosis, do not reduce; incarcerated = surgery consult; strangulation = surgery and Abx; reducible = consider elective surgery

ANORECTAL

Hemorrhoids

What is the definition of a hemorrhoid?

Dilated internal or external hemorrhoidal venous plexus.

What are some risk factors for the development of hemorrhoids?

Straining; increase in portal pressure (ie, cirrhosis); constipation; low fiber diet; pregnancy

What are some important points for the following types of hemorrhoids:

Internal hemorrhoids

Originate above the dentate line; relatively insensitive area—no/little pain; rarely palpable—painless bleeding common; visualized at 2, 5, and 9 o'clock positions

External hemorrhoids

Originate below the dentate line; in well-innervated area, often painful; usually can be visualized

What are some common signs and symptoms for the following types of hemorrhoids:

Internal hemorrhoids

Painless bright red blood per rectum, most common cause of lower GI bleed in younger population

External hemorrhoids

Tender palpable mass often due to thrombosis

What are some considerations in the management of the following types of hemorrhoids:

Internal hemorrhoids

Often resolves on its own; increase dietary fiber and fluids; stool softeners, bulk laxatives, and sitz bath; refractory bleeding = IV fluid/packing/surgery

External hemorrhoids

Analgesics/sitz bath/stool softeners; acute thrombosis: excision of clots

What are some indications for surgical intervention?

Refractory bleeding or pain; incarceration/strangulation

Anorectal Abscess

What is the definition of an anorectal abscess?

Abscess that typically develops in one of the potential spaces near the rectum/anus most often due to obstruction of glands at the base of the anal crypts.

Name some potential spaces where an anorectal abscess can occur:

Perianal, intersphincteric, and ischiorectal

What are some other causes of an anorectal abscess?

Inflammatory bowel disease; radiation injury; cancer; trauma; TB

What is a common complication of an anorectal abscess?	Fistula formation
What are some common signs and symptoms of an anorectal abscess?	Dull aching pain that is worse with bowel movements and relieved after, sometimes palpable mass on exam, fever, and obvious discomfort whenever patient sits.
What are some considerations in the management of an anorectal abscess?	Simple perianal abscess = ED drainage; most require surgical intervention; most individuals do not require Abx
What are the indications for the use of Abx?	DM, immunocompromised patient, and valvular heart disease

Anal Fissure

What is the definition of an anal fissure?	Linear tears of the epithelium within the anal canal, typically due to recurrent diarrhea or passage of large hard stools.
What are some important points about an anal fissure?	Majority are located in the posterior midline; number one cause of painful rectal bleeding; IBD and TB are other causes
What are some signs and symptoms of an anal fissure?	Severe pain with defecation, often with a history of constipation, and linear tear of the posterior midline on exam. Pain is so intense; patients often try to avoid defecation.
What are some considerations in the management of an anal fissure?	Symptomatic relief to allow healing; topical analgesic, topical nitroglycerin, sitz baths, and dietary fiber; refractory cases often require surgical referral and excision
What is the recurrence rate, even with treatment?	Up to 50%

Fistula-In-Ano

What is the definition of a fistula-in-ano?	Abnormal communication between anus and the skin.

What is fistula-in-ano often caused by?	Commonly from ischiorectal or perianal abscess
What conditions are fistula-in-ano associated with?	TB; cancer; IBD
What are some of the signs and symptoms of fistula-in-ano?	Persistent blood-stained purulent discharge or an abscess if it becomes blocked.
What is the primary treatment for fistula-in-ano?	Surgical incision

Anal Foreign Bodies

How do anal foreign bodies usually occur?	Placement of object into anus; transit from GI foreign body
What important distinction must be made in regard to location of the foreign object?	Whether the object is below or above the rectosigmoid junction (difficult to visualize and remove if above).
What age group commonly present with anal foreign bodies?	20 to 30 years of age (anal eroticism)
What are some important points to know about anal foreign bodies?	Often present late due to embarrassment; suspected in psychiatric patients with anal symptom; attempted self-extraction = risk of perforation
What are some signs and symptoms of anal foreign bodies?	Anal pain, bleeding, pruritus, and F/C with rigid abdomen in perforation
What are some commonly used diagnostic tests for anal foreign bodies?	Abdomen x-rays; upright CXR if perforation suspected; rigid proctosigmoidoscope
What are some considerations in the management of anal foreign bodies?	ER removal if the object is low riding; retractors, snares, forceps may be used; consider serial observation after removal; surgical consult if evidence of perforation

Proctitis

| What is the definition of proctitis? | It is inflammation of the rectal mucosa within 15 cm of the dentate line that typically affect adult males. |

What are some signs and symptoms of proctitis?	Passage of blood and mucus, tenesmus, and abdominal cramping.
What are some common causes of proctitis?	Idiopathic; infectious (HSV-1 and-2); radiation; ischemia
What is the diagnostic study of choice to evaluate proctitis?	Proctosigmoidoscopy
What are some complications of proctitis?	Fistula; fissures; strictures
What are some considerations in the management of proctitis?	Analgesic relief; Abx if cause is infectious (ie, HSV-1); sitz bath for relief

Rectal Prolapse

What is the definition of rectal prolapse?	It is when rectal mucosa or full-thickness rectal tissue slides outside the anal orifice.
What is the pathophysiology of rectal prolapse?	Initially begins as an internal prolapse that progresses to an external prolapse outside the anal orifice.
What are some common causes of rectal prolapse?	Straining (ie, constipation); weakness of the pelvic floor; neurologic disorder
What two age groups are commonly affected with rectal prolapse	1. Pediatric (up to 90% resolve on their own) 2. Elderly (most require corrective surgery)
What are some signs and symptoms of rectal prolapse?	Fecal incontinence, painless mass on exam, and rectal bleeding.
What are some complications of rectal prolapse?	Ulceration; bleeding; necrosis
What are some considerations in the management of rectal prolapse?	Most rectal prolapses can be reduced; emergent surgery if evidence of ischemia; stool softeners if reduction is successful

Pilonidal Sinus

What is the definition of a pilonidal sinus?	Abscess that forms at the superior edge of the buttock in midline.

What is pathophysiology for the development of a pilonidal sinus?	Ingrowing hair that penetrates the skin and induces a foreign body reaction.
What are some signs and symptoms of a pilonidal sinus?	Recurrent pain and purulent discharge
What are some considerations in the management of pilonidal sinus?	Incision and drainage of abscess; surgical intervention for excision; consider Abx if immunocompromised; tend to recur

DIARRHEA

What is the definition of diarrhea?	Loose watery stools that occur more than three times per day that typically is self-limited, but can lead to dehydration and electrolyte imbalance.
What are some important causes of diarrhea?	Infection (bacterial/viral/parasitic); food intolerance; medication reaction; intestinal disease (ie, celiac disease); functional bowel disorder (ie, IBS)
List common parasite-induced diarrhea:	*Giardia lamblia; Entamoeba histolytica; Cryptosporidium; Necator americanus*
What are some important things to know about viral-induced diarrhea?	Causes the majority of all acute episodes; Norwalk and rotavirus most common; peak during winter months; adenovirus also common
What are some signs and symptoms of viral-induced diarrhea?	Low-grade fever, vomiting, diarrhea, mild abdominal cramping, and sometimes an upper respiratory infection (URI) prodrome beforehand
What are some common modes of transmission?	Sick contact; contaminated food
What are some considerations in the management of viral-induced diarrhea?	Treatment is supportive; ensure adequate hydration; typically self-limited
What are some important points to know about bacteria-induced diarrhea?	Accounts for about 25% of acute diarrhea; classified as invasive or toxin-producing

What are some examples of invasive bacteria?

Salmonella; Shigella; Vibrio; Campylobacter

What are some examples of toxin-producing bacteria?

Bacillus cereus; Staphylococcus aureus; Clostridium difficile

What does a wet mount of stool typically show?

Fecal leukocytes (typically + with bacteria); WBCs (use of methylene blue)

What are some important points and treatment for the following bacterial-induced diarrhea:

Vibrio cholera

Typically from contaminated water/seafood; incubation about 5 days; profuse watery diarrhea is the hallmark; Tx: IV hydration and Abx-fluoroquinolone

Vibrio parahaemolyticus

Invasive bacteria—typically from bad seafood; range from mild to explosive diarrhea; Tx: supportive care; usually self-limiting

Staphylococcus aureus

Number one common cause of food-related diarrhea; presentation from preformed toxins; often in protein-rich food such as meat; incubation in hours; Tx: supportive; usually self-limiting

E coli serotype 0157:H7

Common cause of hemorrhagic colitis; often from contaminated beef and milk; incubation in about a week; diarrhea, vomiting, and severe abdominal pain; associated with HUS; Tx: supportive—typically a week to resolve

E coli (enterotoxigenic)

Very common cause of traveler's diarrhea; often in contaminated food and water; presents like V cholera; Tx: supportive; Abx can shorten course

Shigella

Includes *S flexneri* and *S dysenteriae*; highly infectious and usually from fecal-oral; high-grade fever, bloody mucoid stool, and abdominal pain is common; Tx: typically resolve in a week, highly infectious, and supportive care

Salmonella

Includes *S typhi* and *S typhimurium*; often from contaminated food or pets; immunocompromised patients most at risk; variable presentation (ie, typhoid fever); Tx: mild cases supportive care; more severe cases may require Abx

| *Campylobacter* | Very common cause of bacterial diarrhea; often in food (poultry) and water; more common in the pediatric population; incubation is about 4 days; fever, HA, abdominal pain, and watery bloody stool; Tx: Abx in severe cases; associated with HUS and Guillain-Barre syndrome |

CLINICAL VIGNETTES—MAKE THE DIAGNOSIS

61-year-old man with long history of alcohol abuse presents with progressive difficulty in swallowing which was initially to foods only, but now to liquids; PE: unremarkable exam

Esophageal carcinoma

17-year-old woman who recently finished her course of tetracycline presents with odynophagia, but is otherwise healthy; PE: unremarkable exam

Inflammatory esophagitis

3-year-old child is brought in by her mother due to recent onset of dysphagia and gagging, otherwise the child is healthy with no other complaints; PE: unremarkable exam, clear oropharynx

Swallowed foreign body

17-year-old man with no PMH presents with abdominal pain that was initially around the umbilicus, but now has progressed to the RLQ associated with nausea and vomiting after the onset of pain; PE: RLQ tenderness and (+) Rovsing sign

Appendicitis

51-year-old elderly man with arthritis presents with epigastric pain that is often relieved by intake of food, but is otherwise healthy; PE: epigastric tenderness, but no rebound

Peptic ulcer disease

41-year-old woman with an Hx of recent ERCP presents with epigastric pain radiating to her back associated with nausea and emesis; PE: epigastric tenderness; labs: elevated lipase

Pancreatitis

17-year-old woman with a history of bulimia presents with chest pain with dysphagia that occurred soon after her bout of emesis; PE: unremarkable exam

   Mallory-Weiss syndrome

31-year-old obese woman presents with RUQ pain along with fever and nausea, patient has a history of gallstones; PE: fever, tachycardia, RUQ tenderness, and yellowish sclera on examination of eye; labs: elevated alkaline phosphate and LFTs

   Ascending cholangitis

71-year-old woman with an Hx of HTN, afib, and DM presents with a sudden onset of diffuse abdominal pain along with nausea and vomiting; PE: pain out of proportion on exam, guaiac positive stool, and rebound; labs: elevated lactate

   Mesenteric ischemia

21-year-old woman presents with 2 days of lower GI bleeding and describes the toilet bowl as being bright red after each bowel movement, other then a history of constipation, patient is otherwise healthy; PE: unremarkable exam and guaiac positive stool

   Internal hemorrhoids

61-year-old man presents with LLQ pain with nausea, vomiting, and urinary changes for 2 days; PE: LLQ tenderness and no rebound on exam; labs: elevated white count

   Diverticulitis

28-year-old man with recent discharge from hospital now presents with diffuse watery diarrhea and crampy abdominal exam: PE: low-grade fever and mild tenderness of abdomen

   Pseudomembranous enterocolitis

30-year-old man with history of HIV presents with tenesmus, abdominal cramping, and passage of blood and mucus for 3 days; PE: tenderness on rectal exam

   Proctitis

CHAPTER 8

Genitourinary Emergencies

ACUTE RENAL FAILURE

What is the definition of acute renal failure (ARF)?

It is deterioration of renal function that results in accumulation of waste and loss of internal homeostasis.

What are some considerations about the kidney?

Kidney receives 25% of the cardiac output; outer medulla is susceptible to hypoxia; with decreased renal blood flow (RBF), increased susceptibility to toxins

What is the primary way to assess renal function?

Glomerular filtration rate (GFR) (via creatinine clearance)

What are three types of acute-renal failure?

1. Prerenal
2. Renal
3. Postrenal

What are some important causes of prerenal azotemia?

Hypovolemia (ie, diuretics/dehydration); third space sequestration (ie, pancreatitis); sepsis; decreased cardiac output

What is the typical urine status in patients with prerenal azotemia?

Oliguric; avid reabsorption of sodium and water; BUN/creatinine (BUN/Crea) ratio of 20:1; U/A typically shows no evidence of damage; fractional excretion of sodium <1%

What are some important causes of renal azotemia?

Acute tubular necrosis; thrombosis; glomerular disease; vascular disease; acute interstitial nephritis

What are common causes of acute tubular necrosis (ATN)?

Ischemia—most common; pigments (ie, myoglobin); nephrotoxic agents

What are some common nephrotoxic agents?

IV contrast dye; nonsteroidal anti-inflammatory drugs (NSAIDs); angiotensin-converting enzyme inhibitors; antibiotics (ie, penicillin)

What is the typical urine status in patients with renal azotemia?

Inability to concentrate urine (dilute); have evidence of damage (ie, casts); high urine sodium (>40 mEq/L)

What are some important causes of postrenal azotemia?

Ureteral obstruction (ie, stones); bladder obstruction; urethral obstruction (ie, strictures)

What are some important tests to consider differentiating the type of ARF?

Urinalysis; ultrasound; postvoid residual urine; urine and serum Na and creatinine; urine osmolality; urine eosinophils

What are some considerations in treatment for each of the following causes of ARF:

    Prerenal

Rapid volume replacement; find the cause of hypoperfusion and correct it; initial fluid administration of isotonic saline is appropriate in most cases

    Renal

Increase the urine flow; if cause is a nephrotoxic agent, remove it; maintaining balance of fluid/electrolytes; dialysis if indicated

    Postrenal

Relieve obstruction; catheter until obstruction is relieved

What are some considerations for each of the following complications of ARF:

    Hypocalcemia

It is common in setting of ARF; typically asymptomatic; intravenous (IV) calcium chloride if symptomatic

    Hypermagnesium

It is common in setting of ARF; typically asymptomatic

Hyperkalemia	Potentially the most life-threatening; death due to cardiac dysrhythmias; important to obtain serum K and ECG; treat (IV glucose/insulin, bicarb, etc)
Metabolic acidosis	It is also common in the setting of ARF; typically asymptomatic
What are some indications of dialysis in the setting of ARF?	Hyperkalemia; uremia (ie, encephalopathic); creatinine >10 mg/dL or BUN >100 mg/dL; clinically significant fluid overload/acidosis; particular nephrotoxins (ie, ethylene glycol)

CHRONIC RENAL FAILURE

What is the definition of chronic renal failure (CRF)?	The irreversible and gradual loss of renal function that results in inability to regulate homeostasis and concentrate urine.
What are the two most common causes of CRF?	1. Diabetes 2. Hypertension
What are some other causes of CRF?	Glomerulonephritis; polycystic kidney disease; Alport syndrome
What are some important things to know for each of the following stages of CRF:	
Stage I	Decreased renal function <50% GFR; at least ½ of renal function is gone; homeostasis and excretion intact
Stage II	Renal insufficiency with 20 to 50% GFR; mild anemia due to decreased erythropoietin (EPO); mild azotemia
Stage III	Renal failure with 5 to 20% GFR; severe anemia; azotemia; electrolyte imbalance (ie, hyperkalemia)
Stage IV	Renal failure <5% GFR; multiple organ system effects
What is the treatment for CFR?	Kidney transplant; peritoneal dialysis; hemodialysis (also for ARF)
What are some complications associated with hemodialysis?	Infection of vascular access; thrombosis of the vascular access; hemorrhage

NEPHROLITHIASIS

What is the definition of nephrolithiasis?

Supersaturation of a mineral within the ureters that result in urinary changes and ureter spasms.

What are some important things to know about nephrolithiasis?

More common in males between 20 and 45; there is a hereditary predisposition; over 90% of stones <5 mm will pass; recurrence can be as high as 50%

What is the most common type of kidney stone?

Calcium oxalate (about 75% of all stones)

What are some possible causes of calcium stones?

Hyperparathyroidism; sarcoidosis; neoplasm

What are some important things to note for each of the following stone types:

Struvite stone

After calcium stones, the next most common; radiopaque; associated with urea-splitting *Proteus*

Uric acid stones

Next common after calcium and struvite; radiolucent; common in patients with gout and leukemia

Xanthine stones

Rare; radiopaque; deficiency of the enzyme xanthine oxidase, which results in the production of xanthine and hypoxanthine rather than uric acid as an end product of purine metabolism

Cystine stones

Radiopaque; familial associated

What are some signs and symptoms of nephrolithiasis?

Unilateral flank pain that is often colicky, can also have pain in the back with radiation to the groin (labia/ testicles), urinary symptoms (hematuria, dysuria, etc.), and nausea/vomiting (N/V).

What is another important diagnosis to consider in a person who presents for the first time with flank pain and is elderly with history of uncontrolled HTN?

Ruptured/leaking abdominal aortic aneurysm

What are some important laboratory tests to consider and common findings:

Complete blood count (CBC)   Usually normal

U/A   Hematuria (can be absent in up to 25%); urinary pH >7.6 (suspect *Proteus*)

Urine culture   Positive if infection is present

BUN/Crea   To assess renal function

What are some important diagnostic tests to consider?   CT: diagnostic study of choice; intravenous pyelogram (IVP): for anatomical/functional assessment; ultrasound (U/S): for pregnant women and children

What are some considerations in the management of nephrolithiasis?   Proper fluid hydration; opioids with ketorolac (optimal pain control); antiemetic for sustained emesis; tamsulosin may result in faster expulsion of small distal stones.

What are some common indications for admission of a patient with nephrolithiasis?   Evidence of active infection (fever/pyuria); inability to tolerate oral intake; stone >5 mm (unlikely to pass on its own); renal insufficiency

URINARY TRACT INFECTIONS

What is the definition of a urinary tract infection (UTI)?   Presence of bacteria in the urinary system.

What are some important things to know about UTI?   One of the most common bacterial infections; 50% of women will have at least one UTI; sexual activity increases risk of UTI

What are the three most common organisms associated with UTI?   1. *E coli* (up to 80% of all UTIs)
2. *Chlamydia*
3. *Staphylococcus saprophyticus*

What are some signs and symptoms of UTI?   Dysuria, urge to urinate, increased urination frequency, nocturia, and suprapubic heaviness (should not have systemic effects such as fever)

What are some other differentials to consider in a woman who presents with UTI?

Pelvic inflammatory disease (PID); vulvovaginitis

What are some features of a complicated UTI?

Resistant species; male; children or elderly; pregnant female; associated condition such as pyelonephritis; underlying anatomical abnormality of the GU system

List some methods used to collect a proper urine sample:

Catheterization; midstream clean catch; suprapubic aspiration (infants)

What are some common microscopic findings in a U/A of a patient with UTI?

Pyuria (>10 WBC/HPF in women and 1-2 for men); significant bacteriuria; nitrate positive (specific but not sensitive)

When is it appropriate to obtain a urine culture?

Infants; men; pregnant females; associated complications

What are some considerations in the management of a UTI?

Bactrim or nitrofurantoin are first-line; fluoroquinolone if UTI is complicated; treatment time ranges from 3 to 7 days for cystitis, and up to 14 days for pyelonephritis; pyridium if dysuria is intolerable

What is another important consideration in a patient who presents with a UTI?

Consider STDs in sexually active patients

What is the definition of pyelonephritis?

It is infection of the kidney most commonly as a result of a UTI with ascending infection.

What are some risk factors for the development of pyelonephritis?

Recurrent UTI; immunocompromised person; vesicoureteric reflux

List the classification of pyelonephritis:

Acute pyelonephritis; chronic pyelonephritis (chronic infection); reflex nephropathy (typically obstruction)

What are some signs and symptoms of pyelonephritis?

High-grade fever and chills in the setting of a UTI typically with flank/back pain and nausea/emesis.

What are some complications of pyelonephritis?

Chronic pyelonephritis; perinephric abscess; sepsis; ARF

What are some considerations in the management of pyelonephritis?	If mild and can tolerate PO—fluoroquinolone may discharge with follow-up; low threshold to admit if elderly or if severe
What are some indications for admissions in patients with pyelonephritis?	Uroseptic; children and elderly; unable to tolerate PO and persistent emesis; immunocompromised

MALE GENITAL PROBLEMS

What are the three cylindrical bodies of the penis?	1. Two corpora cavernosa 2. Corpus spongiosum
What is the primary blood supply of the penis?	Internal pudendal artery to the superficial/deep penile arteries
What is the average size of the testis?	4 to 5 cm × 3 cm
What are the two investing layers of the testis?	1. Tunica albuginea 2. Tunica vaginalis
What are some important components of the physical exam?	Visual inspection; palpation of the scrotum for fluid; milk the penis for discharge; rectal exam (check prostate); check for inguinal hernias

Common Genital Infections

What are some common organisms responsible for urethritis?	Gonorrhea and chlamydia (most common); *Trichomonas vaginalis*; *Ureaplasma urealyticum*
What are some signs and symptoms of urethritis?	Discharge and dysuria, but can be asymptomatic
How is the diagnosis of urethritis usually made?	Gram stain
What is the treatment of choice?	Directed against gonorrhea (ie, ceftriaxone); directed against chlamydia (ie, doxycycline); metronidazole if suspected trichomonas infection
What is orchitis?	Inflammation of the testis

What are some common causes of orchitis?	Systemic infections (ie, mumps); direct extension such as epididymitis
What are some signs and symptoms of orchitis?	Testicular swelling and pain that typically does not include urinary symptoms
Does mumps-induced orchitis require treatment?	No—typically resolves
What are some considerations in the management of orchitis?	Urology consultation; it is rare when compared to torsion/cancer
What are some common etiologic causes of acute bacterial prostatitis?	Usually gram (–) bacteria such as *E coli*, *Proteus*, and *Pseudomonas*
What are some signs and symptoms of acute bacterial prostatitis?	Urinary symptoms (ie, dysuria), pelvic/back pain, systemic signs of infection such as fever/chills; PE: swollen/tender prostate
What should one be careful not to do during a rectal exam?	Massaging the prostate
What will a urinalysis commonly show?	Evidence of cystitis
What are some considerations in the management of acute bacterial prostatitis?	Antibiotic therapy; analgesics, stool softeners, and hydration; urology consultation if evidence of urinary retention
What are some common causes of penile ulcers?	Herpes simplex, chancroid, syphilis, and granuloma inguinale
How is the diagnosis of syphilis commonly made?	Positive VDRL or RPR confirmed by *Treponema*-specific tests
What is the antibiotic of choice for syphilis?	Penicillin, doxycycline, and tetracycline
What is the cause of a chancroid?	*Haemophilus ducreyi*
What is the antibiotic treatment of choice for a chancroid?	A macrolide (ie, azithromycin)
What is the cause of granuloma inguinale?	*C granulomatous*
What are some antibiotics commonly used to treat granuloma inguinale?	Doxycycline or trimethoprim-sulfamethoxazole (TMP-SMX)

What is Fournier gangrene?	Known as idiopathic scrotal gangrene
What are some common clinical features of Fournier gangrene?	Often febrile and toxic with a painful erythematous penis/scrotum
What groups are more commonly affected with Fournier gangrene?	Elderly; diabetics; immunocompromised
What are some common etiologic causes of Fournier gangrene?	*Typically mixed: E coli, Streptococcus, Bacteroides fragilis, etc*
What are some considerations in the management of Fournier gangrene?	Broad-spectrum antibiotics; urologic consult for debridement; supportive management
What is phimosis?	Inability to retract foreskin behind the glans.
What is the most common cause of phimosis?	Chronic infection of the foreskin that results in scarring.
What can be done if phimosis appears to be causing vascular compromise?	Dorsal slit of the foreskin and circumcision for definite treatment.
What is paraphimosis?	Inability to pull the foreskin over the glans.
What is the primary concern of paraphimosis?	Vascular compromise
What can be done in an emergent situation if vascular compromise is evident?	Manual reduction; if not effective dorsal slit and circumcision for definitive treatment
What age group is epididymitis more common in?	Young adults
What are some signs and symptoms of epididymitis?	Gradual onset of unilateral testicular pain, dysuria, fever, and tenderness of epididymis on exam.
What is Prehn's sign?	Relief of testicular pain by elevating it
What are some common etiologic causes of epididymitis?	*E coli, Pseudomonas,* and *Chlamydia*
What are some common diagnostic studies to consider in epididymitis?	CBC; urethral culture and gram stain; urinalysis

What are some considerations in the management of epididymitis?	Antibiotic coverage (ceftriaxone/doxycycline); fluoroquinolones no longer recommended in several areas due to resistance. Stool softeners; analgesics with ice
What age groups are commonly affected with testicular torsion?	Bimodal distribution: neonates and 12 to 18 years of age
What are some important elements in the history of a patient who presents with testicular torsion?	Recent physical exertion (ie, sports/sex); history of testicular pain with relief after; history of cryptorchidism
What are some signs and symptoms of testicular torsion?	Acute onset of unilateral testicular pain often with nausea/vomiting; PE: affected testicles are high riding with loss of cremasteric reflex
What diagnosis can testicular torsion be confused with?	Epididymitis
What is the diagnostic test of choice for testicular torsion?	Color Doppler ultrasound
What are some considerations in the management of testicular torsion?	Urgent urology consult for surgery; surgery within 6 hours: 80 to 100% salvage rate; analgesics prior to surgery; salvage rate is 20% after 10 hours and 0% after 24 hours

Hematuria

What is the primary emergent concern when dealing with hematuria?	Urinary obstruction
What are some common causes of hematuria?	Painful—ureterolithiasis, trauma, UTI Painless—bladder cancer, BPH, medications, GU tumor
Describe the management of hematuria with signs of urinary obstruction.	Attempt to quantify degree of obstruction (ED ultrasound), relieve obstruction (3-way foley catheter with irrigation), UA, INR (if on warfarin).

CLINICAL VIGNETTES—MAKE THE DIAGNOSIS

31-year-old woman with PMH of afib presents with a sudden onset of left flank pain and hematuria; Abdominal CT: wedge-shaped lesion of the left kidney

Renal infarct

21-year-old man presents with dysuria and increased frequency of urination, patient is sexually active; PE: suprapubic tenderness; U/A: (+) nitrate and leukocyte esterase

Urinary tract infection

25-year-old man presents with sudden onset of right flank pain along with nausea, vomiting, and hematuria; PE: right CVA tenderness and in severe pain; U/A: (+) blood; U/S: shows right hydronephrosis

Nephrolithiasis

22-year-old man presents with hemoptysis, dark urine, and general fatigue for 3 days; PE: unremarkable exam; labs: anti-GBM antibodies and urine that shows blood

Goodpasture syndrome

81-year-old man with DM presents to the ER via EMS with fever and appears ill; PE: unremarkable except an erythematous penis that is very tender to the touch with evidence of a prior wound in the scrotum

Fournier gangrene

13-year-old man with a recent history of sore throat presents with low-urine output and swelling of lower legs; PE: periorbital edema; labs: elevated BUN/Crea and urine that shows blood

Poststreptococcal glomerulonephritis

25-year-old woman presents fever, chills, and left flank pain for about 2 days; PE: left CVA tenderness; U/A: (+) nitrate and leukocyte esterase

Pyelonephritis

19-year-old man with no PMH presents with fever, dysuria, and pelvic/back pain; PE: remarkable for a tender and swollen prostate

Bacterial prostatitis

81-year-old man with a long history of smoking presents with frank blood on urination, also with recent weight loss: PE: unremarkable exam; U/A: gross blood

Bladder cancer

61-year-old man presents with a 2-week history of nocturia, urinary hesitance, and weak stream during urination, otherwise healthy; PE: rectal exam showed diffusely enlarged prostate; labs: normal prostate-specific antigen (PSA)

Benign prostatic hyperplasia

13-year-old boy with PMH of undescended testis presents with sudden onset of right testicular pain associated with nausea and vomiting; PE: tender/swollen right testicle with (–) cremasteric reflex

Testicular torsion

61-year-old woman with a history of long-standing hypertension and DM presents with altered mental status; labs: significant for a potassium of 6, BUN of 99, creatinine of 7 with a GFR <5%

Chronic renal failure

20-year-old man presents with a gradual onset of unilateral testicular pain, fever, and dysuria for about 4 days, patient does admit to having unprotected sex; PE: tenderness of the penis on exam that is relieved when raised

Epididymitis

CHAPTER 9

Orthopedic Emergencies

GENERAL PRINCIPLES

What are some important principles of performing a closed reduction?

Displaced fractures should be reduced to minimize soft tissue complications

When applying splints, pad all bony prominences

Reduction of fractures often require axial traction and reversal of the mechanism of injury

Immobilize the joint above and below the injury

Describe the following common splinting techniques:

1. **Sugar-tong:**

U-shaped slab applied to the volar and dorsal aspects of the forearm for distal forearm fractures

2. **Coaptation splint:**

U-shaped slab applied to the medial and lateral aspects of the arm which encircles the elbow and is used as an upper extremity splint for humerus fractures

3. **Ulnar gutter splint:**

A slab that is applied to ulnar aspect of the forearm as temporary immobilization for fractures of the fourth or fifth metacarpals or phalanx

4. **Thumb spica splint:**

Temporary immobilization for confirmed or suspected fractures of the scaphoid (navicular) bone of the wrist

What is an important concern when applying a cast immediately to an acute fracture?

Swelling in a confined space leading to compartment syndrome

What are some other complications of splints and casts?	Loss of reduction Joint stiffness Compartment syndrome Pressure necrosis
Why is it important to cast a fracture in a "position of function"?	To avoid contractures
What is the position of function for the hand?	"Beer can position" where the MCP is flexed, interphalangeal joints in extension as if the patient is holding a can
What is an open fracture?	It is a fracture (osseous disruption) that results in soft tissue damage and breaks the skin resulting in open communication.
What is the primary concern with an open fracture?	Aside from neurovascular damage, infection of the bone (osteomyelitis)

Gustilo and Anderson Open Fracture Classification

Grade I:	Simple transverse or short oblique fracture with clean skin opening <1 cm
Grade II:	Laceration >1 cm long with more extensive soft tissue damage
Grade III:	Extensive soft tissue damage which may include muscles as well as neurovascular damage

What are some important considerations in the management of open fractures?	Avoid probing in the wound Orthopedic consultation for possible washout and/or operative intervention Antibiotic coverage Tetanus
What is the antibiotic of choice for open fractures?	Will depend on the grade of injury, but general overage is as follows: Grade I and II-First-generation cephalosporin (ie, cefazolin) Grade III-Aminoglycoside *Add penicillin with soil contamination such as farm injuries

Define the following types of nerve injury:

Neurapraxia	Is the contusion of a nerve, with disruption of the ability to transmit impulses

Axonotmesis	Is a more severe crush injury to a nerve. The injury to nerve fibers occurs within their sheaths. Because the Schwann tubes remain in continuity, spontaneous healing is possible but slow
Neurotmesis	Is the severing of a nerve requiring surgical repair
What is the difference between a dislocation and subluxation?	Subluxation is partial loss of continuity and dislocation is complete loss of continuity

BASIC PEDIATRIC ORTHOPEDIC PRINCIPLES

Table 9-1 Salter-Harris Classification of Epiphyseal Fractures[*]

Type I:	Fracture through the epiphyseal plate with separation of the epiphysis (good prognosis)
Type II:	Fracture of the metaphysis with extension through the epiphyseal plate (most common with a good prognosis)
Type III:	Fracture of the epiphysis with extension into the epiphyseal plate which is a total intra-articular fracture (open reduction often required)
Type IV:	Fracture through the metaphysis, epiphysis, and epiphyseal plate (open reduction often needed and despite perfect reduction still may get growth disturbances
Type V:	Crush fracture of the epiphyseal plate most commonly in the knee and ankle; radiographs can appear normal; poor prognosis due to interruption of the blood supply

[*]Higher the type, worse the prognosis. Applied in the pediatric population

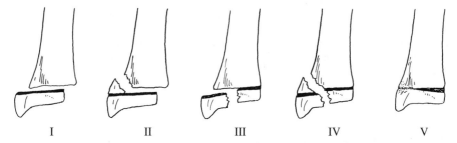

Figure 9-1. Reproduced, with permission, from Tintinalli JE, Kelen GD, Stapczynski JS, et al. Tintinalli's Emergency Medicine: A Comprehensive Study Guide. 6th ed. New York: McGraw-Hill, 2004. Fig. 267-7.

What are some important distinguishing factors between the pediatric and adult musculoskeletal system?	1. Presence of a physis or growth plate 2. Presence of a thick periosteum that is easily stripped from the bony cortex 3. Growing bone is more pliable, more porous, and less dense than adult bone

Define the following types of pediatric fractures?

Greenstick fracture:	Bone and one cortex are disrupted; the periosteum on the fracture's compression side remains intact.
Plastic deformation:	Bone is bowed with no obvious cortical disruption.
Torus fracture (also known as buckle fracture):	Buckling of bone without cortical disruption; it tends to occur because of compression failure of the bone at the metaphyseal-diaphyseal junction.
Complete fracture:	The fracture propagates completely through the bone; included are transverse, spiral, oblique and comminuted fractures.

What are some examples of fracture patterns that may be concerning for abuse?	An isolated diaphyseal fracture Any fracture for children less than 1 year of age Fractures in different stages of healing Multiple or bilateral fractures Rib and skull fractures
What heritable connective tissue disorder may sometimes be mistaken for abuse?	Osteogenesis imperfecta

HAND AND WRIST INJURIES

What is the primary purpose of treatment when dealing with hand injuries?	Restoration of function rather than appearance
Which body part injury is one of the most often seen in the ED?	Hand and fingers

Define the following terms:

Dorsal surface:	The back of the hand
Volar surface:	The palmer surface

Radial and ulnar:	The border of the hand on their respective side
Digits 1-5:	Starting from thumb to the little finger
What are the three joints that make up the finger?[*]	1. Metacarpophalangeal (MCP) 2. Proximal interphalangeal (PIP) 3. Distal interphalangeal (DIP) [*]Thumb has an MCP and one IP joint
What are the two motions that interphalangeal joints are capable of?	Flexion and extension
Name the eight carpal bones:	1. Trapezoid 2. Trapezium 3. Capitate 4. Scaphoid 5. Hamate 6. Triquetral 7. Pisiform 8. Lunate
What is the primary goal in the case of an amputated digit?	Preservation of the digit with ice water (isolated from the ice with a bag to prevent further tissue injury)
What are some possible contraindications for reimplantation?	• Severe crush injury • Contamination • Underlying disease which would make reimplantation difficult (such as diabetes) • Prolonged warm ischemia
With which digit should all attempts be made for reimplantation, given the potential for significant loss of function?	Thumb
What is the Volkmann ischemia?	Compartment syndrome of the upper extremity leading to deformity and contractures.
What are some causes of compartment syndrome in the setting of hand/wrist fractures?	• Crush injury to forearm • Supracondylar fracture • Fracture of the ulna or radius
What are the six Ps of compartment syndrome?	Pain out of proportion on the exam Paresthesia Paralysis Pallor Poikilothermia Pulselessness (late finding)

What is the compartment pressure where surgical decompression is indicated? >30 mmHg

What nerve runs deep to the flexor carpi ulnaris and through Guyon's canal? Ulnar nerve

Name some examples of muscles that are innervated by the ulnar nerve:
- Interosseous muscles
- Hypothenar eminence
- Lumbrical muscles

What area of the hand does the ulnar nerve provide sensation to? The dorsal and volar aspect of the little finger and ulnar half of the ring finger.

What are some motor tests that one can perform to test the ulnar nerve? Abduction of the fingers against resistance

Name some examples of muscles that are innervated by the radial nerve: Extensor muscles

Triceps

Brachioradialis

Supinator

What area of the hand does the radial nerve provide sensation to? Dorsum of the radial aspect of the hand, dorsum of the thumb, and the dorsal aspect of the middle and index fingers.

What are some motor tests that one can perform to test the radial nerve? Extension of the wrist

Name some examples of muscles that are innervated by the median nerve:
- Flexor muscles such as flexor carpi radialis
- Pronator quadratus
- Opponens pollicis

What area of the hand does the median nerve provide sensation to? Dorsal aspect of the tips of the index and middle finger along with radial side of the hand and volar aspect of digits 1-3.

What are some motor tests that one can perform to test the median nerve? Opposition of the thumb

What is the most commonly injured carpal bone? Scaphoid bone

What is the most common mechanism by which scaphoid injuries occur? Fall on outstretched hand

What are the signs and symptoms of a scaphoid injury? Pain in the area of the anatomic snuff box as well as referred pain to the anatomic snuff box with compression of the thumb.

What are some radiographic views to obtain to evaluate a potential scaphoid fracture?	Lateral and an AP view. Additionally, one may also obtain a dedicated scaphoid view
Does a normal radiograph rule-out a scaphoid injury?	No—Initial x-ray may not show a fracture. Follow-up MRI may be required.
What are the complications of a missed scaphoid fracture?	Avascular necrosis, non-union, and malunion
What is the reason for avascular necrosis with scaphoid fractures?	The vascular supply is distal
What are some considerations in the management of scaphoid fractures?	• Treat all suspected scaphoid fractures as a potential fracture despite normal radiographs • Immobilization in a thumb spica cast • Displaced fractures often require an open reduction-internal fixation (ORIF)
Name the next two most common carpal bone fractures:	Lunate and triquetrum carpal bone
What is Kienböck disease?	Avascular necrosis of the lunate bone.
What is the general rule with all carpal bone dislocations?	All should be referred to an orthopedic surgeon
Name the most common wrist dislocation:	Perilunate dislocation
What is the best view on a radiograph to evaluate for a possible perilunate dislocation?	Lateral view
What is a "Boxer's fracture"?	Metacarpal neck fracture of the fifth and/or fourth digit.
What is the most common mechanism for a Boxer's fracture?	Punch with a clenched fist
Is a Boxer's fracture unstable?	Yes—most are unstable
What are some findings that may require operative intervention?	Any rotational deformity Significant angulation Neurovascular compromise
What is the most common type of MCP joint dislocation?	Thumb

What are two types of MCP dislocations? Complete dislocation and subluxation

What are some complications of an MCP joint dislocation? Avulsions
Volar plate injury

What is the treatment of choice of an MCP joint subluxation? Usually managed with a closed reduction, whereas a complete dislocation often require ORIF

What is skier's thumb or gamekeeper's thumb? Ulnar collateral ligament tear.

What is mechanism by which a skier's thumb may occur? Often due to forceful radial deviation of the thumb at the MCP joint

What are some exam findings for a skier's thumb? Thumb grasp is weak, as well as tenderness along the ulnar aspect of the thumb

What is the treatment for a skier's thumb? Based on degree of joint stability—If greater than 10 to 20 degree of laxity=surgical repair

What is a Colles fracture? It is a transverse fracture of the metaphysis of the distal radius with a dorsal displacement of the distal portion.

What is a common mechanism of injury of a Colles fracture? Fall on an outstretched hand

Which nerve injury is associated with a Colles fracture? Median nerve

What is the treatment of choice for a non-displaced Colles fracture? Immobilize with a coaptation or "sugar-tong" splint and refer to orthopedics
A displaced fracture will often require operative intervention

What is a Smith fracture? It is a transverse fracture of the distal radial metaphysis with volar displacement of the distal fragment.

What is a "jersey finger"? Injury to the flexor digitorum profundus tendon often when a player grabs a shirt and fingers get caught.

How do you test for a flexor digitorum profundus tendon injury? Extend and immobilize the MCP and PIP and instruct the patient to flex at the DIP.

How do you test for a flexor digitorum superficialis tendon injury?

Hold the uninjured finger in extension and flex the injured finger.

Does a normal test of the flexor tendons rule-out an injury?

No—Even with a 90% full-thickness laceration one can have normal range of motion.

What are some physical exam findings that may be suggestive of a flexor tendon injury?

The strength of motion and merely not being able to range the affected digit

Change in the resting posture of the digit

What is the treatment for a partial flexor tendon injury?

Controversial but most would apply a conservative approach with splinting

What are a mallet finger and a Boutonniere deformity examples of?

Extensor tendon injury

What is a mallet finger?

It is a disruption or laceration of the extensor tendon at the DIP joint.

What is the mechanism of injury of a mallet finger?

Blow against the tip of an extended finger with sudden forced flexion.

What is a delayed complication of an untreated mallet finger?

"Swan neck deformity" where there is hyperextension of the PIP and flexion deformity of the DIP

What are the treatment options for a mallet finger?

Can split the DIP in extension if no associated fracture

If there is a fracture, may either splint or pin the fragment

What traumatic injury causes a Boutonniere deformity?

Rupture of the central slip of the extensor tendon at the PIP

What is the mechanism of injury of a Boutonniere deformity?

Direct blow to the PIP joint

What is the treatment option for a Boutonniere deformity?

Splint the PIP in extension with orthopedic referral

What is De Quervain tenosynovitis?

Inflammation of the extensor tendons due to overuse of the thumb.

What bedside test can confirm this diagnosis?

A positive Finkelstein's test-pain on ulnar deviation of the wrist with the thumb in a flexed position.

What are some treatment options for De Quervain tenosynovitis?

Splint in a position of function with use of NSAIDs

Can most high-pressure injection injuries be discharged for follow-up with normal radiographs and exam?

No—Surgical emergency (appearance is almost always benign appearing but a devastating injury)

What is the mechanism of injury of high-pressure injections?

Typically a paint or grease gun that causes a small (1-2 mm) wound in the hand and the substance travels down the tendon sheath.

What is the overall prognosis of high-pressure injuries?

Poor—Up to 60% often have some form of amputation

What are some considerations in the management of high-pressure injection injuries?

Radiographs of the affected area; update tetanus status; empiric antibiotics; and immediate orthopedic consultation for debridement

What is a herpetic whitlow?

A viral infection (most commonly HSV) of the distal finger causing painful vesicle formations.

What is the diagnostic test of choice for a herpetic whitlow?

Clinical diagnosis but can confirm with Tzanck smear

What are some considerations in the management of a herpetic whitlow?

Analgesics for pain control; antiviral medication (ie, acyclovir); dry dressing and instructions to avoid touching others with affected part

What is a pitfall in the management of herpetic whitlow?

Incision and drainage as if it was an abscess

What should always be a consideration of a patient who presents with a laceration over an MCP joint?

"Fight bite" or a punch to another's mouth

What are some complications of a fight bite?

Deep palmer space infection with resultant loss of function or amputation.

What is the general rule when managing fight bites?

Treat all suspected fight bites aggressively; radiographs to evaluate for fractures; wound cultures; empiric antibiotics; irrigate; orthopedic consult for possible washout

What is a paronychia?

Lateral nail fold infection.

What are the two most common agents involved with a paronychia?

S aureus and strep

What bedside procedure can be used to provide drainage and relief?	Can remove a portion of the nail bed
What is a felon?	Infection within the pulp space of a fingertip.
What is the causative agent in most cases of a felon?	*S aureus*
What are complications of an untreated felon?	Osteomyelitis and flexor tenosynovitis
What is the treatment of choice of a felon?	Incision and drainage
Explain how to perform an incision and drainage of a felon:	1. Central longitudinal incision one-half centimeter from the distal to the flexion crease 2. Extend into the pulp space
What is the typical mechanism of injury for flexor tenosynovitis?	Most commonly from a puncture wound
What are the four Kanavel signs of flexor tenosynovitis?	1. Pain with passive extension of the finger 2. Symmetric swelling of the finger 3. Finger held in slight flexion 4. Tenderness with percussion along the flexor tendon sheath
What are some considerations in the management of flexor tenosynovitis?	Hospitalization with intravenous antibiotics and emergent orthopedic or hand consultation for operative drainage.

SHOULDER INJURIES

What is the most common dislocation seen in the emergency department?	Shoulder dislocations
Which is the most common type of shoulder dislocation: posterior or anterior?	Over 95% of all shoulder dislocations are anterior
What are some common causes of posterior shoulder dislocations?	Seizures or electric shocks are often in the history. Also possible is a direct blow to the anterior shoulder.

What is the most common subtype of posterior shoulder dislocation?

Subacromial account for the majority

What is the mechanism of injury with anterior shoulder dislocations?

Often due to external rotations or excessive abduction or extension

Name the following types of anterior shoulder dislocations:

Subglenoid

Head of the humerus is inferior to the glenoid fossa

Subcoracoid

Most common

Intrathoracic

Very rare

Subclavicular

Very rare as well

What are some common physical exam findings of an anterior shoulder dislocation?

Flattening of the normal contour of the shoulder, prominent acromion, the affected arm is often held in external rotation with slight abduction

What is the standard x-ray series to obtain with a suspected anterior shoulder dislocation?

AP, transscapular, and an axillary view especially if a posterior shoulder dislocation is suspected

Are nerve injuries common with anterior shoulder dislocations?

No

What is the most common nerve injured with a suspected anterior shoulder dislocation?

Axillary nerve

What are the physical exam findings of a possible axillary nerve injury?

Sensory loss over the lateral aspect of the shoulder and weakened abduction

Is axillary nerve involvement permanent?

No—often due to neurapraxias which recover

Can nerve injury occur during the post-reduction period?

Yes—important to document nerve exam before and after any reduction

What is the most common complication of an anterior shoulder dislocation?

Recurrence

What is a Bankart's fracture?

It is a fracture of the anterior glenoid lip.

What is a Hill-Sachs deformity?

Compression fracture of the posterolateral aspect of the humeral head.

What is the treatment of choice for anterior shoulder dislocations?

Closed reduction using a combination of traction and scapular manipulation.

Name some techniques used for reduction and briefly describe each:

- Traction-countertraction: applying a force in the other direction while one exerts gentle traction of the affected arm in a downward motion
- Stimson technique: patient lies in a prone position with a weight attached to the affected arm which exerts a downward force

What is the most important factor to ensure a successful reduction?

Patient must be relaxed!

What are some techniques to enhance muscle relaxation?

One can use an intra-articular block or conscious sedation

Name some commonly used agents for conscious sedation:

- Fentanyl/midazolam
- Ketamine
- Etomidate
- Propofol

What are some important considerations in any post-reduction maneuver performed?

- Post-reduction films
- Document a neurovascular examination post-reduction!
- Proper orthopedic follow-up
- Immobilization

What is the treatment of choice for a posterior shoulder reduction?

Closed reduction

What are some considerations when attempting a closed reduction for a posterior shoulder dislocation?

- It is rare with more complications associated such as fracture and nerve injury
- Early orthopedic involvement should be considered
- Can be difficult to reduce and may require operative reduction (open or under general anesthesia)
- Any evidence of neurovascular involvement mandates immediate orthopedic involvement

What injury should one suspect with a fall on an outstretched hand?

Acromioclavicular (AC) separation

What is the most common mechanism of injury with an AC separation?

Fall on the affected shoulder with the arm adducted

What are some signs and symptoms of an AC injury?

Swelling with tenderness over the AC joint, gross deformity with high degree injury, and pain with upper extremity movement.

What view is preferred with a suspected AC injury?	AP view of both clavicles
What is the classification of AC injuries and their respective management?	
Type I/First degree:	It is essentially a sprain with conservative management
Type II/Second degree:	Subluxation with sling and orthopedic follow-up
Type III/Third degree:	Immobilization versus operative intervention
Type IV/Fourth degree:	Most require operative intervention
What is the classification of sternoclavicular (SC) joint injuries and their respective management?	
Type I/First degree:	It is essentially a sprain with conservative management
Type II/Second degree:	Subluxation with sling and orthopedic follow-up
Type III/Third degree:	Dislocation that requires immediate orthopedic consultation
What type of SC joint injury requires immediate attention?	Posterior dislocations due to high risk of life-threatening such as great vessel laceration.
Are scapular fractures common?	No—often due to high-energy trauma such as motor vehicle crashes (MVCs)
What is the real concern for any scapular fractures?	Associated injuries
What are some important associated injuries to consider with all scapular fractures?	Lung injuries, rib fractures, and shoulder injuries
What areas of the scapula are commonly fractured?	Glenoid, body, and neck of the scapula
What is the general rule in the management of scapular fractures?	Most can be managed conservatively with a sling.
When is open reduction and internal fixation (ORIF) indicated?	Angulated fractures as well as severe displacement
What is a common upper extremity fracture to consider in the elderly population?	Proximal humeral fracture

What is the most common mechanism of injury?	Fall on an outstretched arm
What is a common classification system used for proximal humeral fractures?	Neer classification (classification based on amount of displacement of four segments that include greater/lesser tuberosity and anatomic/surgical neck)
What are some complications of a proximal humeral fracture?	Neurovascular injuries such as axillary nerve, avascular necrosis of the head, and adhesive capsulitis
What is the most complication of a proximal humeral fracture?	Adhesive capsulitis
What is adhesive capsulitis?	Known as frozen shoulder, this can be avoided with early mobilization

ELBOW AND RADIAL/ULNAR INJURIES

What comprises the elbow?	Three bones comprise the elbow which consists of the distal humerus, proximal ulna, and proximal radius.
Is a posterior fat pad sign seen on a lateral x-ray of the elbow normal?	No—never normal
What does a posterior fat pad often indicate?	Distension of the joint capsule by an effusion and probable fracture.
What is the most common type of elbow dislocation?	Posterior, in which the radius and ulnar are dislocated posteriorly to the distal humeral head.
What is the most common mechanism of injury seen with a posterior elbow dislocation?	Fall on an abducted and extended arm
What are some physical exam findings seen with a posterior elbow dislocation?	Prominent olecranon along with swelling with 45° of joint flexion
What is the best view on x-ray to obtain to best demonstrate a posterior elbow dislocation?	Lateral view
What are some associated injuries to consider with a posterior elbow dislocation?	Fractures, ulnar/median nerve damage, and brachial artery injury

What is the treatment of choice for a posterior elbow dislocation?	Closed reduction (should be performed by orthopedics) unless neurovascular compromise in which case reduction should be attempted without delay.
What are some important maneuvers when attempting a closed reduction?	Immobilize the humerus, traction distally at the wrist with elbow in flexed position, apply posterior pressure to distal humerus.
What are other considerations in the management of a posterior elbow dislocation?	Document a repeat neurovascular exam after reduction Immobilize the elbow in a long-arm posterior splint Consider delayed neurovascular compromise
What is the mechanism of injury for an anterior elbow dislocation?	While the elbow is flexed, a blow to the olecranon occurs
What are some physical exam findings seen with an anterior elbow dislocation?	Arm is often held in an extended position
What are some associated injuries to consider with an anterior elbow dislocation?	Fractures, ulnar/median nerve damage, and brachial artery injury but a much higher incidence when compared to a posterior elbow dislocation.
What are some important maneuvers when attempting a closed reduction?	Immobilize the humerus, traction distally at the wrist, and apply backward/downward pressure to the proximal forearm.
What are other considerations in the management of an anterior elbow dislocation?	Document a repeat neurovascular exam after reduction Immobilize the elbow in a long-arm posterior splint Consider delayed neurovascular compromise
What is a Nursemaid's elbow?	Radial head subluxation
What population does this commonly occur in?	Often in children less than 4-6 years of age
What is the mechanism of injury which occurs with a radial head subluxation?	While the arm is in pronation there is an abrupt longitudinal traction applied to the hand or forearm resulting in the annular ligament being pulled over the radial head.

What is the typical clinical presentation for a radial head subluxation?	The elbow is often flexed and the arm held in pronation.
Is radiographic imaging typically required for a suspected radial head subluxation?	Often not required unless history is not clear
Describe the technique with closed reduction.	With one hand grasp the affected arm as if ready to give a hand shake and with the other hand place thumb on radial head. Supinate and flex the arm with a click that is often heard when successful.
What is the most common mechanism of injury with an olecranon fracture?	Often due to a direct blow
What are some physical exam findings with an olecranon fracture?	Often will have tenderness and swelling in that area as well as difficulty in extending elbow
What nerve is typically associated with an olecranon fracture?	Ulnar nerve
What are some considerations in the management of an olecranon fracture?	If nondisplaced can immobilize elbow in 30° flexion; fractures with >2 mm displacement often require ORIF for repair
Name two types of supracondylar fractures:	Extension (more common) Flexion
What is the mechanism of injury with a supracondylar extension fracture?	A fall on an outstretched hand with the elbow in extension
Describe a supracondylar extension fracture?	The distal humeral fracture is displaced posterior
What are some complications of this type of fracture?	Potential brachial artery and median nerve damage Compartment syndrome
What are some considerations in the management of a supracondylar extension fracture?	May be immobilized if nondisplaced ANY displaced fracture requires reduction and ORIF Always document a repeat neurovascular examination
What nerve is most likely to be injured in a supracondylar flexion fracture?	Ulnar

Name the two articular surfaces of the condyles located at the distal humerus:	Capitellum (lateral) Trochlea (medial)
Name the two nonarticular surfaces of the condyles located at the distal humerus:	Medial and lateral epicondyle
What are some considerations in the management of a condylar fracture?	Nondisplaced or minimal displaced fractures can often be immobilized in 90° flexion whereas displaced fractures will often require ORIF especially articular surface fractures
What is a common mechanism of injury of a radial head fracture?	Fall on an outstretched hand
What are some common physical exam findings with a radial head fracture?	Swelling and tenderness over the radial head with increased pain with supination
What radiographic finding can be seen with a radial head fracture?	Posterior fat pad sign
What is the treatment for a nondisplaced fracture?	Sling immobilization where displaced/ comminuted fractures may require early ORIF
What is a Galeazzi fracture?	Fracture of the distal radial shaft with an associated distal radioulnar dislocation.
What is the treatment of a Galeazzi fracture?	ORIF
What is a Monteggia's fracture?	A fracture of the proximal third of the ulna along with dislocation of the radial head.
What nerve is most commonly injured?	Radial nerve
What is a nightstick fracture?	Isolated fracture of the shaft of the ulna
What are some indications of ORIF for a nightstick fracture?	Displacement greater than 50% of the diameter of the ulna or greater than 10° angulation

PELVIS INJURIES

Name the bones that comprise the pelvis:	1. Innominate (ilium, ischium, and pubis) 2. Sacrum 3. Coccyx
Name the two major nerve roots that run through the pelvis:	Lumbar and sacral
What is the line that divides the lower (true) pelvis from the upper (false) pelvis?	Ileorectal line
Name important structures that may be damaged with any injury to the lower pelvis:	• Anus • Nerve roots • Bladder/urethra • Colon • Rectum
Name the three leading causes of pelvic fractures:	1. Motor vehicle crashes 2. Falls 3. Crush injuries
What is the normal width for the following areas of the pelvis on an AP view of the pelvis?	Sacroiliac (SI) joint 2-4 mm Symphysis pubis <5 mm

Describe following classification for pelvic fractures:

	AP Compression
Type I	Disruption of the pubic symphysis <2.5 cm of the diastasis with no significant posterior pelvic injury
Type II	Tearing of the anterior sacroiliac and disruption of the pubic symphysis >2.5 cm
Type III	Complete disruption of the pubic symphysis and posterior ligament complexes
	Lateral Compression
Type I	Posterior compression of the SI joint without any ligament disruption
Type II	Rupture of the posterior SI ligament with internal rotation of the hemipelvis on the anterior SI joint
Type III	Meets criteria for type II along with evidence of AP compression injury to the contralateral hemipelvis

Define the following signs in relation to pelvic fractures:

Earle sign:

A large hematoma or tenderness along the fracture line is felt on rectal exam

Roux sign:

The distance between the greater trochanter and pubic spine is decreased on one side when compared to the other side

Destot sign:

Superficial hematoma above the inguinal ligament

What is the most common pelvic fracture?

Pubic rami

What is a "straddle injury"?

It is from a fall on the crotch with the legs apart that result in bilateral fracture of both the inferior and superior pubic rami.

What is the primary cause of death in patients with pelvic fractures?

Hemorrhage

About how much blood can be found in the retroperitoneal space?

Up to 5 L

What is an initial management step to consider in patients with an unstable pelvic fracture?

Application of a MAST (Military Anti-Shock Trouser) in addition to the normal resuscitation

What are some other interventions utilized in unstable pelvic fractures?

External fixation and angiographic embolization

What is the most commonly associated pelvic injury?

Urethral injuries

What are some delayed complications that may occur with pelvic fractures?

Thromboembolic complications

Chronic pain

Malunion

How are hip dislocations classified?

Based on the final position of the femoral head

Are anterior or posterior hip dislocations more common?

80 to 90% of hip dislocations are posterior

What is the most common mechanism of a posterior hip dislocation?

Most common scenario is a motor vehicle crash where direct force is applied to the flexed knee which pushes the femoral head through the posterior capsule.

What is the physical exam finding of a posterior hip dislocation?	Leg is often shortened, adducted, and internally rotated
What are some other associated injuries with a posterior hip dislocation?	Knee injury Sciatic nerve injury Associated acetabular fracture
What are some different types of anterior hip dislocations?	Superior pubic Superior iliac Inferior
What are some possible mechanisms of injury of an anterior hip dislocation?	Motor vehicle crash Fall
What is the physical exam finding of an anterior hip dislocation?	Limb is adducted, externally rotated, and extended
Which nerve injury is associated with anterior hip dislocations?	Femoral nerve
Which nerve injury is associated with posterior hip dislocations?	Sciatic nerve
Aside from nerve injury, what is the primary concern with a hip dislocation?	Avascular necrosis
What is the treatment of choice for all hip dislocations?	Early reduction
What are some types of hip fractures?	• Femoral head • Femoral neck • Trochanteric • Intertrochanteric • Subtrochanteric
Does the ability to ambulate rule-out a hip fracture?	No
Does a negative radiograph rule-out a hip fracture if pain is still present?	No
What is the most significant complication of a femoral neck fracture?	Avascular necrosis
What is an important differential to consider in a child who presents with fever and limp?	Septic arthritis
What is a diagnosis of exclusion sometimes considered in the above case?	Transient synovitis (always consider septic joint as a missed case is devastating)

Which organism is most commonly involved with septic joint?	*S aureus*
What is the diagnostic test of choice?	Arthrocentesis
What are some characteristic findings of a positive tap with arthrocentesis?	80,000-200,000 WBCs and a high PMNs predominance
What is slipped capital femoral epiphysis (SCFE)?	Irregular widening of the epiphyseal plate with associated swelling of the joint capsule that results in slippage.
What age and gender does SCFE commonly occur in?	Typically an obsess male in the adolescent years
What are some radiographic findings of SCFE on radiograph?	Often described as an ice cream cone (the femoral head being the ice cream) slipping off the cone
What are important radiographic views to obtain when evaluating for a possible SCFE?	AP and frogleg lateral view
Once an SCFE is diagnosed, that are some considerations in the management of SCFE?	Make the patient immediately non-weight-bearing Immediate orthopedic referral
What is Legg-Calve-Perthes disease?	Osteochondrosis of the femoral head

KNEE INJURIES

Which muscle allows extension of the knee as well as acting as the primary stabilizer?	Quadriceps tendon (Vastus lateralis/intermedius/medialis and rectus femoris)
Name some structures that are responsible for the stability of the lateral knee:	Lateral collateral ligament Iliotibial tract Popliteus muscle
Name some structures that are responsible for the stability of the medial knee:	Medial collateral ligament Pes anserinus Medial joint capsule
Which ligament is more commonly injured: medial or lateral collateral ligament?	Medial collateral ligament

Which ligaments control anteroposterior as well as rotary stability of the knee?	Anterior and posterior cruciate ligament
What is the most common fracture of the knee?	Tibial plateau fracture
What is the most common mechanism of a tibial plateau fracture?	Valgus stress with axial loading
What is the most common type of patellar fracture?	Transverse fracture
What is the mechanism of injury with a patellar fracture?	Direct impact to the patellar
What are some signs and symptoms of a patellar fracture?	Swelling in the affected region along with tenderness; pain on extension of the knee
What are some radiographic views to consider with a patellar fracture?	AP, lateral, and sunrise view
What are some considerations in the management of a patellar fracture?	Most nondisplaced fractures can be managed with immobilization in full extension whereas wide displacement requires surgical intervention.
Which population does patellar subluxation/dislocations generally occur in?	Female adolescents with some type of chronic patellofemoral problem such as patellae alta.
Which is the most common type of patellar dislocation?	Lateral
What is the most common mechanism of injury with a patellar subluxation/ dislocation?	Impact to the patellar while in flexion or extension
What are some considerations in the management of a patellar subluxation/ dislocation?	Obtain other radiographs to rule-out other injuries in the surrounding area Reduction Immobilization in full extension
Which knee injury is considered an orthopedic emergency?	Knee dislocation
What is the most common mechanism of a knee dislocation?	Motor vehicle crash

What is the most common type of knee dislocation?	Anterior/posterior dislocations are the most common (as opposed to medial/lateral, or rotary)
What are some associated injuries to consider with a knee dislocation?	Popliteal artery injury which is the biggest concern; peroneal (fibular) nerve injury Ligament injury Proximal tibial fracture
What test must be considered with all potential knee dislocations?	An arteriogram
What is a pitfall with knee dislocations?	Not fully evaluating the knee even with spontaneous relocation (they should still undergo full vascular evaluation)
What is an immediate action required for knee dislocations?	Immediate relocation by longitudinal traction
What are some other considerations in the management of a knee dislocation?	A thorough neurovascular exam should be performed before and after reduction After reduction, knee should be immobilized in a posterior splint at 15° flexion
What are some indications for immediate surgical intervention?	Failure to reduce knee dislocation Any open dislocation Any popliteal injury, preferable within 6 hours

LOWER LEG INJURIES

What are the four compartments of the lower leg?	Anterior compartment Lateral (peroneal) compartment Superficial posterior compartment Deep posterior compartment
What is a concern with a lower extremity injury given the many compartments?	Compartment syndrome
Which compartment is compartment syndrome most common in?	Anterior
Which fracture is associated with an anterior compartment syndrome?	Proximal tibia fracture

What is another important cause of anterior compartment syndrome (although it can also be seen with other compartments)?

Strenuous exercise

What are some considerations in the treatment for compartment syndrome?

Early diagnosis-high index of suspicion

Early surgery involvement

Measure compartment pressure if possible (>30 mmHg)

Name three groups of ligaments that provide support to the ankle:

Medial collateral ligament (deltoid ligament)

Lateral collateral ligament (Calcaneofibular, anterior talofibular, and posterior talofibular)

Ligaments of syndesmosis

Which ligament is most commonly sprained?

Up to 90% are lateral collateral ligament sprains

What is the mechanism of injury for lateral ligament sprains?

Inversion with internal rotation

What is the most frequently injured ligament with a lateral ligament sprain?

Anterior talofibular

What is the mechanism of a medial collateral ligament sprain?

External rotation with eversion

What is the classification commonly used for sprains and some associated physical findings?

First degree:

Mild tenderness and swelling; able to bear weight and no loss of function

Second degree:

Moderate swelling and tenderness; pain with stress maneuvers of the ankle

Third degree:

Significant swelling and tenderness along with inability to bear weight and significant loss of function

What is a Maisonneuve fracture?

A proximal fibular fracture that can occur with rupture of the deltoid ligament.

What are some considerations in the management of an ankle sprain?

All sprains should be initially managed with RICE (rest/ice/compression/elevation)

Crutches can be considered if difficulty in bearing weight

Management of third degree sprains are controversial and ranges between conservative versus operative

What are five types of ankle dislocations?

1. Posterior (common)
2. Medial (common)
3. Lateral
4. Anterior
5. Superior

What fracture are most ankle dislocations associated with?

Malleolar fractures

What are some considerations in the management of ankle dislocations?

Immediate reduction with a thorough neurovascular exam

Early orthopedic involvement for possible operative intervention if any neurovascular compromise

If reduction is successful, post-reduction film and a posterior splint

What is a consideration of ankle injuries that occur in the pediatric population?

Since the ligaments are stronger than bone, fractures at the epiphyseal plate can occur

What are three parts that comprise the foot?

1. Forefoot (phalanges and metatarsals)
2. Midfoot (navicular, cuneiforms, cuboid)
3. Hindfoot (talus and calcaneous)

What separates the hindfoot from the midfoot?

Chopart joint

What separates the midfoot from the forefoot?

Lisfranc joint

What is the most frequently fractured tarsal bone?

Calcaneous

What is a common cause of a calcaneous fracture?

Compression injury landing on the foot

What are some signs and symptoms of a calcaneous fracture?

Swelling/tenderness in the region along with inability to bear weight

What are some other injuries to consider with calcaneous fractures?

Up to 10% can be bilateral

Associated dorsolumbar spine compression injury

What are some considerations in the management of calcaneous fractures?

Most non-displaced fractures respond to conservative management

Intra-articular or displaced fractures may require operative intervention

What are some mechanisms of injuries with Lisfranc fracture?

Compression

Rotational (twisting the body about a fixed foot)

Axial loading (fall on a plantar-fixed foot)

What are some radiographic findings that may indicate disruption of the Lisfranc joint?

Separation between the base of the first and second metatarsals

Fracture through the base of the second metatarsal

Is conservative management appropriate in most cases of a Lisfranc fracture?

No—unstable fracture, require early orthopedic involvement for reduction

What is a Jones fracture?

Transverse fracture of the fifth metatarsal at the proximal aspect.

What is the mechanism of injury with a Jones fracture?

A load that is applied to the ball of the foot laterally.

What is a dancer's fracture?

Avulsion fracture of the base of the fifth metatarsal.

What is the treatment for a Jones fracture?

While a dancer's fracture often will heal well with conservative management, a Jones fracture has a poor rate of union so often require orthopedic consultation.

CLINICAL VIGNETTES—MAKE THE DIAGNOSIS

13-year-old mildly obese boy presents with a history of right knee pain. He does mention worse pain while playing soccer, however, denies any actual trauma; PE: examination of both knees is unrevealing. What is also crucial to exam for any pediatric knee complaint?

A thorough examination of the hips as well

35-year-old man with no past medical history presents from prison with bilateral thigh pain. He admits to doing a series of squats to the point he could not move his legs, but denies any obvious trauma such as assault; PE: examination of both lower extremities reveal pain out of proportion but intact sensation and pulses. What diagnosis must be considered and intervention?

Compartment syndrome with consult for possible release of compartments

16-year-old woman presents with two linear lacerations above the MCP joints. She states that she fell down a flight of stairs and sustained the lacerations from that fall; PE: Two 1-cm lacerations above the MCP joint of both the 2nd and 3rd digit. What diagnosis and interventions must be considered?

"Fight bite" or human bite to the MCP joint which requires immediate orthopedic consult for possible wash-out

31-year-old man was brought in by an air medical transport team for an MVC. Patient was an unrestrained passenger who required extrication at the scene and a reported death of the driver. The patient has been hypotensive and tachycardia with no response to crystalloids. On arrival patient is intubated and has obvious gross deformity of his pelvis. What immediate intervention is required while the patient is being evaluated for other injuries?

An external pelvic binder and may also require embolization in addition to any other interventions

8-month-old infant is brought in for possible head trauma. The parents mention that the infant probably rolled out of the crib, but otherwise note no other events. Radiographs: non-displaced linear skull fracture. What should be a consideration?

Abuse

81-year-old woman presents to the ED after a mechanical fall on a patch of ice directly on to her left hip. She has difficulty walking but no deformity on examination but does complain of some pain with range of motion. Her radiographs are normal. Can she be sent home?

Assume a fracture of the hip despite "normal" radiographs if patient still has pain on exam

CHAPTER 10

Endocrine Emergencies

DISORDERS OF GLUCOSE REGULATION

What is the most common cause of coma associated with diabetes?

Hypoglycemia due to excessive insulin use

What is the definition of hypoglycemia?

Commonly defined as a blood glucose concentration of less than 50 mg/dL with cognitive impairment (note the clinical presentation is more important than a number).

What are some signs and symptoms of hypoglycemia?

*Primarily manifest as CNS dysfunction

Tachycardia

Tremulousness

Diaphoresis

Mental status change

Seizures

Focal neurologic deficits that can mimic a stroke

Note: many early signs may be masked by beta-blockers

List some hormones that play an important role in glucose regulation:

Glucagon

Epinephrine

Growth hormone

Cortisol

Name some causes of hypoglycemia:	Addison disease
	Akee fruit (Jamaican vomiting sickness)
	Ethanol
	Thyroid dysfunction
	Malnutrition
	Medications
List medications that commonly cause hypoglycemia:	Beta-blockers
	Quinine
	Salicylate
	Insulin
	Sulfonylureas
What is Whipple triad?	Diagnostic features of insulinoma of the pancreas:
	1. Signs and symptoms of hypoglycemia
	2. Blood sugar concentration below 50 mg/dL
	3. Recovery from an attack following the administration of glucose
What are some critical actions in the management of hypoglycemia?	Serial glucose concentrations (glucometer often not reliable below 50 mg/dL)
	If patient is awake, oral replacement is preferred
	Intramuscular glucagon may be used if intravenous access in not obtainable
	Administer 25 to 75 g of intravenous dextrose ($D_{50}W$) (1-3 ampules)
	Children: 0.5 to 1 g/kg glucose as $D_{25}W$ IV (2-4 mL/kg)
	Neonates: 0.5 to 1 g/kg glucose as $D_{10}W$
What are some indications to admit a patient who is hypoglycemic?	Overdose of long acting insulin
	Overdose of any sulfonylureas

Diabetes

List the four major types of diabetes mellitus:	Type 1 (insulin-dependent)
	Type 2 (non-insulin-dependent)
	Gestational diabetes
	Impaired glucose tolerance

What are some characteristic features of Type 1 diabetes?

Abrupt cessation of insulin production

Over 90% of type 1 diabetes has an autoimmune component

Parental insulin is required to survive

Ketosis is more common in Type 1 diabetes

What is the primary morbidity in diabetes?

Vascular complications

List important causes of mortality in diabetes:

Cardiovascular disease

Cerebrovascular disease

Diabetic ketoacidosis

List some criteria to diagnose diabetes:

Any random serum glucose concentration of >200 mg/dL

A fasting serum glucose concentration of >126 mg/dL

Glycosylated hemoglobin (HgA1C) >6.5%

Name an important measurement to assess glucose control:

Glycosylated hemoglobin (4-6% is normal limit)

What is the definition of diabetic ketoacidosis (DKA)?

Diabetic ketoacidosis is a state of absolute or relative insulin deficiency leading to the excessive breakdown of fatty acids into ketone bodies. The situation is aggravated by ensuing hyperglycemia, dehydration, and acidosis-producing derangements.

What are some metabolic derangements that occur with DKA?

Relative or absolute lack of insulin

Excessive stress hormones (ie, cortisol)

Overproduction of free fatty acids

What are three commonly seen ketone bodies?

1. Acetoacetate
2. β-hydroxybutyrate
3. Acetone

Does the urine dipstick detect all ketone bodies?

No—it uses the nitroprusside reaction which does not measure β-hydroxybutyrate

What is the typical acetoacetate/ β-hydroxybutyrate ratio in diabetic ketoacidosis?

1:2-10 (can be as high as 1:35). This means that dipstick measurements may underestimate the true level of ketosis.

List important precipitating factors of DKA:

Infection

Lack of insulin

Trauma

Surgery

Myocardial infarction

Cerebrovascular accident

What are some signs and symptoms of DKA?

Nausea

Vomiting

Abdominal pain

Partial motor seizures

Visual change

Lethargy

Coma

Fruity breath

Kussmaul respirations

What percentage of undiagnosed diabetics will present as diabetic ketoacidosis?

25%

What are Kussmaul respirations?

It is a form of hyperventilation in metabolic acidosis where breathing is first rapid and then shallow as the acidemia worsens, becoming deep/slow/gasping. A physiological respiratory compensation for metabolic acidosis.

What are some clinical features in the history of a patient who presents with DKA?

Weight loss

Polyuria/polyphagia/polydipsia

Weakness

Emesis

Abdominal pain

What are some commonly used diagnostic tests in DKA?

Complete blood count

Chemistry panel

VBG or ABG

Ketone bodies (serum or urine dipstick)

Calcium/magnesium/phosphorus

*Also consider an infectious work-up or a cardiac work-up if there is clinical evidence that this is the precipitant

What particular electrolyte is important to monitor in DKA?

Potassium—Patient may initially be hyperkalemic due to insulin insufficiency, but level will rapidly fall and may become hypokalemic with insulin therapy.

What is the correction factor of sodium in the presence of marked hyperglycemia?

The sodium may be approximated by adding 1.5 mEq/L to the sodium value for every 100 mg/dL glucose increase above normal. This correction is required because the osmotic action of the glucose draws free water into the intravascular space, diluting the sodium concentration.

What are some important confirmatory laboratory results in DKA?

pH: <7.3

Bicarbonate: <10 mEq/L

Serum glucose concentration: >350 mg/dL

What are some considerations in the management of DKA?

ABCs and IV-O_2-monitor

Insulin

Correct fluid losses (often have significant volume deficits)

IV infusion of low-dose insulin

Early potassium replacement

Consider use of bicarbonate (if pH <7.0)

What is the dose of regular insulin in patients with DKA?

0.1 U/kg of intravenous regular insulin (sometimes also given as a bolus followed by an infusion/h)

When should one consider switching from 0.9% normal saline to D_5W 0.45% NS?

Often switched when glucose concentration is less than 300 mg/dL

What is the concern in aggressive correction of serum osmolarity in children?

Cerebral edema

What are some complications that may occur in the treatment of DKA?

Volume overload from aggressive fluid resuscitation

Hypokalemia

Hypoglycemia

Alkalosis from excessive bicarbonate use

What is the primary cause of mortality in elderly patients with DKA?

Sepsis

What is hyperglycemic hyperosmolar non-ketotic coma (HHNC)?	Often characterized by hyperosmolarity, marked hyperglycemia, and dehydration with associated altered mental status that often progresses to coma.
Is acidosis and ketosis a common finding in HHNC?	As the name implies, it is not a common finding
What is the etiology of HHNC?	Severe dehydration that is commonly from sustained hyperglycemic with diuresis. Often occurs in elderly patients with poor glycemic control
What are the signs and symptoms of HHNC?	Severe dehydration, altered mental status, and hyperosmolarity Hypotension or orthostatic hypotension Seizures Coma (in <20% of patients)
What are some characteristic laboratory findings in patients with HHNC?	Often will have a serum glucose concentration >600 mg/dL Serum osmolarity >350 mOsm/L
What are some critical actions in the management of a patient with HHNC?	Similar to patients with DKA with attention to volume status and use of insulin Evaluation for the precipitant of HHNC is also critical
What is the general disposition for patients who present with HHNC?	Most are admitted for glucose control, electrolyte correction, and intravenous volume replacement, often in an intensive care setting.

DISORDERS OF THYROID AND ADRENAL GLAND FUNCTION

Thyroid Dysfunction

What is the normal physiologic mechanism of thyroid hormone production?	Hypothalamus → Thyroid-releasing gland Anterior pituitary gland → thyroid-stimulating hormone (TSH) Thyroid gland → T_3 and T_4

What is the defining feature of these particular endocrine disorders?	Often present with chronic and non-specific symptoms that can be difficult to recognize early in the course of the disease process.
Which form of the thyroid hormone is more potent?	T_3 is the biologically active hormone whereas T_4 is a prohormone (some intrinsic activity)
What is the most common form of hyperthyroidism?	Graves disease
What is Graves disease?	Autoimmune condition in which auto-antibodies are directed against the TSH receptor resulting in increase of thyroid hormone production.
What is de Quervain thyroiditis?	Also known as subacute thyroiditis, it is viral disease that presents with pharyngitis, fatigue, and myalgias followed by fever and neck pain. The disease course begins with symptoms of hyperthyroidism, but later progresses to a hypothyroid state, and eventually self-resolves.
What are some signs and symptoms of hyperthyroidism?	*Hypermetabolic state with increased beta-adrenergic activity Increased beta-adrenergic activity resulting in: Heat intolerance Palpitations Fatigue Increased bowel movements Moist skin Insomnia Tremulous hands CNS hyperactivity
What are some characteristic physical findings in a patient with hyperthyroidism?	Tachycardia Exophthalmos Palpable goiter
What is thyroid storm?	Thyroid storm is a decompensated state of thyroid hormone-induced severe hypermetabolism involving multiple organ systems.

What are four diagnostic criteria used to diagnose thyroid storm?

Temperature >37.8°C

Central nervous system dysfunction

Cardiovascular (tachycardia, dysrhythmias)

Gastrointestinal (ie, diarrhea)

What is important to note about the temperature of a patient who presents with thyroid storm?

Hyperthermia that is often out of proportion–which can mimic heatstroke with temperatures greater than 105°F.

Name the screening test of choice in the diagnosis of thyroid storm:

TSH-depressed or undetectable

What are other diagnostic tests to consider in thyroid storm?

Free T_4 and free T_3

Liver function tests

Complete blood count

Chemistry panel

What are some common precipitants of thyroid storm?

Infection

Graves disease

Trauma

Medication

Myocardial infarction

What are some critical actions in the management of thyroid storm?

Early recognition is critical!

Medications to reduce the production, release, conversion, and peripheral action of thyroid hormone (Thioamides, Glucocorticoids, beta-blockers)

Cardiac monitoring (atrial fibrillation may occur)

Cooling measures as needed (although ASA is contraindicated as it releases protein bound thyroid hormone)

IV fluid replacement to compensate for increased insensible and GI losses

Identify and treat the precipitant

What is the first-line treatment of thyroid storm?

Thioamides such as methimazole and propylthiouracil (PTU)

What is the mechanism of action of thioamides?

Inhibition of thyroid peroxidase

What is the role of beta-blockers in the management of thyroid storm?

Blockade of peripheral hyperadrenergic activity

What is the beta-blocker of choice?

Propranolol (also blocks conversion of T_4 to T_3)

What is primary hypothyroidism?

Intrinsic failure of the thyroid gland—most common cause

What are some common causes of primary hypothyroidism?

Partial thyroidectomy

Radioactive ablation

Autoimmune (ie, Hashimoto thyroiditis)

Iodine deficiency

Medications (ie, lithium)

What is secondary hypothyroidism?

Hypothyroidism due to dysfunction of the pituitary or hypothalamus gland.

What are some common causes of secondary hypothyroidism?

Pituitary tumor

Sarcoidosis

Sheehan syndrome

What are some common signs and symptoms of hypothyroidism?

Hypometabolic state:

Cold-intolerance

Hypoventilation

Fatigue

Constipation

Weight-gain

Memory loss

Irregular menstruation

Scaly skin

Muscle cramps

What is the definition of myxedema coma?

A life-threatening decompensation of hypothyroidism with hypothermia and altered mental status as the hallmark. The thyroid hormone level may be normal or only slightly low range, but represents a failure to adequately respond to a stressor or period of increased need.

What is an important point to know about myxedema coma?

True emergency with up to 45% mortality

More common in women

Who is commonly affected with myxedema coma?

Elderly women

List some common causes of myxedema coma:	Trauma Congestive heart failure Medications (beta-blockers) Sepsis
What are some important diagnostic tests to consider in the evaluation of myxedema coma?	TSH Free T_4 to T_3 An infectious work-up (CBC, blood cultures, etc) is indicated
What are some considerations in the management of myxedema coma?	Supportive care is the cornerstone Correction of electrolyte disturbances Vasopressors for hypotension if indicated Hydrocortisone for adrenal insufficiency Antibiotics for underlying infection Search for underlying trigger
What is the concern with aggressive thyroid hormone replacement?	Risk of cardiac arrhythmias and infarction
What is the agent of choice for thyroid hormone replacement?	The most effective choice is unclear, often an intravenous form of T_4 or T_3 (more potent), should involve consultation with endocrinology.
What is the disposition for patients who present with myxedema coma?	Intensive care admission Require endocrinologist consult

Adrenal Gland Dysfunction

What are the two major regions of the adrenal gland?	Adrenal medulla Adrenal cortex
What major hormones does the adrenal medulla produce?	Catecholamines
What three major hormones does the adrenal cortex produce?	Mineralocorticoids (Aldosterone) Glucocorticoids (Cortisol) Sex Hormones (Androgens)
What are some common causes of primary adrenal insufficiency (Addison disease)?	Infections (ie, TB) Infiltrative (ie, metastatic) Medications Idiopathic atrophy

What deficiency in hormones does primary adrenal failure lead to?

Only a deficit in aldosterone and cortisol

What deficiency in hormones does secondary adrenal failure lead to?

Only cortisol (Aldosterone release is regulated by the angiotensin system)

What is the name of the syndrome of bilateral adrenal hemorrhage secondary to meningococcemia?

Waterhouse-Friderichsen syndrome

What are some common causes of secondary (pituitary dysfunction) adrenal insufficiency?

Pituitary tumor

Head trauma

Infections

Infiltrative disease (ie, sarcoidosis)

What is the most common cause of adrenal suppression?

Iatrogenic steroid use (chronic)

What are some signs and symptoms of adrenal insufficiency?

Weakness

Fatigability

Lethargy

Postural hypotension/syncope secondary to aldosterone deficiency

Nausea

Abdominal pain

Emesis

True or False: hyperpigmentation can be seen in Addison disease?

True—Addison disease will result in increased production of ACTH, as well as the closely related melanocyte stimulating hormone, resulting in increased production of melanin

What may be the only diagnostic clue to adrenal insufficiency/failure?

Hypotension refractory to fluids

What are characteristic laboratory findings in adrenal insufficiency?

Hyponatremia and hyperkalemia

Hypoglycemia

Azotemia

What is the diagnostic test of choice?

Varies if it is chronic versus acute presentation but a serum cortisol concentration is the mainstay (important what time of day the test is done)

What is important test to obtain to distinguish between primary versus secondary adrenal failure?	ACTH
What is adrenal crisis?	Patients who have underlying chronic adrenal insufficiency and are exposed to any stress.
What are some common stressors that can put a patient into adrenal crisis?	Infections Trauma Surgery Pregnancy
What are some common clinical features of adrenal crisis?	Typically weak and very ill appearing Gastrointestinal affects (ie, diarrhea) Hypotension (often unresponsive to volume expanders) Delirium
What are some critical actions in the management of adrenal crisis?	Supportive care Aggressive fluid replacement Hydrocortisone replacement

CLINICAL VIGNETTES—MAKE THE DIAGNOSIS

18-year-old man with history of type I diabetes mellitus presents with diffuse abdominal pain, nausea, and vomiting along with confusion; PE: shallow rapid breathing; labs: glucose >300 and metabolic acidosis

Diabetic ketoacidosis

21-year-old woman presents with heat intolerance, fatigue, increased bowel movements, palpitations, and tremulous hands for months, but otherwise doing well; PE: exophthalmus, tachycardia, palpable goiter; labs: decreased TSH, increased free T_4 and T_3 levels

Graves disease

34-year-old man is brought in by EMS for altered mental status and only knows that the patient is on a sulfonylurea; PE: tachycardia, diaphoresis, and tremulousness

Hypoglycemia

24-year-old woman presents with weight loss, progressive weakness, nausea; PE: hyperpigmentation of skin; labs: hyponatremia and hyperkalemia

Primary adrenal insufficiency (Addison disease)

21-year-old man on lithium presents with a 2-week history of polyuria and polydipsia; U/A: urine osmolality <100 mOsm/kg, hypernatremia, and urine specific gravity of <1.005

Diabetes insipidus

72-year-old woman currently on thyroid hormones presents via EMS with obtundation; vital signs were as follows: blood pressure, 117/53 mm Hg; pulse, 40 beats/min; respiratory rate, 10 breaths/min; temperature, 94°F (38.4°C); labs: TSH is high

Myxedema coma

CHAPTER 11

Hematology and Oncology

SELECTED ONCOLOGIC EMERGENCIES

Superior Vena Cava Syndrome

What is the definition of superior vena cava syndrome?	It is the compression of the superior vena cava which results in obstruction to the return of venous blood.
What are some common mechanisms by which obstruction occurs in superior vena cava syndrome?	Direct compression from an adjacent mass (neoplasia, goiter, aortic aneurism) Infiltration Thrombosis Indwelling central venous catheters
What type of malignancy is the most common cause of superior vena cava syndrome?	Lung cancer
Where does the superior vena cava arise from?	Superior vena cava arise from brachiocephalic (innominate) veins, which in turn arise from the internal jugular and subclavian veins.
What are some signs and symptoms of superior vena cava syndrome?	Early morning swelling of various areas of the upper body, plethora of the face, cough, congestion, and venous neck distension.

What life-threatening diagnosis that can be similar in presentation must also be considered?	Cardiac tamponade
What are some diagnostic tests to consider?	Chest radiograph Tissue biopsy
What are some findings on a chest x-ray?	Mass Pleural effusion (commonly right side) Widening of the superior mediastinum (commonly right side)
What is the current management of superior vena cava syndrome?	Radiation treatment Chemotherapy In recurrent superior vena cava syndrome: intravascular stent

Fever in the Oncology Patient

Name some important causes of fever in the oncology patient:	Infection (most causes are infectious in origin) Chemotherapy Transfusion Tumor necrosis
What is the definition of neutropenia?	Absolute neutrophil count (ANC) of less then 1000 cells/mm^3, <500 cells/mm^3 is considered severe
How do you calculate the ANC?	The total white blood cell count multiplied with the percent of neutrophils and bands.
What is considered a fever in a patient with cancer?	Greater than 38°C (101.4°F)
Should antibiotics be held until a source of the fever is discovered?	No—fever in a neutropenic patient is considered a medical emergency

What are some important diagnostic studies to consider when evaluating a cancer patient?

Complete blood count with differential cell count

Chemistry panel

Coagulation panel

Two sets of blood culture

Chest radiograph

Urinalysis

Culture from any indwelling catheters

What is the concern in obtaining a rectal temperature in neutropenic patients?

Risk of tearing the mucosa and introducing an infection

Name the three common gram positive bacteria involved infection in neutropenic patients:

Staphylococcus aureus, Staphylococcus epidermis, and *Streptococcus viridans*

What is a common fungal pathogen in neutropenic patients?

Candida albicans

What are some choices in antibiotic treatment in the management of a neutropenic fever?

An antipseudomonal penicillin, an aminoglycoside, and vancomycin; meropenem

Acute Tumor Lysis Syndrome

What is the definition of acute tumor lysis syndrome?

It is a set of metabolic derangements that occur with death of rapidly growing tumors.

When does tumor lysis syndrome commonly occur?

It can occur 1 to 5 days following use of radiation or chemotherapy of responsive tumors.

What are some signs and symptoms of tumor lysis syndrome?

Nausea, vomiting, lethargy, fluid overload, muscle cramps, cardiac arrhythmia, or seizure <72 hrs after chemotherapy.

List some examples of tumors tumor lysis syndrome has been associated with:

Burkitt lymphoma

Acute leukemias

What are some metabolic derangements that occur with tumor lysis syndrome?	Hyperkalemia Hyperuricemia Hyperphosphatemia Hypocalcemia
What is the pathophysiology of hyperkalemia and hyperphosphatemia?	Released during cell death
What is the pathophysiology of hypocalcemia?	Results from hyperphosphatemia driving calcium precipitation. Also results from renal failure.
What is the pathophysiology of hyperuricemia?	Typically results from increased production (from metabolism of nucleic acids released during cell death) or decreased excretion (renal failure).
List some examples of renal disease as a consequence of hyperuricemia:	Nephrolithiasis Gouty nephropathy Acute hyperuricemic nephropathy
Name some important issues in the management of hyperuricemia:	Fluids, allopurinol, and alkalinization of the urine should be initiated prior to treatment of cancer.
What are some signs and symptoms of acute tumor lysis syndrome?	ECG changes of hyperkalemia (peaked T waves) and hypocalcemia (prolonged QTc) Renal failure
What are some critical actions in the management of tumor lysis syndrome?	Early recognition prior to initiation of therapy Intravenous hydration is a critical intervention Supportive care with use of hemodialysis In the setting of hyperkalemia, would institute standard therapy and use calcium with ECG changes consistent with hyperkalemia

Hypercalcemia

What is important about hypercalcemia in the setting of cancer?	It is the most common life-threatening metabolic disorder

Name two proposed mechanisms of hypercalcemia:

1. Metastatic bone involvement with increased calcium release
2. Tumor-produced hormone-like substances have been associated with hypercalcemia (PTH)

List some non-cancer causes of hypercalcemia:

Acute adrenal insufficiency

Drugs (thiazide diuretics, lithium, and calcium carbonate)

Hyperparathyroidism

Hypervitaminosis (A and D)

Renal insufficiency

What are some signs and symptoms of hypercalcemia?

"Moans, bones, groans, and psychic overtones"

Symptoms can be attributed to mental status change, kidney stones, bone pain, and dehydration

What calcium concentration is considered a medical emergency?

A serum calcium level above 14 mg/dL

What is the significance of *corrected calcium* level?

Changes in albumin concentration affects the measured total serum calcium level, but does not affect the biologically available calcium concentration.

What is the mainstay in the treatment of hypercalcemia?

Hydration

List other options utilized in the management of hypercalcemia:

Loop diuretics (avoid thiazides)

Bisphosphonates

Corticosteroids (should be used in conjugation with oncology)

Calcitonin

Dialysis in severe cases may be indicated

Hyperviscosity Syndrome

What is hyperviscosity syndrome?

It is an increased blood viscosity resulting in sludging in the microcirculation.

What is the most common cause of hyperviscosity syndrome?

Waldenström macroglobulinemia (lymphoma with high IgM production)

What other conditions can hyperviscosity occur in?	Polycythemia vera Leukemoid reaction
What is the clinical triad of hyperviscosity syndrome?	Visual disturbances (blurred vision, vision loss) CNS symptoms Mucosal bleeding
What are some laboratory tests to consider?	Complete blood count Coagulation studies Chemistry panel
What is an important test to consider with suspected dysproteinemias?	Urine and serum protein electrophoresis
Name the definite treatment for hyperviscosity syndrome:	Fluids followed by diuresis Emergency plasmapheresis

Neoplastic Cardiac Tamponade

What is the most common cause of malignant cardiac tamponade?	Malignant pericardial effusion
Name some tumors associated with neoplastic cardiac tamponade:	GI primary tumors Lung cancer Breast cancer Radiation pericarditis
What are some signs and symptoms of cardiac tamponade?	Beck Triad (JVD, hypotension, diminished heart sounds) Rapid and shallow breathing may be present Facial plethora Pulsus Paradoxus Kussmaul signs (increased JVD during inspiration)
What are characteristic ECG findings in cardiac tamponade?	Sinus tachycardia Low-voltage Electrical alternans (very specific) Non-specific ST-T wave changes
What is the diagnostic test of choice that can be done in the emergency department?	Ultrasound

Name the life-saving technique of choice in acute cardiac tamponade:

Pericardiocentesis

Once the patient has been stabilized, name some other modalities used to treat cardiac tamponade?

Pericardial window
Pericardiectomy
Pericardial sclerosis

SELECTED HEMATOLOGIC EMERGENCIES

Disorders of Hemostasis

What is hemostasis?

It is an intrinsic balance between thrombosis and excessive bleeding.

What are the major components of hemostasis?

Platelets
Vascular integrity
Coagulation factors
Fibrinolysis

What are some components for bleeding disorders?

Abnormal platelet function or count; missing factors in the coagulation cascade; excessive fibrinolysis; inflammation of blood vessel walls

What are some important points for the following laboratory tests used to evaluate hemostasis:

   Bleeding time (BT)

Normal time 3 to 8 min

Defects in the coagulation cascade does not affect this test

Measures integrity of platelet function and vascular wall

Also increased BT in von Willebrand (vWF) disease and uremia

Aspirin and non-steroidal anti-inflammatory drugs can affect BT

   Platelets

Normal is 150,000 to 400,000 per mm^3

One platelet is present per 10 to 20 RBCs

The platelet count does not give any information about function

Decreased count: disseminated intravascular coagulation (DIC), uremia, idiopathic thrombocytopenic purpura (ITP), etc

Increased count: consider malignancy

Less than 20,000 per mm^3: life-threatening bleeding possible

Prothrombin time	Normal time is 10 to 12 s
	Measures the extrinsic (factor VII) and common pathway
	Normal PTT but elevated PT: factor VII deficiency
	Coumadin/Vitamin K/liver disease: < factor VII
Internationalized normalized ratio (INR)	PT ratio: normal value 1
	Monitor anticoagulation in Coumadin (both PT and PTT will be increased, but PT is a more sensitive measurement to follow)
	INR 2 to 3 for most patients (ie, afib)
	INR 2.5 to 3.5 for patients with mechanical valves
Partial thromboplastin time (PTT)	Normal time is 25 to 35 s
	Measures integrity of the intrinsic and common pathway
	Elevated in heparin use, Coumadin use, hemophilia, DIC, and von Willebrand disease (Factor VIII normally complexes with vWF)
Fibrinogen	Final substrate in the coagulation cascade
	DIC and severe liver disease common cause of low levels
	It is an acute phase reactant
List some important ancillary tests to obtain to assess potential bleeding disorders:	Complete blood count (including a smear)
	Coagulation panel (PT, INR, and PTT)
	Fibrinogen level
	Factor levels
	Thrombin time
	Mixing studies
	Dilute Russell Viper Venom Time
Is the measurement of hemoglobin/ hematocrit in the setting of an acute blood loss accurate?	No—reductions in hemoglobin/ hematocrit are not always seen due to slow equilibrium time

What are some clinical features that help to distinguish disorders of the coagulation pathway from platelet disorders?

Normal BT (except in patients von Willebrand disease)

Often a deep soft tissue hematoma

Occurs predominantly in men (congenital form of the disease)

What are some causes of an elevated PT?

Acquired forms include severe liver disease and Coumadin use

What is one of the oldest hereditary bleeding disorders?

Hemophilia

What are two types of hemophilia and their associated factor deficiency?

Hemophilia A: lack of factor VIII

Hemophilia B: lack of factor IX

What is the more prevalent form?

Hemophilia A

If a male hemophiliac mates with a normal woman what would be the outcome of his children?

Sons would all be normal and all daughters would be carriers

What is the factor affected in hemophilia A?

Factor VIII that is present in normal levels but have decreased activity

What are some major sites of bleeding in hemophilia A?

Urinary tract system

Intracranial space

Joints

What is the major source of morbidity?

Joint destruction

What are some important elements in the bleeding history of hemophilia?

Hematomas

Hemarthrosis

Prolonged bleeding from dental procedures

Spontaneous hematuria

Epistaxis

Note: Platelet function is normal, so bleeding time is not affected

What are characteristic laboratory findings in hemophilia?

Prolonged PTT

Normal BT, PT, and platelets

What is the treatment of choice in bleeding for patients with hemophilia A?

Factor VIII

Desmopressin (DDAVP)

Cryoprecipitate (not used often)

What is hemophilia B known as?

Christmas disease

What are some important things to know about hemophilia B?

Sex-linked recessive disorder

Deficiency of factor IX

Much less common than hemophilia A

What is the treatment of choice in bleeding for patients with hemophilia B?

Factor IX concentrate

Fresh frozen plasma (FFP)

What is von Willebrand disease (vWF)?

Autosomal dominant with either quantitative or qualitative disorder in vWF.

What is the primary defect in each of the following forms of vWF disease?

Type I A low level of the vWF factor; mildest and most common form

Type II Qualitative disorder of vWF

Type III Virtual absence of vWF; most serious, but rare form

What are some common clinical features of vWF disease?

Mucocutaneous bleeding is the defining feature (ie, epistaxis)—bleeding is milder then hemophilia A

What are classic laboratory findings in a patient with vWF disease?

Increased BT

Increased PTT

Normal platelet count and function

Normal PT

What are the treatment options available for vWF disease?

Factor VIII

FFP (in extreme circumstances)

Cryoprecipitate

DDAVP

What is disseminated intravascular coagulation (DIC)?

It is a form of acquired life-threatening coagulopathy with a multitude of causes, in which excessive small vessel thrombosis causes consumption of fibrinogen and results in excessive bleeding tendency.

What are some laboratory findings in DIC?

Prolonged PT, PTT, and thrombin time

Low platelet and fibrinogen

Peripheral smear often show schistocytes

What is important to know about managing DIC?

Reversing the triggering mechanism

If bleeding is the primary feature, replace blood product as appropriate, but supportive care is typically adequate

Platelet Disorders

What are some common initial symptoms of platelet disorders?	Gastrointestinal bleeding and epistaxis
What are some physical manifestations of platelet dysfunction?	Petechiae and purpura
What are some major causes of thrombocytopenia?	Splenic sequestration Decreased production (chemotherapeutic drugs) Destruction of platelets (Immune thrombocytopenia, DIC)
What is the platelet count in thrombocytopenia?	Less than 100,000/mm; spontaneously bleeding can occur when platelets are below 20,000/mm
What is immune thrombocytopenia?	It is an increased peripheral destruction of platelets caused by an antiplatelet antibody that is seen in a number of diseases.
List some common causes of immune thrombocytopenia:	Heparin-induced thrombocytopenia (HIT) Systemic lupus erythematosus Quinine and quinidine Sulfonamides Idiopathic thrombocytopenic purpura (ITP)
What is idiopathic thrombocytopenic purpura (ITP)?	Many consider it to be a diagnosis of exclusion if no other causes can be found, there is an acute and chronic form
What are some important features of the acute form of ITP?	More common in children ages 3 to 6 years A viral prodrome is common Platelet count usually to less than 20,000/mm^3 Greater than 90% rate of spontaneous remission

What are some important features of the chronic form of ITP?

More common in female adults

Often manifest as easy bruising and mucosal bleeding

Relapse is common

Overall long term mortality is less than 1%

What is eltrombopag?

It is a thrombopoietin-receptor agonist that increase platelet counts and have been used in refractory ITP.

What is thrombotic thrombocytopenic purpura (TTP)?

It is due to subendothelial deposits of fibrin and platelet aggregates in capillaries and arterioles that is very similar to hemolytic uremic syndrome (HUS).

What is the most common cause of TTP?

It is idiopathic in most cases

What medication is commonly associated with TTP?

Quinine

What is the classic pentad of TTP?

Neurologic symptoms

Renal disease

Microangiopathic hemolytic anemia

Thrombocytopenic purpura

Fever

Is this pentad commonly seen?

No—appears in less than 30 to 40% of cases

What is the survival rate of untreated TTP?

It is almost universally fatal without treatment

What is the mainstay in the treatment of TTP?

Plasmapheresis is the treatment of choice

Steroids

Splenectomy is refractory cases

What is the platelet count typically seen in thrombocytosis?

600,000 to 1,000,000/mm^3

What is the differential diagnosis of thrombocytosis?

Polycythemia vera

Chronic myelogenous leukemia

Reactive

Myelofibrosis

Red Blood Cell Disorders

What is the definition of anemia?	Absolute decrease in the number of red blood cells (RBCs) which depends on the age and the sex of the patient.
Name the three major components of hemoglobin:	Porphyrin Iron Globin
What are some important features of erythropoietin (EPO)?	It is a glycoprotein Kidney is responsible for most of the production of EPO It is stimulated by tissue hypoxia and hemolysis
List important causes of intravascular RBC destruction:	Oxidant stress Malaria ABO incompatibility Mechanical destruction from artificial valves or congenital bi-leaflet aortic valve
What are some signs and symptoms of anemia?	Tachycardia Syncope Tachypnea Pallor Dyspnea Fatigue
What are some factors that may influence the clinical findings in anemia?	Age Medication (ie, beta blockers) Cardiovascular status
What are some laboratory tests to consider in acute anemia?	Complete blood count Type and screen/cross Coagulation panel Urinalysis for free hemoglobin Peripheral smear LDH Haptoglobin

What are some other laboratory tests to consider in chronic anemia?	Total iron-binding capacity Folate Vitamin B_{12} Iron Reticulocytes Direct antiglobulin (Coombs test)
How is the reticulocyte count interpreted?	Increased corrected reticulocyte count indicates increased RBC destruction Normal or low corrected reticulocyte count indicates decreased RBC production
What does the direct antiglobulin (Coombs) test evaluate?	Detects antibody or complement on human RBC membranes.
What does the indirect test measure?	Serum antibody titers
Name two common examples of intrinsic causes of hemolytic anemia:	Glucose-6-phosphate dehydrogenase deficiency Pyruvate kinase deficiency
Name three major sub-classification based on red blood cell indices:	
Normocytic	Aplastic anemia Myelophthisic anemia Chronic inflammation
Macrocytic	Folate deficiency Vitamin B_{12} deficiency
Hypochromic microcytic	Iron deficiency Thalassemia
What are the normal values for the following red blood cell indices?	
Mean corpuscular volume	81-100 fL
Mean corpuscular hemoglobin	26-34 pg
Mean corpuscular hemoglobin concentration	31-36%
What is the most common cause of anemia in women of child-bearing age?	Iron-deficiency anemia
What are some laboratory tests to consider in iron-deficiency anemia?	Serum ferritin, fasting level of serum iron, and total iron-binding capacity.

What is the treatment of choice for iron-deficiency anemia?	Ferrous sulfate
What is the definition of thalassemia?	Decreased synthesis of globin chains secondary to a genetic autosomal defect.

List each type of hemoglobin and their corresponding globins:

Normal adult (HbA)	Two α chains and two β chains ($\alpha_2\beta_2$)
HbA$_2$	$\alpha_2\delta_2$
Hemoglobin (HbF)	$\alpha_2\gamma_2$

Name three common variations in thalassemia:	Homozygous β-chain thalassemia (thalassemia major)
	Heterozygous β-chain thalassemia (thalassemia minor)
	α-Thalassemia
What does therapy mainly consist of?	Blood transfusion
What is sickle cell anemia?	HbS that is inherited from both parents where virtually all the RBCs will only contain HbS
What are some important features of sickle cell disease?	Characterized by abnormal hemoglobin—HbS
	High prevalence in African Americans (up to 10% of patients with sickling disorders are not African American)
What is the genetic defect in sickle cell anemia?	Replacement of glutamic acid by valine at the sixth position
What are some characteristic features of HbS?	RBC sickling responsible for majority of symptom
	Sickled RBCs are more easily hemolyzed
	RBCs sensitive to hypoxia (ie, sickling)
What is sickle cell trait?	Occurs when a child inherits HbS from one parent and HbA from another parent, so most RBCs will contain both types.

What are some clinical features of sickle cell trait?	Generally asymptomatic
	Spontaneous bleeding
	Decreased ability to concentrate their urine
What are some complications of sickle cell trait?	Splenic infarction
	Vaso-occlusive crisis
	Death
Are these complications common in patients with sickle cell trait?	Rarely occur unless extreme hypoxia
What are some signs and symptoms of sickle cell anemia?	Anemia
	Jaundice
	Hand-foot syndrome (swelling of foot/hand)
	Frequent infections
	Vision problems
What particular pathogens are patients with sickle cell anemia more prone to?	Salmonella
	Haemophilus influenzae
	Streptococcus pneumoniae
	Encapsulated organisms due to functional asplenia
What are some important complications to consider with significant morbidity and mortality in all patient with sickle cell anemia?	Aplastic crisis
	Vaso-occlusive crisis (ie, pain crisis)
	Acute chest syndrome
	Cerebral vascular accident
	Renal papillary necrosis
	Priapism
List some precipitating factors for a vaso-occlusive crisis:	Infection
	Cold exposure
	Trauma
	Dehydration
	Spontaneous
What is the pathophysiology of a vaso-occlusive crisis?	It is tissue ischemia caused by sludging and microvascular obstruction as a result of sickled cells.

What are some signs and symptoms of a vaso-occlusive crisis?

Deep pain that can appear in a variety of locations which can mimic various conditions such as renal colic or pulmonary embolus.

What are some important aspects of management of vaso-occlusive crisis?

Hydration

Adequate analgesia

Consideration of other potential causes of pain (ie, not always vaso-occlusive!)

What is one of the leading causes of death in patients with sickle cell anemia?

Acute chest syndrome

What are the signs and symptoms of acute chest syndrome?

Cough and dyspnea

Fever

Chest pain

Infiltrates on the chest radiograph

What are other important differentials to consider in patients who may present with acute chest syndrome?

Pneumonia

Pulmonary embolism

Myocardial infarction

What are some important aspects of management of acute chest syndrome?

Primarily supportive care with emphasis on hydration, analgesia, and proper ventilation along with empiric antibiotics as indicated

What is an important complication of sickle cell anemia to consider in patients who present with an acute drop in hemoglobin in the setting of a post-infection?

Aplastic anemia

What may hydroxyurea be used in patient with recurrent vaso-occlusive crisis?

It is believed to cause an increase in hemoglobin F (made up of 2 alpha globins, and 2 gamma globins. Since no beta globin is involved sickling does not occur).

What is polycythemia?

It is an increase in the number of RBCs also known as erythrocytosis

Can be classified as primary or secondary

What is an example of primary polycythemia?

Polycythemia vera

What are some causes of secondary polycythemia?	Hypoxia (ie, high-altitude acclimatization)
	Pulmonary disease
	Hemoconcentration secondary to dehydration
At what hematocrit can complications of polycythemia occur?	Typically when the hematocrit rises above 60%
List some known complications of polycythemia:	Thrombosis
	Hemorrhage
What are some signs and symptoms of polycythemia?	CNS symptoms such as headache, vertigo, and dizziness
	Bleeding
	Facial plethora
	Conjunctival suffusion
What are some treatment options for polycythemia?	Phlebotomy with a goal hematocrit of less than 60%
	Consideration for the use of low-dose aspirin (prevent thrombotic complications)

CLINICAL VIGNETTES—MAKE THE DIAGNOSIS

8-year-old boy presents with a long history of intermittent epistaxis along with prolonged bleeding whenever he goes for any dental procedures, patient's mother is now concerned since patient is having recent hematuria; labs: prolonged PTT, but normal PT time as well as platelet count

Hemophilia A

17-year-old woman with no known PMH presents to the ER with concern of nose bleeding that has become frequent; labs: abnormal PTT and BT, but normal platelet count and PT

von Willebrand disease

6-year-old boy is brought in by his mother due to concerns of frequent episodes of epistaxis about two days after an upper respiratory illness; labs: CBC otherwise unremarkable except for platelet count of 5,000

Idiopathic thrombocytopenic purpura

23-year-old African American man with sickle cell disease presents with a recent cold and excruciating pain in his limbs; PE: unremarkable with no evidence of acute ischemia of extremities

Vaso-occlusive crisis

41-year-old African American man with sickle cell disease presents with chest pain and shortness of breath; chest radiograph: left lower infiltrate

Acute chest syndrome

71-year-old woman with a history of untreated squamous cell lung cancer presents with fatigue, constipation, and back pain; ECG shows a shortened QT interval

Hypercalcemia

81-year-old man with recently treated cancer presents with weakness, flank pain, dysuria, and abdominal pain; labs: elevated potassium, LDH, BUN/creatinine, and uric acid

Tumor lysis syndrome

65-year-old woman with history of HTN, breast cancer, and CAD presents with recent onset of urinary retention and lower extremity weakness; PE: bilateral leg weakness with positive Babinski sign

Spinal cord compression

76-year-old man with history of bronchogenic cancer now presents with dyspnea and cough for about 1 month which is becoming more progressive; PE: obvious venous distension of face and JVD

Superior vena cava obstruction

56-year-old woman with breast cancer in the past presents with chest pain and dyspnea for the past 2 weeks which is getting progressively worse; PE: distant heart sound, pulsus paradoxus, and JVD; ECG: low-voltage QRS complex

Malignant pericardial effusion

CHAPTER 12

Infectious Diseases

INFLUENZA AND HERPES VIRUSES

Influenza Virus

What are influenza viruses?	Single-stranded RNA viruses that fall within the orthomyxovirus family with three types—A, B, and C.
Name two surface glycoproteins that are responsible for the pathogenicity of the influenza virus:	1. Hemagglutinin (H)—initiates infection 2. Neuraminidase (N)—degrades mucus
Which strain of influenza virus is responsible for pandemics?	Influenza A causes worldwide epidemics every 10 to 20 years. Influenza B causes major outbreaks and influenza C causes mild respiratory tract infections.
What is the avian "bird" flu?	Avian flu (H5N1) resulted in the death of millions of chickens in 2003-2004, but only 10 people died.
What is the swine flu?	Swine flu is a subspecies (H1N1/09) of the common flu virus. It is unique because it is highly contagious and can be lethal to pregnant women and those with underlying medical conditions.
What is antigenic drift?	Minor mutations in the RNA genome that code for N or H molecule causing a change in antigenicity.
What is antigenic shift?	Occurs when a host is infected with two different influenza viruses, producing a new virus with little antigenic similarity to the old.
When does the flu generally occur in the United States?	The fall and spring

What are some signs and symptoms of the flu?

Headache, fever, chills, myalgia and malaise often with rhinorrhea, sore throat, enlarged cervical lymph nodes, and a dry cough.

What is the typical time course for the flu?

Fever that lasts for 2 to 4 days with rapid recovery, although cough and malaise may last longer.

What are some complications of an influenza infection?

Secondary bacterial pneumonia; pneumonitis; croup; chronic obstructive pulmonary disease (COPD) exacerbation; Reye syndrome (if ASA used)

How can influenza virus be rapidly detected?

Detection of antigen with monoclonal antibodies or detection of viral neuraminidase with a colored substrate.

Name two medications currently approved for the treatment of influenza A:

1. Rimantadine
2. Amantadine

What are some points with regard to rimantadine and amantadine?

Should be started within 48 hours of symptoms; amantadine is renally cleared; rimantadine is hepatically cleared

Name two medications approved for treatment of influenza A and B:

1. Zanamivir (inhaled)
2. Oseltamivir (oral)

What is the flu vaccine?

It is made annually and contains two strains of influenza A and one strain of influenza B.

Is there a live flu vaccine?

Yes—in 2003 a live vaccine containing mutants of influenza A and B was approved. It must be administered nasally where it induces IgA response.

Which groups should receive the influenza vaccine?

Anyone with cardiopulmonary disease; immunocompromised patients; healthcare workers; patients over 65

What is Reye syndrome?

Encephalopathy and liver degeneration with aspirin administration following viral infection.

Herpes Virus

What are some important facts about the herpes virus family?	They are an ubiquitous group of DNA viruses; ability to remain in a host as a lifelong latent infection that can reactivate; commonly transmitted by close contact.
What is the pathophysiology of herpes simplex virus (HSV) exposure?	Infects and replicates in epithelial cells, causing lysis of the cell leading to an inflammatory response and the characteristic HSV rash. Epstein-Barr and cytomegalovirus are in the herpes virus family, but do not cause the typical rash.
What is the general appearance of a HSV rash?	Clusters of small, thin-walled vesicles on an erythematous base.
What are some signs and symptoms of oral HSV?	Primarily caused by HSV-1, but can be caused by HSV-2 that range from asymptomatic to pharyngitis or gingivostomatosis with fever and cervical adenopathy.
How is oral HSV diagnosed?	Typically made clinically, although viral cultures can be used (takes days)
What is the oral distribution of the lesions?	Painful oral lesions or ulcers all over the mouth
What is the recurrence rate of oral lesions?	Virus becomes latent in the trigeminal nerve ganglia. Recurrences vary from 60 to 90%, but tend to be milder
What are some triggers for an HSV recurrence?	Stress; trauma; sunburn
What role does acyclovir play in oral HSV?	Shown to shorten course if given within 72 hours of symptoms and can be used as prophylaxis in severe cases.
What are some important points about genital herpes?	Majority caused by HSV-2; recurrent lesions can cause intrauterine infections; C-section if active lesions are present during a pelvic exam
What is the most common manifestation of ocular HSV?	Ulcerative keratoconjunctivitis
What is the most feared complication of ocular HSV?	Recurrent infections leading to blindness

What are some signs and symptoms of ocular HSV?

Herpetic vesicles on the conjunctiva or the lid margin and fluorescein staining that shows dendritic ulcerations.

What are some considerations in the management of ocular HSV?

Consultation with ophthalmology; administration of IV acyclovir; avoid the use of topical steroids

What is one of the most common viral encephalitis?

HSV encephalitis (usually HSV-1)

What portion of the brain is typically involved?

Temporal lobes

What are some signs and symptoms of HSV encephalitis?

Often a viral prodrome which may be followed by HA, fever, altered mental status, and even focal seizures

What does a lumbar puncture often show?

Nonspecific—elevated WBC count with an increase in mononuclear cells, protein, and red cells.

What is the test of choice for diagnosing HSV encephalitis?

PCR

What is the treatment of choice for suspected HSV encephalitis?

Intravenous acyclovir

What is an HSV infection of the finger known as?

Herpetic whitlow

What is the concern of a patient who is immunocompromised with HSV?

Dissemination or severe HSV infection

What are some complications of HSV in an immunocompromised patient?

Proctitis, esophagitis, colitis, and pneumonitis

What is the cause of chickenpox?

Varicella-zoster virus (VZV)

What is some important epidemiologic information about VZV?

Chickenpox is the primary infection; zoster (shingles) is reactivation of VZV; prior to vaccine, over 90% of primary infections occurred to those <10 years

What is the dermatologic hallmark of chickenpox?

Erythematous papular lesions in various stages throughout the body

What are some signs and symptoms of chickenpox?

Prodrome of fever, HA, and malaise followed by clear vesicles on an erythematous base which eventually scab over

What are some serious complications of chickenpox?	Cerebellar ataxia; pneumonitis; encephalitis
Who is oral acyclovir recommended for?	Patients older than 14 years of age; patients on chronic ASA therapy
Who should receive IV acyclovir?	Patients suffering from varicella encephalitis/pneumonitis
What treatment is indicated for immunocompromised patients?	Oral acyclovir and varicella zoster immunoglobulin (VZIG)
What is herpes zoster (shingles)?	Reactivation of latent VZV infection with a lifetime incidence of 25%, especially in the elderly
What are some signs and symptoms of shingles?	Vesicular lesions similar to chickenpox in a single dermatome that may persist for up to a month
What is herpes zoster ophthalmicus (HZO)?	Involvement of the ophthalmic branch of cranial nerve (CN) V which can threaten vision and also cause a lesion on the tip of the nose (Hutchinson sign)
What is the most common complication of shingles?	Postherpetic neuralgia
What are some signs and symptoms of postherpetic neuralgia?	Severe pain and occasional involvement of the anterior horn cells leading to transient weakness
What is the initial treatment for postherpetic neuralgia?	Systemic analgesia such as narcotics; carbamazepine may work as a second-line treatment
What is the role for the use of antivirals in shingles?	If used within 72 hours, may decrease the duration of the disease
What is the primary cause of infectious mononucleosis?	Epstein-Barr virus (EBV)
How is EBV typically spread?	Close contact such as kissing, EBV cannot survive outside the host for long
What is the pathophysiology of infectious mononucleosis?	1 to 2 month incubation period where the EBV replicates in B lymphocytes resulting in the production of anti-EBV antibodies and heterophil antibodies.

What are some signs and symptoms of infectious mononucleosis?	Fever, HA, exudative pharyngitis, hepatosplenomegaly, atypical lymphocytosis, and bilateral cervical lymphadenopathy.
What are some complications of infectious mononucleosis?	Splenic rupture; thrombocytopenia; autoimmune hemolytic anemia; meningitis; encephalitis
How is the diagnosis of EBV typically made?	Clinical features of EBV along with atypical lymphocytes and (+) monospot test are generally confirmatory
What are some epidemiologic features of CMV?	Ubiquitous virus found worldwide; causes primary infection and often exists as a latent infection; not easily spread by casual contact
What are some signs and symptoms of CMV infection?	Often asymptomatic in healthy people, but can appear as flu-like symptoms such as fever, chills, and myalgia.
When should CMV infection be suspected in healthy adults?	Mononucleosis-like illness, but heterophil antibody negative
What are some complications of CMV infection in healthy individuals?	Guillain-Barré syndrome; hepatitis; hemolytic anemia; pneumonitis; thrombocytopenia
In what population group can CMV be particularly devastating?	HIV; transplant recipients
What is the most common CMV infection in patients with advanced HIV?	CMV retinitis
What are some CMV infections to consider in transplant recipients?	Hepatitis; colitis; CNS disease
What is the most serious CMV infection in transplant patients?	CMV interstitial pneumonitis
What are some ways in which transplant patients can contract CMV infection?	Blood products or transplant organ; reactivation of latent infection
When does CMV infections most commonly occur in transplant recipients?	Within 3 months of transplantation
What are two medications used in CMV infections?	1. Ganciclovir 2. Foscarnet

Which herpes viruses have been suspected of causing cancer?

1. Epstein-Barr with the Burkitt lymphoma and nasopharyngeal carcinoma
2. HHV-8 with Kaposi sarcoma

HIV/AIDS

What are some important points about the HIV virus?

Cytopathic retrovirus of the lentivirus family; very labile outside the body; two major subtypes: HIV-1 and HIV-2; selectively attacks CD4$^+$ T-cells

What are some risk factors for the development of HIV infection?

Intravenous drug use; vertical transmission; unprotected sex

What is the most common presentation of acute HIV infection?

Fever, pharyngitis, fatigue, rash, and headache

Why is the diagnosis of HIV infection initially difficult?

Nonspecific presentation, which often resembles flu-like symptoms. Followed by a relatively asymptomatic "window" period with low blood titers.

What is seroconversion?

Detectable antibodies in response to HIV that usually occurs between 4 and 8 weeks, but can be delayed for up to a year.

What is the average time frame from initial HIV infection to the development of AIDS?

8 to 10 years

What are some conditions that may indicate AIDS?

Kaposi sarcoma; *P (carinii) jiroveci* pneumonia; brain toxoplasmosis; cryptococcosis; *Mycobacterium avium* complex; CD4$^+$ T-cell count <200 cells/μL

What is the standard and most common way to diagnosis HIV infection?

Detection of the antibodies to the virus by Western blot assay or ELISA

How often should testing be performed?

Testing is often done at 6 weeks, 3 months, and 6 months after exposure

What are two useful things to know when a patient with HIV presents to the ED?

1. CD4$^+$ T-cell count
2. HIV viral load

What are some numbers to keep in mind about CD4$^+$ T-cell count and HIV viral load?

CD4$^+$ T-cell count of <200 and HIV load >50,000 is often associated with progression to AIDS-defining illness and an indication to start antiretrovirals

What are some differentials to keep in mind about HIV-infected patients who present with fever based on CD4$^+$ T-cell count:

   CD4$^+$ T-cell count >500

Cause of fever similar to healthy patients who are non-immunocompromised

   CD4$^+$ T-cell count 200–500

Early bacterial respiratory infection

   CD4$^+$ T-cell count <200

P (carinii) jiroveci pneumonia; *M avium* complex; CMV; *M tuberculosis*

What is the most common cause of serious opportunistic viral disease in HIV-infected patients?

CMV

What is the most common cause of fever that is noninfectious in origin?

Drug fever; neoplasm

What is an important diagnosis to keep in mind about HIV-infected patients with a history of intravenous drug abuse (IVDA)?

Infective endocarditis

Name the three most common causes of CNS disease in HIV-infected patients?

1. *Toxoplasma gondii*
2. AIDS dementia
3. *Cryptococcus neoformans*

What are some signs and symptoms that are indicative of CNS disease?

Altered mental status, seizures, headache, and focal neurologic deficits

What should an ED evaluation include for HIV-infected patients who present with neurologic symptoms?

CT of the head and LP, especially if the CD4$^+$ T-cell count <200 cells/μL

What is important to know about toxoplasmosis in patients with AIDS?

Most common cause of focal encephalitis

What is the treatment of choice for patients with suspected toxoplasmosis?

Sulfadiazine; pyrimethamine; decadron for brain swelling/edema

What should be given for HIV-infected patients who have positive toxoplasmosis antibodies and CD4$^+$ T-cell count <100 cells/μL?

Trimethoprim-Sulfamethoxazole (TMP-SMX)

What are some presenting symptoms of cryptococcal CNS infection?	Diffuse meningoencephalitis; focal cerebral lesions
How is the diagnosis of cryptococcal CNS infection commonly made?	CSF cryptococcal antigen, culture, and staining with India ink; LP will often have a very high opening pressure
What is the preferred treatment for patients with cryptococcal CNS infection?	Amphotericin B; fluconazole
What are some other important CNS infections to consider?	Bacterial meningitis; CMV; HSV; neurosyphilis; TB
What is the most frequent and serious ocular opportunistic infection of HIV-infected patients?	CMV retinitis
What is the treatment of choice for patients with CMV retinitis?	Ganciclovir
What are some important pulmonary infections to keep in mind with HIV-infected patients?	Bacterial pneumonia; CMV infection; TB; *P (carinii) jiroveci* pneumonia (PCP); *C neoformans*; neoplasms
Which disease is the most serious complication and common cause of death in HIV-infected patients?	*Pneumocystis (carinii) jiroveci pneumonia* (PCP). Causative organism has been renamed *P jiroveci* [pronounced "yee-row-vet-zee"]
What are some signs and symptoms of PCP?	Nonproductive cough, fever, and shortness of breath with diffuse interstitial infiltrates on CXR
What physiologic changes are observed with PCP infections?	Hypoxemia with an increased alveolar-arterial oxygen gradient; respiratory alkalosis; impaired diffusing capacity; changes in total lung capacity and vital capacity
What is the medication of choice for PCP?	21 day course of TMP-SMX; pentamidine as second line
What are some signs and symptoms of TB in HIV-infected patients?	Fever, hemoptysis, weight loss, night sweats, and anorexia
What is the CD4+ T-cell count where TB is more common?	CD4+ T-cell count 200-500 cells/μL
Does a negative PPD test in an HIV-infected patient rule out TB?	No—can be negative due to immunosuppression. This is known as "anergy."

What is a common treatment option for HIV-infected patients with TB?	Isoniazid
What are some common oral/esophageal complaints in HIV-infected patients?	Oral candidiasis (most common); HSV; oral hairy leukoplakia
What is the most frequent GI complaint in HIV-infected patients?	Diarrhea
What are some common causes of diarrhea in HIV-infected patients?	Shigella; *Isospora belli; E coli; Cryptosporidium*
What are some common generalized cutaneous conditions in HIV-infected patients?	Seborrheic eczema; pruritus; xerosis
What is the appearance of Kaposi sarcoma?	Painless dark papules/nodules that do not blanch.
What are some other important causes of skin lesions to consider?	HSV; zoster; scabies; syphilis
If a patient presents with acute HIV infection, should the treatment be initiated in the ED?	A number of studies, including HIV genotype analysis, must be performed before starting antiretroviral therapy. There are many side-effects to the medications and no immediate clinical benefit.
What are some important treatment goals for HIV-infected patients?	Prolongation and improvement of life; reduction of viral load; improved CD4$^+$ T-cell count; maintain drug regiment with minimal ADR
What are three main classes of drugs used in the treatment of HIV?	1. Protease inhibitors 2. Nucleoside reverse-transcriptase inhibitors 3. Nonnucleoside reverse-transcriptase inhibitors

SEXUALLY TRANSMITTED DISEASES

What are some important elements to establish when evaluating a patient for sexually transmitted diseases (STDs)?	Pregnancy status; sexual practice; evaluate for sexual abuse; evaluate for domestic violence
What infection commonly coexists with gonorrhea?	*Chlamydia trachomatis*

What are some facts about chlamydial infections?

Common cause of nongonococcal infection; often asymptomatic in patients

What are the 3 serotypes of *Chlamydia trachomatis*?

[D-K] : sexually transmitted causing genital infection; neonatal conjunctivitis

[A, B, C] : trachoma, invasion of the conjunctival epithelium

[L1, L2, L3] : lymphogranuloma venereum, painless lesion progressing to genital elephantiasis

What are some signs and symptoms of chlamydial infections?

Urethritis, dysuria, vaginal discharge, and proctitis

Name two important complications of chlamydial infections in females if left untreated:

1. Pelvic inflammatory disease (PID)
2. Infertility due to fallopian tube damage

Name some antibiotics commonly used to treat nongonococcal urethritis/ cervicitis:

Azithromycin (single dose); doxycycline

What are some signs and symptoms of gonococcal urethritis/cervicitis?

Males tend to have dysuria and purulent penile discharge while females tend to have more nonspecific symptoms such as lower abdominal pain.

What are some factors that contribute to complications of gonococcal infection?

Poor detection method; subclinical presentation (especially females)

How common is disseminated gonococcal infection if left untreated?

About 5%

What are some signs and symptoms of disseminated gonococcal infection?

Fever, malaise, skin lesions on an erythematous base, and asymmetric arthralgias

What is the standard for the diagnosis of gonococcal infection?

Cervical or urethral culture

Name the antibiotics commonly used to treat gonococcal urethritis/cervicitis:

Ceftriaxone or Ciprofloxacin

What is important to keep in mind about using fluoroquinolones for gonococcal infections?

Increasing resistance in certain areas like California and Asia. CDC no longer recommends using this class of antibiotics.

Name five diseases that are characterized by genital lesions:

1. Syphilis
2. HSV
3. Lymphogranuloma venereum
4. Granuloma inguinale
5. Chancroid

What is the causative organism of syphilis?

Treponema pallidum; the spirochete enters the body through the mucous membrane or non-intact skin

What are the three phases of syphilis and some important points regarding each phase:

Primary

Hallmark: painless chancre; incubation period is about 3 weeks; lesions typically disappear after a month

Secondary

Nonspecific symptoms: fever and malaise; rash that starts at the trunk and moves towards the palms/soles; often resolves spontaneously

Tertiary (latent)

CVS/CNS involvement is characteristic; granulomatous lesions are common; meningitis, dementia, tabes dorsalis, and thoracic aneurysm more likely

What are some methods for diagnosing syphilis?

RPR, VDRL, and dark-field microscopy

What is the treatment of choice for syphilis?

Penicillin; doxycycline for penicillin allergy

What is the causative agent of chancroid?

Haemophilus ducreyi

What are some signs and symptoms of chancroid?

Painful genital ulcer and lymphadenitis/abscess/periadenitis if left untreated

What are some other infections to consider in patients with chancroid?

Syphilis, HSV, and HIV

How is the diagnosis of chancroid typically made?

Typically made clinically

What is the prevalence of chancroid in the United States?

Chancroid is rare in the US, but is found widely in Africa, Asia, and the Caribbean

What are some antibiotics commonly used to treat chancroid?

Single dose of Azithromycin, Ceftriaxone, or Ciprofloxacin

How should fluid-filled lesions be treated?

Incision and drainage of fluctuant buboes is preferable over needle aspiration

What is the causative agent of lymphogranuloma venereum (LGV)?	*C trachomatis*
What are some signs and symptoms of LGV?	Painless primary chancre of short duration, lymphadenopathy, and systemic effects such as fever, arthralgias, and erythema nodosa
How is the diagnosis of LGV commonly made?	Culture and serologic tests
What is the treatment of choice for LGV?	Doxycycline
What are the 3 stages of LGV infection?	Primary stage—usually goes undetected, marked by painless herpetiform ulceration

Secondary stage—unilateral tender inguinal lymphadenopathy

Tertiary stage—years after initial infection patient develops proctocolitis, perirectal abscess, and fistulas |
What is the causative agent of granuloma inguinale?	*Calymmatobacterium granulomatis*
What are some signs and symptoms of granuloma inguinale?	Subcutaneous nodules on penis or labia/vulva area after incubation which progresses to a painless ulcerative lesion with a "beefy" appearance.
How is the diagnosis of granuloma inguinale commonly made?	Difficult to culture; visualization of Donovan bodies on tissue biopsy is characteristic
Is granuloma inguinale highly contagious?	Low infectious capabilities because repeated exposure is necessary for clinical infection to occur. Rare in the US, but common in tropics and subtropics.
What is the treatment of choice for granuloma inguinale?	3 week course of doxycycline and TMP-SMX; ciprofloxacin and azithromycin
What is the causative agent of genital warts?	Human papillomavirus (HPV)
What is the typical appearance of HPV?	Flesh-colored papules or cauliflower-like projections "condyloma acuminatum" that are often painless.

How is HPV commonly diagnosed?	Often clinically, but can be done with PCR
What is an important long-term complication of HPV to consider?	Cervical cancer
What HPV types are commonly associated with cervical cancer?	HPV type 16 and 18
What risk factors are associated with acquisition of HPV?	Increasing number of partners; early age of first sexual intercourse
What is the primary reason for treatment of HPV?	Removal of visible warts for cosmetic reasons
What are some treatment options for visible lesions of HPV?	Cryotherapy; surgical removal; podophyllin resin
Is there a vaccine for HPV?	Yes—a quadrivalent vaccine that protects against HPV types 6, 11, 16, and 18. These four are responsible for 70% of cervical warts and 90% of genital warts.

MALARIA

What is the most deadly vector-borne disease in the world?	Malaria
What is the primary vector for the transmission of malaria?	*Anopheles* mosquito
Name four species that are responsible for malaria:	1. *Plasmodium vivax* 2. *Plasmodium ovale* 3. *Plasmodium malaria* 4. *Plasmodium falciparum*
Which species of *Plasmodium* is the most deadly form of malaria?	*Plasmodium falciparum*
Name some locations in the world where malaria transmission primarily occurs:	Caribbean; Middle East; Central America; Indian subcontinent
Name two species of *Plasmodium* that can lie dormant for months and cause clinical relapse:	1. *Plasmodium vivax* 2. *Plasmodium ovale*

What form of the parasite is injected into the bloodstream when a mosquito takes its bloodmeal?	Sporozoites
What form of the parasite invades the erythrocytes?	Merozoites
What are some signs and symptoms of malaria?	Nonspecific: fever, HA, myalgia, and malaise; PE: splenomegaly and tender abdomen in acute infections
What are some common laboratory findings in malaria?	Elevated ESR and LDH, mildly abnormal kidney and liver function
What is the clinical hallmark of malaria?	Recurrent febrile paroxysm that corresponds to the hemolysis of infected erythrocytes.
What are some complications of malaria if left untreated?	Immune-mediated glomerulonephritis; splenic enlargement or rupture; hemolysis; noncardiac pulmonary edema
What is cerebral malaria?	Most common with infection from *Plasmodium falciparum*: coma, delirium, seizures, and somnolence with up to a 25% mortality
How is the diagnosis of malaria made?	Giemsa-stained thick and thin blood smear—with the first smear being diagnostic in 90% of cases
What are two important questions to address when viewing a blood smear?	1. Is *Plasmodium falciparum* responsible? 2. Degree of parasitemia? (>3% is concerning)
What is the drug of choice for the treatment of malaria due to any species aside from *Plasmodium falciparum*?	Chloroquine
What drug is recommended for the dormant form of *Plasmodium vivax* and *Plasmodium ovale*?	Primaquine
What drug is used for prophylaxis in chloroquine-resistant regions and what are some common side-effects of this medication?	Mefloquine which commonly results in side-effects including severe depression, anxiety, paranoia, aggression, nightmares, insomnia, and seizures.

How long should malaria prophylaxis be continued after returning from a malaria endemic area?	4 weeks
What can the use of primaquine in a patient with G6PD deficiency cause?	Hemolytic anemia
What is the treatment for malaria caused by *Plasmodium falciparum*?	Doxycycline and quinine with or without pyrimethamine-sulfadoxine
What new medication has been approved for the treatment of acute malarial infection?	(Co artem) Artemether/Lumefantrine
What treatment option is available for patients with extensive parasitemia?	Exchange transfusion

SOFT TISSUE INFECTIONS

Cellulitis

What is the definition of cellulitis?	Bacterial invasion of the skin that leads to a local soft tissue inflammatory reaction.
What groups does cellulitis more commonly occur in?	Elderly; immunocompromised patients; diabetics; peripheral vascular disease
Name the two most common groups of bacteria that are involved with cellulitis:	Streptococcus; staphylococcus
What organism is becoming more common as a cause of cellulitis, especially among team athletes, prison inmates, and military personnel?	Community-acquired methicillin-resistant *Staphylococcus aureus* (CA-MRSA)
Name a common cause of cellulitis in children:	*Haemophilus influenzae*
What are some signs and symptoms of cellulitis?	Induration, pain, erythema, and warmth; PE: fever, leukocytosis, and lymphadenopathy as systemic involvement
When is the use of soft-tissue radiography or ultrasound recommended?	If a foreign body is involved as a cause.

What is *elephantiasis nostra*?

Recurrent attacks that can lead to dermal fibrosis, epidermal thickening, permanent swelling, and impairment of lymphatic drainage.

What are some treatment options for cellulitis in an otherwise healthy adult?

Macrolide; amoxicillin-clavulanate; dicloxacillin

What is an exception to an outpatient treatment of simple cellulitis?

Cellulitis of the head or neck where they should be admitted for IV antibiotics or immunocompromised patients with evidence of rapidly spreading cellulitis.

What is erysipelas?

Superficial cellulitis with involvement of the lymphatic system.

What organism is the most common cause of erysipelas?

Group A *Streptococcus*

What are some common ways that erysipelas occurs?

Ulcers; infected dermatoses; toe-web intertrigo

What are some signs and symptoms of erysipelas?

Abrupt onset of symptoms that include high fever, chills, and nausea and with progression of the infection that leads to a shiny, red, and hot plaque; PE: bullae, purpura, and small areas of necrosis can be seen

What is a possible complication of erysipelas that should be considered?

Necrotizing fasciitis

Which bacteria are frequently associated with facial cellulitis?

Haemophilus influenza type B and Streptococcus pneumoniae.

What are some treatment options of erysipelas?

Penicillin G; amoxicillin-clavulanate; imipenem in severe cases; macrolide for penicillin allergy

Which bacteria are commonly associated with dog bites?

Pasteurella canis, S aureus, S pyogenes

When is antibiotic therapy indicated with a dog bite?

Deep puncture, hands, requiring surgical repair, immunocompromised host, venous or lymphatic compromise, crush injury

Which antibiotic is indicated for animal bites?

Amoxicillin/clavulanate

What other infection must be considered with dog and cat bites?

Rabies—a Rhabdoviridae viral infection of the CNS

What is the incubation period for rabies?	5 days to several years
When should postexposure prophylaxis (PEP) be given?	When a dog or cat is a stray or if the animal cannot be observed for 10 days. Any bat exposure should be treated.
What is postexposure prophylaxis (PEP)?	(PEP) consists of wound cleaning, vaccination, and administration of rabies immunoglobulin (HRIG).
When should the vaccine series be administered?	Four doses of vaccine should be administered on days 0, 3, 7, and 14

Cutaneous Abscesses

What are some factors that contribute to the skin's protective function?	Lower pH of 3 to 5; constant desquamation of epidermis; skin continually shedding bacteria
Name some ways in which abscesses can develop:	Abrasions or lacerations; puncture; bites
Which diseases predispose a patient to a higher risk of developing an abscess?	Diabetes, cancer, immunocompromised, autoimmune disease, burn, trauma
How do abscesses typically start?	Local cellulitis
Name some organisms commonly involved with cutaneous abscesses:	Staphylococcal species; streptococci; *Bacteroides*
What is a common site of abscesses when *Staphylococcus* species are involved?	Hair follicles
What is folliculitis?	Bacterial invasion of a hair follicle that causes inflammation.
What is a deeper invasion of the soft tissue surrounding a hair follicle known as?	Furuncle (ie, boil)
What is a carbuncle?	Several furuncles that coalesce to form a large area of infection that contains interconnecting sinus tracts.
What is sufficient to treat most cases of folliculitis and boils?	Warm compresses
What is a common type of folliculitis in young adults?	Acne vulgaris associated with the bacteria Propionibacterium acnes.

What medications are often used to treat acne?	Topical retinoids, topical antibiotics, benzoyl peroxide, systemic tetracycline, and systemic isotretinoin.
What test must be done before prescribing these medications?	Pregnancy test in women. Isotretinoin is a teratogen and tetracycline can cause deficient calcification of fetal teeth.
What are some signs and symptoms of cutaneous abscesses?	Tenderness, erythema, and swelling with an area that may show induration and fluctuance.
What are some signs and symptoms that may indicate systemic involvement?	Fever, lymphadenitis, and localized lymphadenopathy
What is typically done with cutaneous abscesses if it is fluctuant?	Incision and drainage (I&D)
Are antibiotics commonly recommended along with I&D?	I&D is sufficient in most cases
If the abscess is not fluctuant and I&D cannot be done, what is recommended?	Treat with antibiotics as cellulitis
Of all the perirectal abscesses, which is the only one that can be drained safely in the ED?	Perianal abscesses
When are antibiotics recommended in the case of cutaneous abscesses?	Overlying cellulitis; immunocompromised patients
What is a particular concern in patients with underlying structural heart disease?	Bacterial endocarditis
What are some high-risk cardiac conditions where prophylactic antibiotic coverage may be considered?	Prosthetic valves; hypertrophic cardiomyopathy; history of bacterial endocarditis; acquired valvular dysfunction

GAS GANGRENE

What agent is commonly implicated as a cause of gas gangrene?	*Clostridium* species
Name two species of *Clostridium* that are identified as causing gas gangrene:	1. *Clostridium perfringens* (80-90% of cases) 2. *Clostridium septicum*

What is important to note about clostridial myonecrosis?	It is a rapidly progressive and serious disease that threatens both life and limb and it is the deepest of the necrotizing soft tissue infections.
What is the primary pathophysiologic mechanism by which the *Clostridium* species cause myonecrosis?	Production of various exotoxins, α-toxin in particular, that causes a variety of problems such as tissue necrosis, cardiodepressant, and hemolysis.
In what environment does *Clostridium* species thrive?	Anaerobic environments that can occur after injury
What are the most common scenarios for developing gas gangrene?	Post-surgery or trauma
Aside from direct inoculation from an open wound, name another route of entry:	Hematogenous spread
In what group is hematogenous spread more common?	Immunocompromised patients, especially those with GI cancers
What is the incubation period of gas gangrene once inoculation occurs?	The incubation period is usually less than 24 hours but has been described to be anywhere from 7 hours to 6 weeks. When symptoms start, clinical deterioration can occur within hours.
What is the most common presentation of gas gangrene in the early stages?	Pain out of proportion to physical findings
What is the hallmark of gas gangrene?	Sepsis with gas production
What are some other signs and symptoms of gas gangrene?	Low-grade fever, tachycardia, irritable, confused; PE: area may have edema with crepitance, brownish discoloration with a malodorous discharge
What can radiographic studies show in the case of gas gangrene?	Gas within the involved area
What are the four hallmarks for the treatment of gas gangrene:	
Resuscitation	Aggressive fluid resuscitation; avoid vasoconstrictors if possible
Surgical debridement	Mainstay for the treatment of gas gangrene; early removal of the infected area is crucial; debridement may range from fasciotomy to amputation

Antibiotic therapy	Includes penicillin; ceftriaxone and macrolides as alternatives; update tetanus status as indicated
Hyperbaric oxygen (HBO)	Initiated soon after debridement; therapy consists of 100% oxygen at 3 atm of pressure for 90 min with three dives in the first 24 hours and 2 per day for 4 to 5 days
What is the most common cause of gas gangrene that is nonclostridial?	Mixed infections with both aerobic and anaerobic organisms
Does the presentation of nonclostridial gas gangrene differ much from one caused by clostridial species?	Not really
What are some species of bacteria involved with nonclostridial gas gangrene?	*Enterococcus*; *Bacteroides*; *Bacillus*; *Staphylococcus*
What are some treatment differences for nonclostridial gas gangrene when compared to clostridial gas gangrene?	Broad-spectrum antibiotic crucial; HBO still utilized

Necrotizing Cellulitis/Fasciitis

What is necrotizing cellulitis?	Superficial form of necrotizing soft tissue infection limited to the skin and subcutaneous fat.
What are some conditions associated with necrotizing cellulitis?	Surgery; trauma; malignancy; diabetes
What are the most common bacteria causing necrotizing cellulitis?	*Clostridial* species, group A hemolytic streptococci and *Staphylococcus aureus*
What are some signs and symptoms of necrotizing cellulitis?	Erythema and pain is the most common complaint; PE: may show blebs or vesicles
What are some considerations in the management of necrotizing cellulitis?	Surgical debridement is crucial, but extensive soft tissue removal not needed; broad-spectrum antibiotics
What is necrotizing fasciitis more commonly known as?	"Flesh-eating bacteria"

What is necrotizing fasciitis?

Widespread necrosis that commonly involves the fascia and subcutaneous tissue, but not underlying muscle as with myonecrosis.

What are some major predisposing factors for necrotizing fasciitis?

Peripheral vascular disease; diabetes; intravenous drug use

What are two forms of necrotizing fasciitis?

1. One caused solely by group A *streptococcus* (GAS)
2. Other caused by mixed organisms, which is the most common form of necrotizing fasciitis

Why does necrotizing fasciitis have the ability to spread so quickly?

Bacterial tissue toxins cause inflammation and thrombosis that leads to an environment favorable for bacterial growth and rapid spread along the fascial plane.

What is the most common presenting complaint for patients with necrotizing fasciitis?

Pain out of proportion of the exam

What is indicated in all suspected cases of necrotizing fasciitis?

Early surgical consultation

What is the treatment of necrotizing fasciitis?

Similar to that of gas gangrene with focus on resuscitation, antibiotic use, surgical debridement, and HBO.

What are some differences between GAS necrotizing fasciitis when compared to necrotizing fasciitis from mixed organisms?

While very similar in presentation and treatment, GAS necrotizing fasciitis tends to be more rapidly progressive with greater likelihood for bacteremia and TSS.

TOXIC SHOCK SYNDROME

What is the etiologic cause of toxic shock syndrome (TSS)?

Staphylococcus aureus

What are some risk groups of TSS?

Menstruating women; postoperative staphylococcal wound; persons who have undergone nasal surgery

What are some signs and symptoms of TSS?	Sudden onset of fever, chills, vomiting, diarrhea, muscle aches and rash; desquamation, particularly on the palms and soles can occur up to 2 weeks after onset
What is particularly worrisome about TSS?	Rapid progression to severe hypotension and multisystem dysfunction
What is the most crucial aspect in the management of TSS?	Aggressive management of circulatory shock
What are some signs and symptoms in the management of TSS?	Identify and treat source of infection; culture all sites; remove all foreign bodies; prompt antibiotic therapy
How is streptococcal toxic shock syndrome different from TSS caused by *S aureus*?	More aggressive form of TSS that often develops in association with severe skin infection
What group of streptococcus is responsible for this form of TSS?	Group A
What are some signs and symptoms of streptococcus TSS?	Similar to TSS caused by *S aureus*, many will have signs of soft-tissue infection with pain
What are some considerations in the management of TSS from streptococcus?	Aggressive exploration/debridement of soft-tissue infection; early circulatory support; prompt antibiotic therapy

OCCUPATIONAL POSTEXPOSURE PROPHYLAXIS

What are three infections that are commonly evaluated in an occupational postexposure such as needle sticks?	1. Human immunodeficiency virus (HIV) 2. Hepatitis B virus (HBV) 3. Hepatitis C virus (HCV)
Give some examples of potential infectious sources:	Contact with mucous membranes with infectious material; percutaneous injury
Name some examples of potential infectious bodily fluids:	Blood; CSF; semen; amniotic fluid; pleural fluid

What are some things to do when evaluating a patient who is exposed to potentially infectious material?

Obtain a thorough history that includes the circumstance, exposure type, etc; wash the wound with water and soap; assess immune status of patient

Can HBV be transmitted by contact with environmental surfaces?

Yes—HBV can survive in dried blood

What is the risk of developing hepatitis if the blood source is HBsAg (+) and HBeAg (–)?

Less than 5%

What is the risk of developing hepatitis if the blood source is HBsAg (+) an HBeAg (+)?

About 25%

What are some factors to consider in the treatment of HBV?

HBV vaccination status of the patient; immunity of the patient; HBV status of the source

What is the postexposure prophylaxis for HBV?

Hepatitis B immune globulin (HBIG); vaccination series: hepatitis B vaccine at the time of evaluation, at 1 month, and at 6 months

Is pregnancy a contraindication for HBV?

No

What is the risk of seroconversion from an HCV (+) source?

1 to 2%

What is the prophylaxis currently available for HCV?

None available

What is the probability of transmission of HIV from a single exposure in the following situations:

Vaginal intercourse — 0.1 to 0.2%

Anal intercourse — 0.1 to 4%

Percutaneous exposure — 0.3%

What is a basic postexposure prophylaxis regiment for HIV exposure?

4 weeks of Zidovudine and Lamivudine or Combivir

When is HIV prophylaxis not indicated?

If exposure to bodily fluids occurs to intact skin or if only a superficial scratch is present. If the HIV+ patient has low titers and high CD4 counts postexposure prophylaxis may not be warranted

INFECTIOUS DISEASE APPENDICES

Table 12-1 Pregnancy Categories

A	Generally acceptable. Controlled studies show no adverse effect to fetus
B	Use may be acceptable. Animal studies show no risk, but human studies not available
C	Use with caution only if the benefits outweigh the risk
D	Use only in life-threatening emergencies, possible risk to fetus
X	Do not use in pregnancy
NA	Information not available

Table 12-2 Antibiotic Use in Pregnancy

Cephalosporins	Category B: generally safe
Penicillin	Category B: generally safe
Metronidazole	Category B: generally safe
Quinolones	Category C: can cause arthropathy in the fetus
Nitrofurantoin	Category B: avoid in third trimester due to possible hemolytic anemia
Tetracycline	Category D: can stain teeth and bone
Sulfonamides	Category B: in first and second trimester
	Category D: can cause kernicterus
Clotrimazole	Category B: generally safe

CLINICAL VIGNETTES—MAKE THE DIAGNOSIS

8-year-old unvaccinated child presents with 2 to 3 day history of "flu-like" symptoms. Mother notes that patient is getting worse with difficulty swallowing as well as fever; PE: cervical adenopathy as well as presence of grey membranous exudate of the throat. What is a possible cause?

Diphtheria

18-year-old woman with no past medical history presents with generalized confusion as well as weakness unable to give an accurate history; PE: hypotensive and tachycardiac with desquamation of her palms and soles. What is the most likely diagnosis?

Toxic shock syndrome

30-year-old man presents with uncontrolled spasm of his back than his intermittent. He otherwise admits he has poor access to healthcare and does recall getting assaulted by some strangers a few weeks prior to his presentation. What intervention should be considered for the likely diagnosis?

Human tetanus immunoglobulin and Td

18-year-old man presents with a progressive rash as well as fever and headache. He does recall a sick contact in his college dorm, but no other sick contacts; PE: diffuse purpura of his skin. What diagnosis must be considered?

Meningococcemia (not necessarily meningitis)

25-year-old man presents with a suspected bat bite. The patient mentions he woke up in the morning to see a bat fly out of his bedroom but is not sure if he was actually bitten. Should he be treated and if so how?

Yes—assume he was bitten. Human rabies immune globulin (HRIG) and vaccine should be given

18-year-old man presents with a request for a HIV test but otherwise has no obvious symptoms. He does admit to high risk activities such as intravenous drug abuse. Are rapid HIV tests both sensitive and specific?

Sensitivity and specificity is approximately 99%

21-year-old medical resident presents to the ED with a needlestick injury. He mentions he was placing a central line in a HIV positive patient when he stuck his finger with a needle. He requests HIV postexposure prophylaxis (PEP), what is a common regiment?

Two-drug therapy options include zidovudine plus lamivudine (Combivir), didanosine plus stavudine, and lamivudine plus stavudine

31-year-old woman recently came back from Cape Cod from vacation. She woke up with a large red rash with a bull's-eye lesion on her back but otherwise no symptoms. What is the most likely diagnosis and treatment?

Early Lyme disease and can be treated with doxycycline

8-year-old girl is brought in by parents with high fever and weakness. They mention she initially developed fever and stiff joints, but noticed some lesions on the ankles and wrists, spreading to the palms and soles. What is the most likely diagnosis and treatment?

Rocky Mountain spotted fever and can be treated with doxycycline or chloramphenicol

CHAPTER 13

Pediatric Emergencies

HIGH-YIELD PEDIATRIC CHARTS

Table 13-1 Vital Signs

Age	Heart Rate	Respirations	Systolic Blood Pressure
Newborn	90-180	30-60	50-70
6 months	85-170	24-40	65-105
1 year	80-140	20-40	70-110
3 years	80-130	20-30	75-114
6 years	70-120	18-25	80-115
8 years	70-110	18-25	85-120
10 years	65-110	16-20	90-130
12 years	60-110	14-20	95-135
15 years	55-100	14-20	100-140
18 years	50-90	14-18	105-150

Table 13-2 Temperature Conversion

F	106	105	104	103	102	101
C	41.1	40.6	40	39.4	38.9	38.3
F	99	98.6	98	97	96	95
C	37.2	37	36.7	36.1	35.6	35

Table 13-3 Seizures

Medication	Dose	Route
Diazepam	0.1-0.3 mg/kg	IV/IO
	0.5 mg/kg initially	Rectal
	0.25 mg/kg	
Lorazepam	0.05-0.1 mg/kg	IV
Phenytoin	20 mg/kg	IV
Phenobarbital	20 mg/kg	IV

IV, intravenous; IO, intraosseous.

Table 13-4 Rapid Sequence Intubation Protocol

Premedicate:		
Atropine	<10 kg	0.1 mg
	>10 kg	0.01 mg/kg
Lidocaine		1 mg/kg
Sedation:		
Etomidate		0.3 mg/kg
Paralysis:		
Rocuronium		1 mg/kg

CARDIOPULMONARY RESUSCITATION

**Name some important risk factors
associated with cardiopulmonary arrest
for each of the following categories:**

Fetal

Congenital infection; acidosis;
prematurity or postmaturity; thick
meconium

Maternal

Poor prenatal care; illicit substance abuse;
premature rupture of membranes
(PROM); infections (ie, HIV)

Intrapartum

Placenta abruption/previa; cord
prolapse; maternal shock; C-section

What are some important things to know about pediatric intubations?

Pediatric intubation differs slightly from adult; know the anatomic differences; know potential complications

What is a Broselow tape?

Quick length-based reference for pediatric resuscitation that includes tube sizes and pediatric medication dosing.

What are some important differences to note for each of the following anatomical variations when compared to adults:

Larynx

More anterior and superior than adults; angle for intubation is more acute; straight blade (Miller) is preferred; infant tongue is larger relative to mouth size

Trachea

Much shorter compared to adults; intubation of right bronchus is more likely; dislodgement of tube is more likely

Cricoid ring

Narrowest region of the airway

What is the formula used to calculate tracheal tube size for children?

Tracheal tube size = $(4 + age)/4$

What is the backup airway of choice in children less than 12 when intubation fails?

Percutaneous transtracheal ventilation (needle cricothyrotomy)

What are some considerations with the use of percutaneous transtracheal ventilation?

Not a definite airway; will progressively get hypercapnia; typically useful for <1 hour

What is the normal rate of breathing in each of the following age groups:

Neonates

About 50 breaths/min

Infants and children <8 years

20 breaths/min

Children >12 years

12 breaths/min

What is an important point with regard to mechanical ventilation in children?

Make sure it is volume-limited and consider hyperventilation in the setting of acute herniation.

What are some considerations in an infant who presents with complete airway obstruction due to a foreign body?

Avoid the Heimlich maneuver; use back blows and chest compressions; avoid blind finger sweeps

What are the two preferred routes of vascular access?

Intravenous (IV) and intraosseous (IO)

What is the primary purpose of establishing IV/IO access in children?

Administration of medications; fluid resuscitation; IO access is not usually effective for significant volume resuscitation

What are some considerations in vascular access?

The preferred site is the largest vein; peripheral access should be attempted first; central access can have significant complications

What are some considerations with IO access?

Typically performed if peripheral access fails; IO is easier and faster than central access; anteromedial proximal tibia is the preferred site

What is an important point about central access in children (typically <6 years)?

Should only be attempted if peripheral and IO access fails by an experienced provider.

What is an alternative way to deliver medication if no access is available?

Tracheal route

What are some considerations with tracheal medication administration?

Only useful for specific drugs; typically use 2-3 × the amount used IV; switch over to IV once available; pharmacokinetics are less reliable

List commonly used medications that can be given through the tracheal route:

LEAN: lidocaine, epinephrine, atropine, and naloxone

What is a commonly used route for vascular access in newborns?

Cannulation of the umbilical artery

Name some commonly used medications in pediatric resuscitation and their primary indications:

Epinephrine

Used for primary arrests in children; can be given IV/IO/tracheal route

Atropine

Not used in acute resuscitation; can be used for increased vagal stimulation; used as premedication prior to intubation

Adenosine

Used for supraventricular tachycardia (SVT) in pediatric patients

Lidocaine

Used to blunt ICP increase during intubation

What are the two common causes of cardiac arrest in children?	1. Respiratory arrest 2. Hypovolemic shock
What are two common dysrhythmias in a pediatric arrest?	1. Asystole 2. Bradyarrhythmias

NEONATAL/INFANT-SPECIFIC CONDITIONS

What are the main categories of the APGAR score:	Activity (muscle movement) Pulse Grimace Appearance Respirations
What is the definition of the APGAR score?	It is a 0 to 10 point scale that is assigned at 1 and then 5 min that is used to evaluate the newborn and has prognostic functions.
What are the key parameters to monitor in deciding if resuscitation should be done?	Respiratory status; heart rate
List important maneuvers to perform during a neonatal resuscitation:	Suction airway of secretions; maintain temperature; supplemental oxygen; cardiopulmonary resuscitation (CPR) (HR <60 beats)
What is meconium?	Thick green substance that lines the intestines of the fetus and is not typically released as a bowel movement until the first few days of life.
Is it possible for meconium to be released into amniotic fluid prior to delivery of fetus?	Yes—leads to increased risk of aspiration
What is the feared complication of meconium aspiration?	Respiratory distress (especially thick meconium); meconium aspiration pneumonia
In what circumstances can meconium be bad for the fetus/newborn?	Meconium found in amniotic fluid; consistency of meconium is thick/green
What is the mortality rate if a newborn has aspirated thick meconium?	30 to 50%

What are some considerations in the treatment of meconium staining?	Bulb suction mouth/nose during delivery; meconium-stained fluid and respiratory depression = tracheal suctioning
What is esophageal atresia?	Birth defect where the esophagus is segmented and cut off.
How common is esophageal atresia?	Occurs 1 in 4000 live births
What other congenital defect does esophageal atresia typically occur with?	Tracheoesophageal fistula
What is the biggest risk factor for the development of esophageal atresia?	Prematurity
What are some signs and symptoms of esophageal atresia?	Coughing/choking when feeding is attempted, recurrent aspiration pneumonia, and inability to pass a catheter into the stomach.
What is the treatment for esophageal atresia?	Surgical correction
What is the definition of necrotizing enterocolitis?	Condition with varying degrees of intestinal necrosis most common in premature newborns with low birth weight.
What risk factors are associated with necrotizing enterocolitis?	Prematurity; infections; hypertonic feeding solutions
When does necrotizing enterocolitis typically occur in the newborn?	First 2 weeks of life
What is the most common physical finding in a newborn who presents with necrotizing enterocolitis?	Abdominal distension with gastric retention
What are some other signs and symptoms in a newborn with necrotizing enterocolitis?	Bloody stools, bilious emesis, and abdominal wall redness and/or tenderness
What are some important signs and symptoms of a newborn that may be septic?	Bouts of apnea, temperature changes, lethargy, and metabolic acidosis
What are some complications of necrotizing enterocolitis?	Necrosis of bowel; perforation; sepsis

What are some diagnostic tests to consider in a newborn with necrotizing enterocolitis?

Plain films (classic finding is pneumatosis intestinalis); cultures (stool, urine, blood, and CSF)

What are some considerations in the management of a newborn with necrotizing enterocolitis?

NPO and NG tube; IV fluids/Abx; surgical consultation

What is an omphalocele?

A defect in the umbilical wall with herniation of intestinal content covered in a peritoneal sac.

What is important to know about omphalocele?

Many of them are associated with other congenital defects

What is a gastroschisis?

A defect in abdominal wall with herniation of intestinal content without peritoneal sac.

What are some complications of omphalocele and gastroschisis?

Obstruction; strangulation; hypovolemia; death

What are some considerations in the management of an omphalocele and gastroschisis?

NG tube for GI decompression; do not attempt to reduce the mass; cover in saline-soaked sterile gauze; IV fluids and Abx for prophylactic coverage; surgical correction required

What is the definition of diaphragmatic herniation?

A congenital defect due to developmental failure of a portion of the diaphragm that allows herniation of intestinal content.

Which is more common? Right-sided herniation or left-sided herniation?

Left-sided herniation far more common than right side

What is important to know about diaphragmatic herniation?

As with most congenital defects, there are typically other defects as well, with GI/GU abnormalities and congenital heart defects being fairly common

What are some signs and symptoms of diaphragmatic herniation?

Symptoms referable to herniation of GI tract into the chest: emesis and respiratory distress as well as bowel sounds over the chest wall

What are some common radiographic findings in diaphragmatic herniation?

Displacement of mediastinal contents (heart); loops of bowel in the chest; lack of distinct diaphragmatic margin

What is an important consequence of diaphragmatic herniation on the lung?	Hypoplastic lung
What are some considerations in the management of diaphragmatic herniation?	NG tube for GI decompression; NPO and IV fluids; surgical correction
What are some different types of neonatal seizures?	Myoclonic; tonic-clonic; focal clonic
What is the most common cause of seizures in children?	Simple febrile seizure
What are some important things to know about febrile seizures?	Up to 5% of children are affected; commonly occur between 3 months and 5 years of age
What are some signs and symptoms of a febrile seizure?	Rapidly ascending fever; generalized seizure less than 15 min duration; no focal neuro deficit
What is another important diagnosis to rule out in the setting of febrile seizure?	Meningitis
What important diagnostic test should be done for suspected meningitis?	Lumbar puncture
What are some considerations in the management of febrile seizures?	Lower the fever; treat the underlying cause of fever; seizure prophylaxis is not recommended
What is another important seizure to consider in children?	Generalized tonic-clonic seizure
What are some signs and symptoms of a tonic-clonic seizure?	Bilateral hemisphere involvement with motor involvement and alteration of consciousness.
When should one consider use of a non-contrast CT of the heads?	Focal neuro deficit; signs of increased ICP; suspected child abuse/head trauma; new onset seizure
What are some considerations in the management of a tonic-clonic seizure?	Most will terminate on their own; benzodiazepines are the mainstay; phenytoin and phenobarbital are second-line agents
What is the preferred benzodiazepine due to its long duration and least effect on respiratory depression?	Lorazepam

What are some important causes of neonatal seizures to consider?

Hypoxia; drug withdrawal; electrolyte imbalance; metabolic (ie, hypoglycemia); CNS infections; neoplasm

List the TORCHS infections:

Toxoplasmosis
Rubella
Cytomegalovirus
Herpes
Syphilis

What are some considerations in the management of neonatal seizures?

Airway, breathing, circulation (ABCs); correct easily reversible conditions (eg, hypoxia); monitor associated problems (eg, acidosis); anticonvulsant therapy

What is the drug of choice in the management of neonatal seizure?

Phenobarbital

What are other classes of drugs to consider if phenobarbital fails?

Benzodiazepine; phenytoin

What are some reasons that benzodiazepine is not first-line treatment in neonates as opposed to adults?

Profound respiratory depression; displacement of bilirubin from albumin

CONGENITAL HEART DISEASE

Is cyanosis ever normal in the newborn?

Yes—but only within the first ½ hour of life

What are the physical findings in a newborn with central cyanosis?

Bluish tongue, peripheral extremity, and mucous membrane

What is the amount of unsaturated Hgb in a newborn with central cyanosis?

Greater than 5 g/dL

At what point is central cyanosis pathologic?

If it persists for greater than 30 min

What are some important causes of persistent central cyanosis in the newborn?

Primary lung disease; cyanotic heart disease; methemoglobinemia

What are the five "Ts" of cyanotic heart disease that result in central cyanosis due to right-to-left shunt?

Tetralogy of Fallot; tricuspid atresia; transposition of the great vessels; truncus arteriosus; total anomalous pulmonary venous return

What particular agent is important to maintain the patency of the ductus arteriosus in newborns with congenital heart defects such as transposition of the great vessels?	Prostaglandin E_1
What is a useful test to do to distinguish right-to-left shunts from other causes of central cyanosis such as sepsis?	Administer 100% oxygen and watch oxygen saturation, if it fails to improve, it points to a right-to-left shunt
What is the most common cyanotic congenital heart disease in children?	Tetralogy of Fallot
What are the four anatomical abnormalities in tetralogy of Fallot?	1. Pulmonary artery stenosis 2. Right ventricular hypertrophy 3. Ventricular septal defect (VSD) 4. Overriding aorta

What are some common findings for each diagnostic test used with tetralogy of Fallot:

ECG	Right ventricular hypertrophy; right axis deviation
CXR	Decreased pulmonary vasculature; boot-shaped heart
CBC	Compensatory polycythemia

What are two most common non-cyanotic congenital heart defects?	1. VSD 2. Aortic stenosis
What are some signs and symptoms of aortic stenosis?	Typically not detected until later in life: angina, congestive heart failure (CHF), and syncope
What are some complications of congenital aortic stenosis?	Sudden death (secondary to dysrhythmias); endocarditis
What are some signs and symptoms of VSD?	Determined by the size of VSD: ranges from asymptomatic to heart failure
What is the most common cause of CHF in neonates and children?	Congenital heart disease
What are some signs and symptoms of CHF?	Rhonchi, rales, hepatomegaly, failure to thrive, and feeding difficulty
What are some other causes of CHF aside from congenital heart disease?	Sepsis; AV malformations; severe anemia; hypoplastic left heart syndrome; infectious myocarditis

What are some considerations in the management of CHF in neonates/children?	Search for and correct underlying cause; supplemental oxygen; use of digoxin and furosemide when needed

AIRWAY EMERGENCIES

Upper Airway

What is epiglottitis?	Epiglottitis is a life-threatening condition that occurs when the epiglottis—a small cartilage "lid" that covers the windpipe—swells, blocking the flow of air into the lungs.
What is the most common cause of epiglottitis?	*H influenzae*
What are some other causes of epiglottitis?	Burns from hot liquids; direct trauma to throat; various infections
What age group is epiglottitis most prevalent?	2 to 6 years of age
Is HIB epiglottitis common today?	No—since the introduction of HIB vaccine, it is not commonly seen. It is still a problem in immigrants and unvaccinated children.
What are some signs and symptoms of epiglottitis?	Typically will be ill-appearing, stridor and drooling with the child leaning forward in tripod position (classic appearance).
What is the diagnostic test of choice in the evaluation of epiglottitis?	Lateral neck film—typically shows enlarged epiglottis, "thumb-print sign"
What are some considerations in the management and evaluation of epiglottitis?	Ensuring intact airway is paramount; ENT should be consulted in severe cases; low threshold for intubation; IV Abx (third generation cephalosporin common); typically ICU admission for monitoring
What is croup?	Inflammation of the upper airway that leads to a cough that sounds like a seal bark, particularly when a child is crying.
What is the most common cause of croup?	Viral (parainfluenza being most common)

What age group is croup most prevalent?	Around 2 years of age (in the fall/winter)
What are some signs and symptoms of croup?	Barky cough worse at night is the hallmark, upper respiratory infection (URI) prodrome, stridor, and hoarseness with a low-grade fever.
What role does a lateral neck film play?	To rule out epiglottitis (although rare)
What are some considerations in the management of croup?	Typically resolves in a week; Abx not used—since viral most of the time; cool mist and hydration; steroids should be given to help resolve; admit if refractory to tx (persistent stridor)
What role does racemic epinephrine aerosol play?	Used for children who have resting stridor and more severe respiratory distress. (Patient must be observed for rebound if this is used).
What is bacterial tracheitis?	Diffuse inflammatory process of the larynx, trachea, and bronchi with adherent or semiadherent mucopurulent membranes within the trachea.
What are some signs and symptoms of bacterial tracheitis?	Often will present as croup, but defining feature is that child will not respond to standard croup tx and will often get quite sick.
What is the most common pathogen implicated in bacterial tracheitis?	*Staphylococcus aureus*
What are some considerations in the management of bacterial tracheitis?	Ensure an intact airway; IV hydration and Abx directed against staph; ENT consult is usually recommended; admit to ICU for monitoring
What is a retropharyngeal abscess?	Infection in one of the deep spaces of the neck with potential for airway compromise.
What are two ways in which the retropharyngeal space can become infected?	1. Direct inoculation via trauma 2. Spread from local infection
What are some common infections that can lead to a retropharyngeal abscess?	URI, otitis, pharyngitis, and sinusitis
What age group is a retropharyngeal abscess most common?	6 months to 5 years of age

What are some complications of a retropharyngeal abscess?

Airway compromise the most important; abscess rupture; spread of infection (ie, sepsis)

What are some signs and symptoms of a retropharyngeal abscess?

Typical picture is an ill-appearing child who is drooling and cannot tolerate PO and will often have a neck mass.

What are some important diagnostic tests to consider in a retropharyngeal abscess?

Lateral neck film-retropharyngeal swelling; make sure film is done during inspiration; CXR-inspect for possible mediastinitis; CT is study of choice

What are some considerations in the management of a retropharyngeal abscess?

ENT involvement for incision and drainage (I&D) of abscess; antibiotics; ICU monitoring in severe cases

What is the most common cause of accidental home death in young children?

Foreign body aspiration

What are some signs and symptoms of foreign body aspiration?

Stridor is common if the obstruction is higher; respiratory wheezing if obstruction is lower; suspect an impacted object in the airway if recurrent PNA

What is the most common location of foreign bodies?

Right mainstem bronchus

What are some common diagnostic tests used in foreign body aspiration?

CXR and MRI can be used to evaluate; bronchoscopy is diagnostic and therapeutic

Lower Airway

What is bronchiolitis?

Acute infectious disease of the lower respiratory tract.

What is the pathophysiology of bronchiolitis?

Narrowing of the bronchi/bronchioles typically due to inflammation of epithelial cells.

What is the most common cause of bronchiolitis?

Viral—RSV most common

What is a common history element in most patients who present with bronchiolitis?

Sick contact or day care exposure

What age group is most commonly affected with bronchiolitis?	Infants of 2 months to 2 years
What are some signs and symptoms of bronchiolitis?	Typically URI-like symptoms before progression to lower respiratory tract symptoms of wheezing, SOB, and possible cyanosis.
What are common diagnostic findings in a CXR?	Patchy atelectasis; hyperinflation of lungs; air trapping
What airway disease do many children with bronchiolitis later develop?	Asthma
What are some considerations in the management of bronchiolitis?	Supportive care; ensure proper hydration; antibiotics not indicated since it is a viral infection; a trial of bronchodilators may be warranted
What are some indications for admission for bronchiolitis?	Respiratory distress, extreme tachypnea; hypoxia; inability to take PO; poor home care, prematurity, infants less than 2 months old
What is the most common chronic disease of the pediatric population?	Asthma
What are some important points about asthma?	The prevalence is rising in the United States; mortality from asthma is also rising; accounts for large amount of ED visits
What is the definition of asthma?	It is a chronic inflammatory disorder characterized by increased responsiveness to a variety of stimuli that results in reversible airway constriction/obstruction.
List important triggers for asthma exacerbation:	Any upper respiratory infection; inhaled irritants (ie, smoke); medications; GERD; cold environment; exercise
What is the pathophysiology for asthma exacerbation?	Triggers that result in an IgE-mediated response that leads to inflammation and bronchial smooth muscle contraction, this eventually results in airway edema and movement of inflammatory cells. The end result is an increased airway resistance.
What are some signs and symptoms of asthma exacerbation?	Respiratory distress, increased work of breathing, tachypnea, tachycardia. Some will only have a chronic dry cough.

Is it reassuring if no wheezes can be heard on exam of an asthmatic with exacerbation?

No—may represent total cessation of airflow

What is PEFR?

Peak expiratory flow rate—typically measured before and after treatment to assess effectiveness.

What are some important points for each of the following categories of exacerbation:

Mild exacerbation

Oxygen saturation above 95% on room air; PEFR >80%; mild wheezing on exam; able to speak in full sentences

Moderate exacerbation

Oxygen saturation in low 90s; PEFR 50 to 80%; wheezing via expiratory phase; difficulty in speaking

Severe exacerbation

Oxygen saturation <90% in room air PEFR <50%; typically using accessory muscles; can only speak one or two words at a time

Name some risk factors associated with poor outcome in asthma exacerbation:

Prior intubation or ICU admission; greater than three hospitalizations per year; recent use or cessation of oral steroids; significant comorbid disease (CAD); lower socioeconomic status

What are some considerations in the management of asthma exacerbation?

ABCs—particularly with O_2 administration; B_2-agonist is the mainstay treatment; anticholinergic used in severe cases; steroids

What are some important points for each of the following used medications in asthma:

B_2-agonist

The mainstay of treatment: nebulizer or inhaler; primary effect is on small airway; albuterol most commonly used; IV use only in very sick patients

Anticholinergic

Ipratropium most commonly used agent; primary effect is on large airways; added to B_2-agonist in more severe cases; atropine not used due to side effect profile

Steroids

Shown to prevent progression and relapse; IV and oral equally effective; should be continued on steroids on discharge

Leukotriene modifiers	Inflammatory mediators used in outpatient; no role in acute management of asthma
Magnesium sulfate	Has bronchodilator properties; used in acute exacerbations as second-line treatment; not particularly effective in mild exacerbations
Ketamine	Induction agent with mild bronchodilator effects; recommended if intubation is to be done
Heliox	Mixture of helium-oxygen (80:20); helps decrease work of breathing; may help in severe exacerbations
What are some considerations for admission in a patient with asthma exacerbation?	Failure to improve after treatment in the ED; poor home care; history of ICU/ intubation for asthma
What are the general guidelines to safely discharge a patient from the ED?	Good patient follow-up; 3 to 4 hours is usually enough to show improvement with medication.

PEDIATRIC GASTROINTESTINAL

Appendicitis

What are some signs and symptoms of appendicitis?	Typically has diffuse periumbilical pain that eventually leads to N/V and RLQ pain. Will often have a low-grade temperature as well.
What are some commonly used diagnostic tests in appendicitis?	Kidney-ureter-bladder (KUB): rarely shows a fecalith; CT with contrast: test of choice; U/S: operator dependent
What are some findings in a child with perforation of the appendix?	High-grade fever, high WBC, and symptoms over 2 days as well as diffuse abdominal pain and peritoneal signs.
What are some considerations in the management of appendicitis?	IV fluids and NPO; broad-spectrum antibiotics prior to surgery; surgical consult

Pyloric Stenosis

| What is the definition of pyloric stenosis? | It is hypertrophy of the pylorus with gastric outlet obstruction. |

What age group is commonly affected with pyloric stenosis?	Male newborns between 2 and 4 weeks
What are some signs and symptoms of pyloric stenosis?	Nonbilious projectile vomiting is the hallmark with failure to thrive and sometimes a palpable right upper quadrant (RUQ) mass can be felt.
What are some tests used to diagnose pyloric stenosis?	U/S and upper GI series; hypochloremic metabolic alkalosis
What are some considerations in the management of pyloric stenosis?	NPO and IV fluids; prompt surgical correction

Incarcerated Hernia

What age group do incarcerated hernias typically occur in?	Under 1 year of age
What are some clinical features of incarcerated hernias?	Emesis with a palpable scrotal/inguinal mass
What other conditions are in the differential diagnosis for incarcerated hernia?	Hydrocele; torsion of testicles; undescended testis
What are some consideration in the management of incarcerated hernias?	Manual reduction, then outpatient surgery; if any evidence of ischemia = immediate surgical reduction

Intestinal Obstruction

What is the clinical hallmark of intestinal obstruction?	Emesis (bilious) with abdominal pain and distension
What are some important causes of intestinal obstruction?	Hernia; intussusception; congenital atresia
What are some common findings on abdominal plain films?	Dilated loops of bowel with air-fluid levels
What are some considerations in the management of intestinal obstruction?	NPO, IV fluids, and NG tube; surgical intervention required

Intussusception

What are some important things to know about intussusception?	Most common cause of obstruction in children; most common age group: 3 months to 5 years; ileocolic intussusception most common; more common in males
What are some signs and symptoms of intussusception?	Emesis, colicky pain, and red jelly stools as well as possible mental status change. PE: may palpate a sausage-shaped mass
What is the most prominent feature of abdominal pain in intussusception?	Periods of intense abdominal pain followed by periods of no pain.

What are some important points for each of the following diagnostic tests:

Abdominal plain films	May show abdominal mass in RUQ; may show dilated bowel with air-fluid levels; free air in perforation
Barium/air-contrast enema	It the test of choice to detect intussusception; therapeutic: reduces in most cases; BE may show coiled-spring appearance

What is the next step to be taken if BE or air-contrast fails to reduce the intussusception?	Surgical intervention
What is the recurrence rate after a successful BE or surgical reduction?	As high as 10% in the first 24 hours

Meckel Diverticulum

What is the definition of Meckel diverticulum?	A Meckel diverticulum is a remnant of structures within the fetal digestive tract that were not fully reabsorbed before birth and leads to a pouch with GI tissue.
What remnant of tissue from the prenatal development of the digestive system is found in Meckel diverticulum?	Gastric tissue most common
What is the "rule of 2s" in Meckel diverticulum?	Peak age of symptoms is 2 years of age; affects 2% of the population; two times more likely in males

What are some signs and symptoms of Meckel diverticulum? — Painless bleeding from rectum, N/V, and sign of obstruction if a volvulus develops.

What are some other considerations in an infant with painless bleeding? — Anal fissures; juvenile polyps; infection

What are three complications of Meckel diverticulum? —
1. Inflammation that mimics appendicitis
2. Bleeding—can be massive
3. Obstruction—volvulus or intussusception

What is the diagnostic study of choice for Meckel diverticulum? — Meckel isotope scanning

What are some considerations in the management of Meckel diverticulum? — Remove if heavy bleeding or pain; surgical intervention if sign of obstruction

Volvulus

What is the definition of a volvulus? — A form of obstruction typically due to malrotation of the bowel during embryonic development.

What age group is more commonly affected with a volvulus? — Greater than 90% present <1 year of age

What are some signs and symptoms of a volvulus? — Failure to thrive, anorexia, intermittent apnea, emesis (bilious) with abdominal distension

What is a feared complication of a volvulus if not promptly treated? — Gangrene with perforation

What are some important points for each of the following diagnostic tests:

Obstructive series — Gastric/duodenal distension (double bubble); relative paucity of lower GI gas

Upper GI contrast series — Study test of choice; "Bird-beak" obstruction at proximal duodenum

Ultrasonography and CT scanning — Used more as adjunctive tests; definitive diagnosis rests on upper gastrointestinal (UGI) study

What are some considerations in the management of a volvulus? — NPO, IV fluids, and NG tube; surgical intervention

INFECTIOUS DISEASE

Bacteremia and Sepsis

What is the pathophysiology of fever?	Typically due to exogenous substance (antigens/bacterial wall components) that result in the release of pyrogens that in turn result in prostaglandin production, this acts on the hypothalamus to raise the hypothalamic set point.
What are some common manifestations of a raised hypothalamic set point?	Chills, shivering, peripheral vasoconstriction, and behavioral activities (using blankets) that result in elevation of body temperature.
What area of the hypothalamus regulates body temperature?	Ventromedial preoptic area; periventricular nucleus
What are some common methods to measure temperature?	Oral; axillary; rectal; tympanic
What method is the most accurate and thus should be used whenever possible?	Rectal
What are some risks for serious bacterial infection that may not be obvious in the pediatric population?	Infants: rectal temp (>38° C) and leukocytosis; neonates with hypothermia (<36°C); fever with a low white count (<5k); fever with a petechial rash
What are some commonly used drugs to treat fevers?	Ibuprofen; acetaminophen
What role does aspirin play in the treatment of fever from viral illnesses?	Should be avoided due to association with Reye syndrome (it is effective and used commonly in some parts of the world).
What is Reye syndrome?	It affects all organs of the body but is most harmful to the brain and the liver, causing an acute increase of pressure within the brain and, often, massive accumulations of fat in the liver and other organs.
What is the most common preceding factor?	Viral illness (ie, chicken pox)

What are some signs and symptoms of Reye syndrome?	Recurrent vomiting, listlessness, personality changes such as irritability or combativeness, disorientation or confusion, delirium, convulsions, and loss of consciousness.
What other conditions is Reye syndrome commonly mistaken for?	Meningitis, diabetes, drug overdose poisoning, and encephalitis.
What is the most common cause of mortality in Reye syndrome?	Brain herniation from swelling
What is the treatment for Reye syndrome?	Treatment is primarily supportive with care focusing on reducing brain swelling.
What is occult bacteremia?	Fever with positive blood cultures in a child who does not have a major identifiable source of infection.
What are the three most common organisms responsible for occult bacteremia?	1. *S pneumonia*—by far the most common 2. *N meningitidis* 3. Salmonella species
What age group is most susceptible to infection?	Between 6 months and 2 years of age
What is the reason for this?	Infants less than 6 months typically have maternal antibodies which decrease leaving infants more susceptible until the age of 2, when they eventually develop their own.
What is the definition of sepsis?	It occurs when bacteria, which can originate in a child's lungs, intestines, urinary tract, or gallbladder, make toxins that cause the body's immune system to produce various cytokines that act on many targets in the body.
What are the three most common organisms responsible for sepsis in the following age group:	
Neonates	*Group B Streptococcus; Listeria monocytogenes; E coli*
Infants	*S pneumoniae; H influenzae; N meningitidis*
What are some signs and symptoms of an infant who is septic?	Ill-appearing, lethargic, periods of apnea and bradycardia, failure to thrive, and often hypothermic (<36°C).

What is the standard workup for neonates/infants who may be septic?	CBC, blood cultures, U/A with urine cultures, stool cultures, CXR, and LP.

Meningitis

What is the definition of meningitis?	It is a serious CNS infection of the meninges with often devastating results in infants and young children if not treated early.
What are two common sources of infections in meningitis?	1. Hematogenous spread—most common 2. Direct spread from a contiguous focus
Why is the diagnosis of meningitis more elusive in infants?	The classic signs/symptoms (stiff neck/headache/fever) are often not present
What are some signs and symptoms of meningitis in infants (<4 months)?	Lethargy, decreased oral intake, irritability, fever or hypothermia, seizure, and bulging fontanelle.
What are the three most common organisms responsible for meningitis in the following age groups:	
Neonates	Group B streptococcus; *L monocytogenes*; *E coli*
Infants/young children	*S pneumoniae*; *H influenzae*; *N meningitidis*
What are other important causes of meningitis to consider aside from bacteria?	Viral; fungal; TB; aseptic
What are some considerations in the management of meningitis?	IV broad-spectrum antibiotics without delay; LP to diagnose and tailor therapy; antiviral if suspicious of herpes
What role do steroids play in the treatment of meningitis?	They may play a role in reducing neurologic sequelae if given early (before or with the first dose of antibiotics)

Otitis Media

What is the definition of otitis media?	Infection of the middle ear with acute onset, possible presence of middle ear effusion, and signs of middle ear inflammation.

What is the pathophysiology of otitis media?

Obstruction of the eustachian tube that results in a sterile effusion with aspiration of nasopharyngeal secretions into the middle ear that leads to acute infection.

Why does otitis media occur more frequently in children?

Infants and younger children have shorter and more horizontal eustachian tube than adults.

Name four of the most common pathogens that cause otitis media:

1. *S pneumoniae*
2. *H influenzae*
3. *Moraxella catarrhalis*
4. Group A streptococcus

What are some signs and symptoms of otitis media?

Exam of ear often shows distortion of tympanic membrane (TM), erythema, decreased mobility of TM on pneumatic otoscopy, fever, poor feeding, and child pulling at ear.

What are some complications to consider in otitis media if left untreated?

Hearing loss, TM perforation, mastoiditis, lateral sinus thrombosis, and meningitis.

What are the main antibiotics used to treat otitis media?

High dose amoxicillin is the mainstay, followed by TMP-SMX or macrolide as secondline treatment.

When should the fever and symptoms begin to subside?

Within a few days after antibiotic is started

Pneumonia

What age group is most commonly affected with pneumonia?

Incidence is greatest in 6 to 12 months of age

What is the primary mode in which pneumonia occurs?

Typically from aspiration of infectious particles, such as from a preceding URI.

What are some important elements in the history of a child with pneumonia?

Comorbid conditions; age; sick contacts (ie, day care); immunizations

What is the most common cause of pneumonia in children (not neonates)?

Viruses—RSV being most common

What are some common bacterial pathogens that cause pneumonia in infants/children?

Mycoplasma; *S pneumoniae*; *C trachomatis; H influenzae*

What are some signs and symptoms of pneumonia in infants/children?	Often will have a preceding URI, cough, fever, and tachypnea are common
What are some important diagnostic studies to consider in pneumonia?	Pulse ox (hypoxia), CBC and blood cultures are often ordered, CXR, and sputum stain.
What are the more likely causes of pneumonia in which the CXR shows diffuse interstitial pattern?	Viral; chlamydial; mycoplasma
What is the more likely cause of pneumonia in which the CXR shows lobar involvement?	Bacterial
What are some consideration in the management of pneumonia?	Bacterial PNA requires specific antibiotic coverage; viral PNA typically requires supportive care; persistent PNA consider foreign body aspiration in children
What are indications for admission in an infant/child who presents with pneumonia?	Respiratory distress; ill-appearing; PNA complications (ie, empyema); hypoxia; outpatient antibiotic failure; social reasons (poor care at home)

Pertussis

What is the causative agent of pertussis (whooping cough)?	*Bordetella pertussis*
What are some important things to know about pertussis?	Highly infectious (via respiratory droplets); incubation time is about 10 days; mortality is highest in first few months
What group is commonly affected by pertussis?	Nonimmunized children
Can adults who received vaccination against pertussis still develop it later in life?	Yes—does not confer life-long immunity
What is the three-stage illness of pertussis:	
Catarrhal	URI prodrome that last for about 2 weeks; highly infectious at this stage
Paroxysmal	Paroxysmal coughing spells; emesis is common with the coughing; can last up to 1 month
Convalescent	Residual cough that can last for months

What is the characteristic finding on CBC in a patient with pertussis?

WBC that can be as high as 50k; lymphocytosis is common

What are some commonly used tests to diagnose pertussis?

Bordet-Gengou medium; PCR; antibody staining

What is the antibiotic of choice to treat pertussis?

Erythromycin (can also be given to close contacts of patients with pertussis)

What is the typical pertussis vaccine regiment?

Before age 7, children should get five doses of the DTaP vaccine; these are usually given at 2, 4, 6, and 15 to 18 months of age and 4 to 6 years of age

What are some complications of pertussis?

PNA; seizure; brain death from hypoxia

Urinary Tract Infection

What are some important things to know about UTI in infants/children?

They are fairly common in the pediatric population; more common in males during infancy; infants/children have few specific symptoms

What is the mechanism of UTI in infants/children?

Ascending infection from perineal contaminants is common, but hematogenous spread is more common in neonates.

What is an important consideration in infants less than 1 year of age who have recurrent UTIs?

Structural problem in the GU tract; vesicoureteral reflux

How common is urosepsis in infants 1 to 3 months in age?

30%

What are some signs and symptoms of neonates with UTIs?

Irritability, emesis, diarrhea, poor oral intake, and possible sepsis (as children get older, their symptoms become more specific for UTI: dysuria and frequency)

What is the most common pathogen in UTIs in this age group?

E coli

What are some possible causes of UTIs in male children?

Meatal stenosis; phimosis; paraphimosis

What are some complications of UTIs?

Pyelonephritis; urosepsis; renal scarring; renal failure

What are three optimal ways to collect urine for a U/A?

1. Midstream collection
2. Suprapubic aspiration
3. Bladder catheterization

What are the typical U/A findings that suggest UTI?

Pyuria: >10 WBCs/HPF; bacteriuria: >100k CFU/mL

What is another diagnostic test that should be obtained for females <3 years and males <1 year?

Urine culture

What are the indications for antibiotic use?

Symptomatic with pyuria/bacteriuria; any evidence of pyelonephritis

What antibiotics are commonly used in the treatment of UTIs?

Trimethoprim-sulfamethoxazole (TMP/SMX); amoxicillin; third generation cephalosporins

What radiographic studies are commonly used to further evaluate UTIs?

Renal ultrasound; voiding cystourethrography; IVP

CHILD ABUSE

What are three common types of abuse in children?

1. Sexual abuse
2. Neglect
3. Physical abuse

How common is sexual abuse in children?

Up to 25% of all females sexually abused; up to 10% of all males sexually abused

In what percent of sexual abuse is the perpetrator known to the victim?

Up to 90% (most often family/relatives)

What are some physical exam findings that are suggestive of sexual abuse?

Vaginal discharge; sexually transmitted disease; scarring/tearing of the hymen; anal fissures

Do sexually abused children always show evidence of abuse on exam?

No—up to 50% may present normally

What are important laboratory tests to conduct in a child who is sexually abused?

Culture for gonorrhea and chlamydia; syphilis; HIV testing

Are health-care providers required to report a sexual abuse?

Yes

What are some physical findings in a child who is suffering from neglect?

Poor hygiene, evidence of failure to thrive such as low weight for age, alopecia, and avoidance.

What is an important consideration in a child who is suffering from neglect?

Suspect physical abuse

What are some important things to do if a child is suffering from neglect?

A skeletal survey for abuse; report to the proper agencies; child is typically admitted

What does the skeletal survey usually consist of?

AP and lateral views of skull/chest/pelvis/spine, and extremities

What are the most common causes of death in children who are physically abused?

Head and abdominal injury

What are red flags in a child's history that should raise the suspicion of physical abuse?

Inconsistent history from caregivers; history that does not match PE; pattern injuries such as choke marks; bruises in certain areas like buttocks

What injury patterns are commonly associated with physical abuse?

Posterior rib fractures; cigarette burns; skull fractures; healing fractures that were not treated; spiral fractures of extremities

What is shaken baby syndrome?

Type of inflicted traumatic brain injury that happens when a baby is violently shaken.

What are some reasons why a baby is more susceptible to being shaken?

Weak neck; proportionally larger head

What are the characteristic injuries that occur in shaken baby syndrome?

Subdural hematoma; retinal hemorrhages/detachment; spinal neck/cord damage; fracture of ribs and bones

What are some signs and symptoms of shaken baby syndrome?

Extreme irritability, lethargy, poor feeding, breathing problems, convulsions, vomiting, and pale or bluish skin.

What age group is most common for shaken baby syndrome?

Typically infants

What are some important diagnostic tests to consider in suspected physical abuse?

CBC/coags—to assess for coagulopathy; skeletal survey; imaging studies such as CT or MRI

What is essential to do in all cases of suspected physical abuse?

Report to police and proper agencies; must not allow child to go back home

CLINICAL VIGNETTES—MAKE THE DIAGNOSIS

A newborn is noticed to be apneic and choking whenever feeding is attempted for the past week, the newborn's history is only significant for prematurity

Esophageal atresia

1-week-old newborn that was born premature is brought to the ED due to concerns of recent abdominal distension with bilious emesis; PE: abdominal tenderness

Necrotizing enterocolitis

5-week-old is brought in due to periods of breathing difficulty as well as bouts of emesis for about a month; PE: remarkable for bowel sounds heard over the left anterior chest

Diaphragmatic herniation

1-year-old is brought in by his frantic mother due to a sudden onset of a generalized seizure that occurred about an hour ago; PE: low-grade temperature, but otherwise unremarkable exam

Simple febrile seizure

3-year-old ill-appearing girl is brought in by her mother for high-fever, history is significant for recent immigration to the United States from Russia; PE: ill-appearing child leaning forward with drooling and stridor

Epiglottitis

4-year-old child presents with low-grade fever, HA, and decreased oral intake; PE: erythema and decreased motility of right tympanic membrane

Otitis media

2-year-old boy is brought in with a 1-week history of a URI, now presents with a barky cough particularly worse at night; PE: child otherwise appears well despite the cough

Croup

An alarmed father brings in his 2-year-old son due to a sudden onset of wheezing, but is otherwise well; PE: unremarkable

Foreign body aspiration

8-year-old child with a long history of allergies is brought in by her mother due to difficulty in breathing soon after soccer practice; PE: bilateral wheezing

Asthma exacerbation

3-year-old girl is brought in by her concerned mother who mentions that her child has intense periods of colicky abdominal pain with periods of no pain as well as red jelly stools

Intussusception

3-year-old boy presents with a 2-day history of nausea, emesis, fever, and irritability; PE: diffuse abdominal pain; labs: elevated WBC

Appendicitis

3-year-old ill-appearing girl with a recent history of sinusitis now presents with a high-grade fever and the inability to swallow; PE: child is drooling and a small mass can be felt on the neck, lateral neck film: retropharyngeal swelling

Retropharyngeal abscess

3-week-old child is brought in by her mother with concerns of inability to keep any nutrition down, she mentions whenever the patient eats, he soon has projectile vomiting; PE: a nontender RUQ mass can be felt

Pyloric stenosis

2-year-old child is brought in with a 2-day history of abdominal pain and distension with the inability to tolerate any feedings; abdominal films: dilated loops of bowel with air-fluid levels

Intestinal obstruction

2-year-old child presents with painless bleeding with nausea and vomiting, but otherwise has no other medical problems; PE: unremarkable

Meckel diverticulum

3-month-old infant is brought in by her mother with lethargy, irritability, fever, and decreased oral intake that has been ongoing for about 2 days; PE: bulging fontanelle

Meningitis

5-year-old child is brought in by her mother for a fall from his bed last night, his medical history is significant for three other fractures to various other areas of the body; PE: fracture of the left clavicle

Child abuse

CHAPTER 14

Obstetric and Gynecologic Emergencies

NORMAL PREGNANCY

Define the following definitions:

Gestational age

Number of completed weeks of pregnancy from the last menstrual period

Gravidity

Total number of pregnancies

Parity

Total number of births (twins count as 1)

Term

Born between 38 and 42 weeks of gestation

Preterm

Born before 38 weeks of gestation

What is the TPAL system?

Indicates number of term, preterm, abortus, and living

What is the general rule with any pregnant patient who presents with vaginal bleeding?

Pathologic until proven otherwise

What are some physiologic changes that occur to each organ system during normal pregnancy:

Respiratory

Increase in tidal volume, minute ventilation, O_2 consumption, and respiratory rate along with a decrease in total lung capacity

Cardiovascular

Increase in circulating volume, heart rate, and cardiac output with a 20% decrease in BP during first trimester. Uterus may compress IVC, reducing preload while supine

Gastrointestinal	Gastroesophageal reflux disease very common, cholestasis, hemorrhoids, and nausea/vomiting
Genitourinary	Increase in renal blood flow, glomerular filtration rate, kidney size, and urinary stasis; decrease in BUN/Crea
Hematology	Increase in plasma volume causes dilutional decrease in hematocrit and white blood cell count. Increase in coagulation factors is a risk for DVT/PE
Endocrine	Increase in glucose level, progesterone, estrogen, T3/T4, thyroid-binding globulin, and prolactin
Uterus	Weight will increase from 80 g to 1,000 g and volume will increase from 10 mL to 5,000 mL
Dermatology	Hyperpigmentation of nipples, abdominal midline, and face; palmar erythema, and spider angiomata due to increased estrogen
What are some important points to know about human chorionic gonadotropin (hCG)?	Detected as early as 9 days after fertilization; normally doubles every 2 days early in pregnancy; very low false-negative rate (<1%); peaks at about 10-weeks gestational age
What are some conditions to consider that can result in a positive pregnancy test?	Intrauterine pregnancy; ectopic pregnancy; recent abortion; trophoblastic disease; germ cell tumors
What are some common causes of very high concentrations of beta human chorionic gonadotrophin (β-hCG)?	Multiple gestations; advanced age; ovarian cancer; trophoblastic disease; germ cell tumors
What is a pregnancy detectable by transvaginal ultrasound?	When the hCG concentration is >1500 IU/L (around 5-weeks)
What are some considerations with a transabdominal sonography?	A small white gestational ring is detectable by about 6 weeks; fetal heart activity by 8 weeks
What are advantages of a transvaginal sonography?	Does not require a full bladder; better resolution; identify a gestational yolk sac at 6 weeks
Name two radiographic procedure associated with a high fetal radiation exposure:	CT abdomen and pelvis; cardiac catheterization

When is the fetal central nervous system most vulnerable to radiation?	8 to 14 weeks

ECTOPIC PREGNANCY (EP)

What differential must be considered in any female who presents with pelvic/lower abdominal pain or syncope?	Ectopic pregnancy, tubal ovarian abscess, ovarian torsion
What are some facts about ectopic pregnancy?	Leading cause of first-trimester death; implantation of fertilized egg outside the uterus; most EPs occur within the fallopian tube
What are some major risk factors for EP?	Pelvic inflammatory disease; use of a intrauterine device; history of tubal surgery; exposure to diethylstilbestrol (DES) in utero
What is the classic triad for the clinical presentation of EP?	Pelvic pain, spotting, and amenorrhea
What are some signs and symptoms of a ruptured EP?	Rebound tenderness, hypotension, and adnexal mass, tachycardia
What are less common clinical features of a ruptured EP?	Syncope, unexplained shock, tenesmus, or shoulder pain
What is the differential diagnosis for a suspected EP?	Ovarian rupture/torsion, abortion, and surgical abdomen
What is the single most important test to do on any female of child-bearing age?	Pregnancy test
How does a pregnancy test work?	Pregnancy tests rely on the detection of β-hCG, human chorionic gonadotropin is a hormone produced by the trophoblast.
Qualitative pregnancy tests are positive at what level?	Serum β-hCG >20 mIU/mL results in a positive urine test; a serum β-hCG >10 mIU/mL results in a positive blood test.
What is a concern of doing a urine pregnancy test?	Dilute urine can be false-negative, especially early in pregnancy
If the bedside urine pregnancy test is negative, but EP is still a consideration, what is the next step?	Quantitative serum test should be done

How is the definitive diagnosis of EP made?	Surgery; visualization during laparoscopy; ultrasound
What is the primary purpose of U/S?	Determine if there is an intrauterine pregnancy (IUP)
If U/S shows an IUP, is EP now excluded?	No—should consider heterotopic pregnancy (although rare, a patient may simultaneously have an IUP and an EP)
What should be noted about transabdominal ultrasound (TA)?	Less invasive; wider field of view and easier orientation; requires a full bladder
What are some findings on ultrasound that may be suggestive of an EP?	Echogenic adnexal mass; free pelvic fluid; ectopic fetal heart activity or fetal pole
What are two reasons to obtain quantitative hCG concentrations?	Correlate a single concentration with ultrasound findings; follow serial concentrations as an outpatient, as the level is expected to double every two days in an IUP
What is the discriminatory zone?	The level of β-hCG at which an IUP can be visualized by U/S and can be reliably differentiated from an EP.
What is the discriminatory zone of TA U/S?	β-hCG >6000 mIU/mL
What is the discriminatory zone of TV U/S?	β-hCG >1500 mIU/mL
What is the diagnostic test of choice for an unstable patient with a suspected ectopic pregnancy?	Laparoscopy
What is the preferred medical management for EP?	Methotrexate (MTX)
What is the mechanism of MTX?	Inhibits dihydrofolic acid reductase: interferes with DNA synthesis
What are some things to keep in mind about the use of methotrexate?	Surgical Tx may be needed if MTX fails; MTX use should be in conjunction with close follow-up
What is the most common surgical method for EP?	Laparoscopic salpingostomy

| What are some considerations in the management of EP? | Medical approach is preferred to surgery, but patient should go to the operating room if unstable; alloimmunization can occur—give RhoGAM to Rh-patients |

EMERGENCIES DURING EARLY PREGNANCY

What are some risk factors associated with pregnancy-related death?	Poor prenatal care; unmarried; advanced maternal age; minority race
What are some leading causes of pregnancy-related death:	Pulmonary embolism; HTN (ie, stroke); hemorrhage
Name some common causes of first trimester bleeding:	Abortion; ectopic pregnancy; gestational trophoblastic disease; cervical infection

Abortion

What is the definition of spontaneous abortion (SAB) or miscarriage?	The loss of pregnancy prior to 20 weeks or delivery of a fetus less than 500 g.
What is the most common cause of SAB?	Chromosomal abnormalities
What are some risk factors associated with SAB?	Poor prenatal care; advanced maternal care; infections
What are important elements in the history to obtain in patients with suspected SAB?	Last menstrual period; degree and duration of bleeding; fever; pain
What is the most common method of surgical evacuation in the first trimester?	Dilation and curettage (D&C)
What are some findings on ultrasound suggestive of an abnormal pregnancy?	No fetal heart tones after 10 weeks' gestational age; 5 mm crown-rump length with no fetal heart tones; no gestational sac at a β-hCG concentration of >3000 mIU/mL; no fetus with gestational sac of 25 mm mean diameter
What is the most important differential to consider in a patient who presents with suspected SAB?	Ectopic pregnancy
What is the most common method of surgical evacuation in the second trimester?	Dilation and evacuation (D&E)

Name the different types of abortion and their treatment:

Threatened abortion

Vaginal bleeding with no cervical dilation; **Tx:** verify live fetus and bed rest

Inevitable abortion

Vaginal bleeding with cervical dilation; no expulsion of products of conception (POC); **Tx:** surgical evacuation

Incomplete abortion

Partial expulsion of POC; **Tx:** typically admit for D&C

Complete abortion

Complete expulsion of POC; **Tx:** none

Missed abortion

Death of fetus and retained POC; **Tx:** surgical evacuation of POC

What are some general management considerations for SAB?

Assess hemodynamic status; administer Anti-D immunoglobulin if the patient is Rh-negative; consider ectopic pregnancy

Gestational Trophoblastic Disease

What is gestational trophoblastic disease (GTD)?

Rare neoplasm of the trophoblastic cells that produce hCG.

Name three types of hydatidiform moles for each description:

Karyotype of product is 69XXY due to two sperms that fertilize egg, fetal parts are present

Incomplete mole

Karyotype of product is 46XX due to sperm that fertilizes an egg with no DNA, no fetal parts

Complete mole

GTD that becomes malignant, penetrates the myometrium, and can potentially metastasize

Invasive mole

What are some signs and symptoms of GTD?

Vaginal bleeding, hyperemesis gravidarum, and hypertension that typically manifest in the first trimester.

What diagnostic abnormalities are typical of GTD?

Very high hCG (>100,000), U/S that shows absence of fetal heart and "snowstorm" appearance

What are some considerations in management of GTD?

D&C and monitor hCG (should trend down); also monitor for possible metastasis (rare); prognosis is generally good

| What is an important complication to consider in GTD? | Choriocarcinoma |
| What are some considerations in the management of choriocarcinoma? | Chemotherapy that typically achieves almost 100% remission |

Hyperemesis Gravidarum

What is hyperemesis gravidarum?	It is excessive nausea and vomiting that leads to dehydration/electrolyte imbalance.
What are some considerations in hyperemesis gravidarum?	It affects about 2% of all pregnancies; the presence of abdominal pain is unusual; associated with weight loss and ketosis; severe cases require admission
What is an important consideration for anyone who presents with hyperemesis gravidarum?	Gestational trophoblastic disease
What are some considerations in the management of hyperemesis gravidarum?	NPO and IV fluids; antiemetics; refractory cases may require termination of pregnancy

EMERGENCIES DURING LATER PREGNANCY

Hypertensive Emergencies

How is hypertension defined during pregnancy?	BP over 140/90 or a 20 mmHg increase in systolic pressure or 10 mmHg increase in diastolic pressure.
Name four types of hypertension that can occur during pregnancy:	1. Chronic hypertension 2. Transient hypertension 3. Preeclampsia 4. Eclampsia
What are some risk factors that determine HTN in pregnancy?	Multiple gestations; nulliparity; age >40; obesity; GTD
What is the definition of preeclampsia?	It is new onset HTN after 20 weeks with proteinuria

What is believed to be the cause of preeclampsia?	Small vessel disease leading to disturbed blood flow to the placenta, kidneys, and CNS

What are important diagnostic tests used to diagnose preeclampsia and their typical findings:

Blood pressure	More than 140/90 (even one reading merits a workup)
Urine protein collection	Urine protein concentration of 0.1 g/L in two random collections or 0.3 g/day in a 24 hour collection
What are some signs and symptoms of preeclampsia?	Headache, edema, abdominal pain, and visual disturbances
What is the definition of severe preeclampsia?	Blood pressure of greater than 160/110 and more than 5 g/day of protein in the urine.
What are some abnormal laboratory findings in severe preeclampsia?	Thrombocytopenia and elevated liver function tests (LFTs)
What is the definition of eclampsia?	It is preeclampsia with the presence of seizures from 12 weeks gestation to 1 month after delivery.
What are important considerations in the management of severe preeclampsia and eclampsia?	Magnesium sulfate for seizure prophylactic; control HTN with hydralazine; induce labor if fetus/mother unstable; delivery is definitive cure
What is the definition of HELLP syndrome?	Hemolytic anemia, Elevated LFT, and Low Platelets

Abruptio Placentae

What is the definition of abruptio placentae (placental abruption)?	It is separation of the placenta from the uterine wall.
What percentage of miscarriages occurs after the first trimester?	20%
What percentage of third trimester bleeding is due to abruption placentae?	Up to 30%

What are some risk factors associated with placental abruption?

HTN; trauma; cocaine use; advanced maternal age; multiparity

What are some sign and symptoms of a placental abruption?

Third trimester bleeding that is typically dark, painful contractions, fetal distress, hypotension.

Will all women with a placental abruption manifest bleeding or pain?

Up to 20% may have no symptoms

What are some complications of a placental abruption?

Fetal or maternal death; disseminated intravascular coagulation; hypovolemic shock

How is a placental abruption typically diagnosed?

Ultrasound

What are some critical actions in the management of a placental abruption?

Admit and resuscitation if in shock; C-section if fetus/mother unstable; induction if stable; RhoGAM as indicated in Rh-patients

What is the main differential diagnosis to consider in patients with a suspected placental abruption?

Placenta previa

Placenta Previa

What is the definition of a placenta previa?

Implantation of the placenta over the cervical os (total, partial, or marginal).

What are some risk factors for placenta previa?

Multiparity; advanced maternal age; smoking

What are some sign and symptoms of a placenta previa?

Late pregnancy painless bleeding

What is important to keep in mind during an exam?

Avoid a pelvic exam until an U/S is done

What are some complications of placenta previa?

Preterm delivery; hypovolemic shock

What are some critical actions in the management of a placenta previa?

Resuscitation if in shock; RhoGAM when indicated; C/S if unstable or fetus is mature; fetal monitoring; the primary goal is to support the patient until the fetus is mature enough for delivery through C/S

Premature Rupture of Membranes

What is the definition of premature rupture of membranes (PROM)?	Spontaneous rupture of membranes before labor. If it occurs preterm, it is PPROM.
How is PROM diagnosed?	Gush of fluid, positive pool ferning pattern when dried on a microscope slide, or Nitrazine test.
What are some considerations in the management of PROM?	Induction of labor if failure to progress in 24 hours and Abx if chorioamnionitis is suspected (increased WBC count, fever, and uterine tenderness).

Preterm Labor

What is the definition of preterm labor (PTL)?	Onset of labor prior to 37 weeks
What are some risk factors for PTL?	PROM; infection; preeclampsia; multiple gestations; tobacco use
What is the most common cause of mortality in PTL?	Lung immaturity
Name some commonly used tocolytics:	Magnesium sulfate, indomethacin, and terbutaline
What are the purposes of tocolytics?	Delay labor to allow administration of steroids for lung maturation
What are some considerations in the management of PTL?	Empiric Abx, hydration, tocolysis, and steroids if fetus less than 34 weeks to increase fetal lung surfactant.

EMERGENCIES DURING POSTPARTUM

What are some important things to know about each emergency and their treatment:	
Thromboembolic disease	Leading cause of maternal death; greatest risk is first few weeks after labor; commonly will have SOB, CP, or shock; **Tx:** heparin or low molecular weight heparin (LMWH), avoid warfarin

Postpartum hemorrhage	Related to one fourth of all postpartum deaths; most occur within the first 24 hours; consider uterine atony/rupture and inversion; **Tx:** if rupture = operative intervention; atony = oxytocin; inversion = manual reduction
Postpartum infection	Most common postpartum complication; fever, tenderness, and discharge (foul odor); **Tx:** drainage, debridement, and Abx
Peripartum cardiomyopathy	Present similar to dilated congestive heart failure (DOE, cough, CP); echo will show massively dilated chambers; poor prognosis if no cause is found; **Tx:** diuretics and fluid restriction
Amniotic fluid embolus	Very acute onset and high mortality; typically permanent neurological sequelae; **Tx:** supportive with high O_2 and monitor for DIC

VAGINAL BLEEDING IN REPRODUCTIVE WOMEN (NONPREGNANT)

Define the following types of vaginal bleeding:	
Abnormal bleeding	Vaginal bleeding outside one's regular cycle
Dysfunctional uterine bleeding (DUB)	Abnormal vaginal bleeding due to anovulation
Menorrhagia	Excessive bleeding or cycles >7 days
Metrorrhagia	Irregular vaginal bleeding
Menometrorrhagia	Excessive irregular bleeding
What are some important elements to gather in the history of anyone who presents with vaginal bleeding?	Menstrual history; last menstrual period (LMP); age of menarche; any pattern of abnormal bleeding; vaginal discharge; if they are pregnant (always do a pregnancy test)
What are important elements to gather in the sexual history of a patient?	Number of sexual partners in the past; contraception use and type; history of venereal disease
What are some important causes of vaginal bleeding to consider in reproductive females who are not pregnant?	Pregnancy; exogenous hormone use; coagulopathy; thyroid dysfunction; polycystic ovary syndrome; leiomyomas; adenomyosis

What are some important causes of vaginal bleeding in menopausal women?	Endocervical lesions; endometrial cancer; exogenous hormone use; atrophic vaginitis
What are some important elements in the physical examination to perform?	A thorough vaginal exam; examine for possible GI or GU bleed
What are some considerations in management of vaginal bleeding in reproductive non-pregnant women?	Make sure patient is not unstable (bleeding); rule out pregnancy; OCPs are often effective to control bleeding; NSAIDs are also effective in management

PELVIC/ABDOMINAL PAIN IN NONPREGNANT WOMEN

What is the single most important test to do on a female who presents with pelvic/abdominal pain?	Pregnancy test
What are some important points to know about each of the following causes of pelvic pain in nonpregnant women:	
Adnexal torsion	It is a surgical emergency; often will have a history of cysts or tumors; exercise or intercourse often precede pain; often sudden onset of unilateral pelvic pain; U/S and early surgical consult is important
Ovarian cysts	They may twist, bleed, or rupture; sudden unilateral pelvic pain is common; must distinguish from possible ectopic; U/S is an important diagnostic tool
Endometriosis	Very common cause of cyclic pain; most common in the third decade of life; often due to ectopic endometrial tissue; often can get a normal pelvic exam
Adenomyosis	Often present with dysmenorrhea; most common in the fourth decade of life; pelvic can show a symmetrical large uterus; analgesic and hormonal Tx often help
Leiomyomas (fibroids)	It is a smooth muscle tumor; most common in fourth decade of life; typically estrogen-growth responsive; U/S will often detect fibroids; analgesic and hormonal Tx often help as well

VULVOVAGINITIS

What is the definition of vulvovaginitis?	It is the inflammation of the vulva/vagina.
What are some signs and symptoms of vulvovaginitis?	Discharge, itching, and odor
What are some differentials to consider?	Infection; foreign body; allergic contact; atrophic vaginitis

List some important points and treatment for each of the following:

Candida albicans	Dysuria, dyspareunia, and itching common; wet prep of KOH to detect (shows hypae); **Tx:** topical azole drugs or nystatin
Trichomonas vaginalis	High association with gonorrhea; is almost always sexually transmitted; associated with adverse outcomes in pregnancy; slide prep will show teardrop trichomonads; **Tx:** metronidazole
Gardnerella vaginalis	Is almost always sexually transmitted; commonly have malodorous discharge; associated with PROM and endometritis; **Tx:** metronidazole
Genital herpes	Commonly caused by HSV-2 serotype; neonatal infection can be devastating; commonly have painful ulcers; avoid normal delivery if active lesions; **Tx:** acyclovir or valacyclovir
Foreign body	Very common in children and adolescents; often have malodorous discharge; children tend to insert tissues and objects; adolescents tend to leave tampons; can grow *E coli*/anaerobes if left too long; **Tx:** remove object
Contact vulvovaginitis	Contact dermatitis due to irritant (ie, tights); typically have erythema and edema; commonly have superimposed infection; **Tx:** R/O infection, remove irritant, and steroids in severe cases

PELVIC INFLAMMATORY DISEASE

What is the definition of pelvic inflammatory disease (PID)?

It is a wide spectrum of infections of the upper female genital tract.

What are the two most common causes of PID?

1. *Neisseria gonococcus*
2. *Chlamydia trachomatis*

What is the pathophysiology of PID?

It is an infection that starts at the cervix and vagina and ascends up the genital tract.

What are some immediate complications of PID?

Salpingitis; endometritis; tubo ovarian abscess

What are some long-term complications of PID?

Infertility; chronic pain; ectopic pregnancy

Name some risk factors of PID:

Multiple sexual partners; history of STD; sexual abuse

What are some signs and symptoms of PID?

Lower abdominal pain, vaginal bleeding or discharge, dyspareunia, but can also be asymptomatic.

What are the minimum CDC criteria for the diagnosis of PID?

Cervical motion tenderness; lower abdomen, adnexal, or uterine tenderness

What are some other diagnostic criteria for PID?

Fever; WBC >10,000/mm^3; elevated CRP or ESR; cervical infection with *N torsion gonorrhea* or *C trachomatis*

What are some common pelvic exam findings in PID?

Cervical motion, uterus, and adnexal tenderness

What is the name of the condition of RUQ tenderness and jaundice in the setting of PID?

Fitz-Hugh-Curtis syndrome

What are some important considerations in the management of PID?

Rule out ectopic pregnancy; cervical swab for culture and stain; empiric treatment for gonorrhea/chlamydia; patient education

What are some criteria for admission?

Ovarian abscess; unable to tolerate PO; peritonitis; failed outpatient management

CLINICAL VIGNETTES—MAKE THE DIAGNOSIS

31-year-old G4P5 who just delivered twins followed by two whole placentas now has copious vaginal bleeding; PE: 800 cc blood in 5 min with boggy uterus. What is the treatment?

Uterine atony. Oxytocin

21-year-old woman with no PMH presents via EMS with a syncopal episode, patient has now regained consciousness and mentions she was treated for an STD 2 years ago; pelvic: cervical motion tenderness; labs: positive pregnancy test. What is the most likely diagnosis, and what are some aspects of the work up?

Ectopic pregnancy. Quantitative HCG, ultrasound

37-year-old G2P1 at 10 weeks presents with severe nausea and emesis along with vaginal bleeding; pregnancy test: β-hCG >100,000 mIU/mL; U/S: no fetal activity and a snowstorm appearance

Gestational trophoblastic disease

67-year-old woman with PMH of HTN, CAD, and DM presents with painless vaginal bleeding, but otherwise has no other associated symptoms such as dysuria or abdominal pain; vaginal exam: no cervical tenderness

Endometrial cancer

19-year-old G0P0 presents with a sudden onset of left-sided pelvic pain soon after her basketball game, aside from a past history of an ovarian cyst, is otherwise healthy

Adnexal torsion

23-year-old G5P0 at 6 weeks presents with painless vaginal bleeding, but is otherwise healthy; pelvic: closed OS

Threatened abortion

41-year-old G2P1 at 21 weeks presents with headache as well as lower extremity swelling; PE: BP of 150/95, +1 lower extremity edema; labs: significant proteinuria

Preeclampsia treatment

6-year-old woman is brought in by her mother for a vaginal malodorous discharge, but is otherwise healthy

Foreign body

34-year-old woman in her third trimester presents after an MVC with vaginal bleeding along with painful vaginal contractions; fetal heart monitoring: late decelerations

Abruptio placentae

19-year-old female in her postpartum period presents with dyspnea and chest pain that she describes as sharp and worse on inspiration; PE: unremarkable

Pulmonary embolism

What diagnostic test is ideal for the patient above?

Testing: both CT of the chest or V/Q scan can carry substantial radiation exposure and choice will depend on gestational age. Should consult radiology about best choice. May just obtain lower extremity dopplers and treat based on this test.

CHAPTER 15

Trauma

GENERAL APPROACH

What is the leading cause of death in people under the age of 45 in the United States?

Trauma: 50 million deaths occur each year, half of which require medical attention

Name the top three trauma-related deaths:

1. Motor vehicle crashes (MVCs)
2. Falls
3. Burns and fire-related death

What are the three peak times for traumatic death and common causes of death for each:

First peak (immediate death)

Laceration of the great vessels; airway obstruction; massive head injury; high C-spine injury

Second peak (minutes-few hours)

Tension pneumothorax; cardiac tamponade; multiple injuries leading to hypovolemia; ruptured spleen; massive hemothorax

Third peak (days-weeks)

Sepsis; pneumonia; multi-organ failure

What constitutes the primary survey?

ABCDE: airway, breathing, circulation, disability (neuro), exposure

What is the single most important intervention to perform on all trauma patients at the scene?

Airway control with C-spine stabilization

What are some techniques to secure an airway in the field?

Endotracheal tube; esophageal tracheal combitube; laryngeal mask airway (LMA)

What is the procedure of choice to secure an airway on the field?	Endotracheal intubation
What is the most reliable method to confirm ET placement?	Visualization of the tube passing the cords
Although pediatric airway management is similar to adults, what are the two differences?	1. Children <9 years; use uncuffed ET tube 2. Children <12 years; needle cricothyrotomy preferred over open cricothyrotomy
What surgical techniques can one use if intubation fails?	Needle cricothyrotomy; open cricothyrotomy
What are some methods used to quickly assess volume status in trauma patients?	Skin color, capillary refill, pulse, mental status
What type of access should be done in any trauma patient?	Intravenous (IV) access with two large-bore IVs for rapid fluid infusion
What is the difference between colloid and crystalloid fluids?	Colloid: contains protein such as albumin and fresh-frozen plasma; crystalloid: normal saline (NS) or lactated ringers
Are there any advantages of colloids over crystalloid fluids?	Small amount of colloid can produce a large change in intravascular volume, crystalloids are just as effective/cheaper
What is the optimal fluid type and amount that should be used for initial resuscitation?	2 L of lactated ringers or normal saline
What is minimal amount of circulating volume loss to produce signs of shock?	30%
What is the first sign of hemorrhagic shock?	Tachycardia and cutaneous vasoconstriction
What is shock?	Shock is when tissue perfusion is decreased to the point that the oxygen demands of the body are not met.
What category of shock is most common in trauma?	Hypovolemic shock (Hemorrhagic)
What is the crystalloid to blood replacement ratio (mL)?	3:1

Table 15-1

Hemorrhagic Shock	Class I	Class II	Class III	Class IV
Blood loss (mL)	0-750	750-1500	1500-2000	>2000
Blood volume loss (%)	0-15	15-30	30-40	>40
Pulse rate (bpm)	<100	>100	>120	>140
Blood pressure	Normal	Normal	Decreased	Decreased
Pulse pressure	Normal	Decreased	Decreased	Decreased
Fluid replacement	Crystalloid	Crystalloid	Crystalloid and blood	Crystalloid and blood
Mental status	Anxious	Anxious	Confused	Lethargic

Name five potential spaces where life-threatening bleeding can occur:	1. Chest 2. Abdomen 3. Pelvis 4. Bilateral femoral fractures 5. External wounds
What clinical index is widely used to assess neurological function?	Glasgow Coma Score (GCS)
Name the three components of GCS:	1. Eye opening 2. Verbal response 3. Motor response
What GCS score is indicative of severe neurological impairment?	8 or less—"eight and it's too late"
Which component of the GCS has the highest prognostic factor?	Motor response
What are some examples of blunt trauma?	MVC, falls, assaults, and automobile v. pedestrian accidents
What are some major factors that determine severity of injury in an MVC?	Ejection from vehicle; size and weight of vehicle; location of victim in vehicle; use of restraints; direction of impact; speed of car at impact
Do lateral impacts or frontal impacts carry a higher mortality in an MVC?	Lateral impacts
What is the mortality rate of a fall from 30 ft?	50%

What is the basic pattern of injury in falls where victims land on their feet?	Calcaneus fracture; acetabular fracture; L1-L2 compression fracture
What are some examples of penetrating trauma?	Guns, knifes, arrows, swords
What are some major determinants of injury in gunshot wounds (GSW)?	Mass of projectile; muzzle velocity; location and trajectory of projectile

HEAD INJURY

What is the most common cause of death from trauma?	Central nervous system (CNS) injury
What is the most common mechanism of injury?	MVC
What are the five layers of the scalp?	Skin Connective tissue Aponeurosis Loose areolar tissue Pericranium
What is the thinnest region of the skull that is most vulnerable to injury?	Temporal region
What are the three layers of meninges?	1. Dura mater 2. Arachnoid membrane 3. Pia mater

Name the regions of the brain:	Cerebrum
	Cerebellum
	Brainstem
	   Midbrain
	   Pons
	   Medulla

What portion of the brainstem controls the reticular activating system?	Midbrain; pons
What portion of the brainstem controls the cardiorespiratory system?	Medulla
What is the Monroe-Kellie doctrine?	The total volume in the intracranial compartment is constant

| Why is the Monroe-Kellie doctrine significant in head injury? | The intracranial space does not tolerate acute increases in pressure, such as tumors, bleeding, or brain swelling, very well and has limited ability to compensate. |

Table 15-2 Intracranial Pressure

Normal	<10 mm Hg
High	>20 mm Hg
Severe	>40 mm Hg

What is the threshold of intracranial pressure at which compression or ischemia can occur?	20 mm Hg
What is the goal for the management of ICP?	Maintaining ICP less than 20 mm Hg and consider the placement of ventriculostomy catheter (can drain and monitor ICP)
What are some indications for ICP monitoring?	GCS of less than 8 or abnormal CT consistent with elevated ICP
What is the hallmark of brain injury?	Altered level of consciousness
Which head-injured patients should a head CT be strongly considered?	Intoxicated, anticoagulated, altered mental status, loss of consciousness, elderly, all but the most minor head-injured patients.

Traumatic Brain Injury

| What is the most important evaluation to do in a person suspected of traumatic brain injury (TBI)? | Serial GCS evaluation |
| What are the three categories of TBI and prevalence? | 1. Mild: 80%
 2. Moderate: 10%
 3. Severe: 10% |

Categories of TBI:

Mild TBI	GCS of 13 to 15: with or without loss of consciousness (LOC)
Moderate TBI	GCS of 9 to 12: may be confused with possible focal neuro deficits
Severe TBI	GCS of 8 or less: can have mortality up to 40% and most survivors have significant disabilities

What are some considerations in the management of TBI?

Rapidly diagnose any mass lesions followed by evacuation; treat any extracranial lesions; avoid any secondary insults such a hypotension, hypoxia, or hypoglycemia

During a physical exam, what particular findings should one look for?

GCS, pupillary changes, extremity movement, and ability to answer questions

What is the initial diagnostic test of choice in the setting of TBI?

Noncontrast CT of the head

What are five key features to look for on head CT?

"Blood Can Be Very Bad"

Blood

Cistern

Brain

Ventricles

Bone

What is the period of risk highest for posttraumatic seizure?

First week after head trauma

What are some risk factors for a posttraumatic seizure?

Cortical contusions, subdural hematoma, penetrating head injury, epidural hematoma, and depressed skull fractures

Does anticonvulsant prophylaxis play a role?

Some recommend that phenytoin be given in the first week

What is the general disposition of those with mild head injury?

Most can be safely observed and discharged if normal neuro function

What role does serial neuroassessment have in mild head injury?

Patients with mild head injury can still develop posttraumatic intra-cerebral hematomas and brain swelling.

What factors are considered when deciding if a patient with mild head injury can return to play sports?

No return to play in current game, step-wise return to play after medical evaluation, and resolution of symptoms

What is a major risk factor for sustaining head injuries?

History of head injuries

What is a cerebral concussion?

Head injury that typically results in transient alteration of neurologic function such as LOC, amnesia, dizziness, disorientation.

What are some other signs and symptoms of a head concussion?

Headache, nausea, vomiting, or confusion that often resolves rapidly.

What is the typical finding on a head CT?

Usually normal

What is a cerebral contusion?

Similar to a concussion, but with more pronounced neurologic findings

What are some signs and symptoms of a cerebral contusion?

More severe neurologic findings such as obtundation or coma

What regions of the brain are typically injured in a cerebral contusion?

Frontal and temporal regions

What are some findings on a head CT?

Lesions at the site of impact (coup contusion) and site opposite the impact (contrecoup contusion)

What is an important delayed complication of cerebral contusions?

Cerebral hematoma or edema

What are some considerations in the management of cerebral contusions?

Typically admit for observation; monitor for signs of greater intracranial pressure; if suspect complication, repeat head CT

What is diffuse axonal injury (DAI)?

Serious diffuse brain injury as a result of traumatic deceleration frequently causing a persistent vegetative state in patients.

What are some signs and symptoms of DAI?

Prolonged coma often with posturing and autonomic dysfunction (poor prognosis)

What does the initial CT show for patients who end up with DAI?

Normal in most cases

What are some later CT findings for DAI?

Intraventricular hemorrhage; hemorrhage within the corpus callosum; small focal areas of low density; edema

What are some considerations in the management of DAI?

Admission with neurosurgery consultation

Penetrating Head Injuries

Distinguish between high-velocity and low-velocity injuries:	High velocity: bullets; low velocity: arrows and knives
Is there a difference in prognosis between high- and low-velocity injuries?	Yes—high-velocity projectiles carry a very high mortality
Why are high-velocity injuries more destructive?	Kinetic energy of the projectile destroys surrounding tissues
What is the initial treatment for high-velocity injuries to the head?	IV antibiotics and anticonvulsants
Injury to which part of the brain carries the highest mortality?	Basal ganglia, brainstem, and posterior fossa
What is the primary factor that determines prognosis in low-velocity injuries?	Location of the brain injury
What is the initial management for a protruding object in the head such as knife or arrow?	Leave it alone! The risk of hemorrhage mandates removal in the OR in a controlled fashion

Skull Fractures

Where do linear skull fractures most commonly occur?	Temporal bone
What is the most important complication to monitor in skull fractures?	Intracranial hematoma

What are the treatment guidelines for the following types of skull fractures:

Open skull fractures	Operative intervention
Depressed skull fractures	Operative intervention to raise fragment
Linear skull fractures (nondepressed)	None
Is surgery generally required for depressed skull fractures?	No
When is surgery typically indicated in depressed skull fractures?	Cerebrospinal (CSF) leak or cosmetic purposes

What are the physical findings associated with basilar skull fractures?	CSF leak (rhinorrhea/otorrhea); periorbital ecchymosis (Raccoon eye); hemotympanum; retroauricular ecchymosis (Battle sign)
Why are CSF leaks significant?	Increased risk of meningitis
Is there a role for prophylactic antibiotic use in CSF leak?	Evidence that it may increase mortality (can use in consultation with neurosurgery)

Hemorrhage

What is the most common artery involved in an epidural hematoma?	Middle meningeal artery
What is the classic clinical scenario for an epidural hematoma?	Initially LOC followed by a lucid period then a coma (only in 1/3 of cases)
What are some signs and symptoms of an epidural hematoma?	Mass effect on brain: contralateral hemiparesis with a fixed dilated pupil on the side of the hematoma.
What is the classic CT finding of an epidural hematoma?	Biconvex lesion; associated temporal/parietal skull fracture
What are some considerations in the management of an epidural hematoma?	Immediate neurosurgical consultation; often requires surgical decompression; consider use of mannitol to decrease ICP if evidence of herniation
What is the mechanism by which subdural hematomas occur?	The bridging veins often tear resulting in intrinsic bleeding and mass effect.
What are some groups that are more susceptible to subdural hematomas?	Alcoholics; elderly (smaller brain volume)
What are some signs and symptoms of a subdural hematoma?	Mass effect: range from headache to lethargy and coma; severity will depend on several factors such as rate of bleeding.
What is the classic CT finding of a subdural hematoma?	Crescent-shaped lesion
What are some considerations in the management of a subdural hematoma?	Immediate neurosurgical intervention; distinguish from chronic subdural, which may not require immediate surgery; also consider reversal of any acquired coagulopathy and seizure prophylaxis in conjunction with neurosurgery

NECK TRAUMA

Why are penetrating neck injuries so dangerous?	The high density of vascular, neurologic, and visceral structures
Name some important structures in the neck:	
Vascular	Carotid, jugular, vertebral, and great vessels
Nerves	Vagus, phrenic, sympathetic trunk, and cranial nerve (CN) V
Others	Esophagus, trachea, thoracic duct, and lung apices
What is the mortality rate of a missed neck injury?	10-15%
Which muscle of the neck, if not violated, can neck injuries be managed non-operatively?	Platysma
What is the first concern in any penetrating neck injury?	Airway injury
What are some factors that determine if a patient should be managed operatively or non-operatively?	Stability, presence of hard signs, and location of the injury (zones)
What are some examples of hard signs which may mandate immediate intervention?	Stridor, bleeding, and expanding hematoma
What are some soft signs?	Hoarseness, dysphonia, hemoptysis, dysphagia, and odynophagia

Table 15-3 Three Zones of the Neck

Zone I	Clavicles to cricothyroid membrane
Zone II	Cricothyroid membrane to angle of mandible
Zone III	Above the angle of the mandible

What mandates exploration?	Zone II injury with hard signs or an unstable patient

What is the standard diagnostic approach in a stable patient who has a neck injury?

Angiography, EGD/barium swallow, and tracheobronchoscopy

What are the three most common mechanisms of blunt injury to the neck?

1. Direct impact (car/all-terrain vehicle)
2. Excessive flexion/extension
3. Compression (hanging)

What are some common causes of airway loss?

Expanding hematoma, thyroid fracture, tracheal fracture, and aspiration

What are some contraindications to orotracheal intubation in neck injury?

Obvious pharynx, larynx, tracheal, or facial injury causing upper airway obstruction

What are some signs and symptoms of a missed esophageal injury?

Fever, tachycardia, and sepsis

What diagnostic test should be done in a patient who has an abnormal GCS with a normal CT in the setting of a neck injury?

Four-vessel angiogram

BONY ORAL-MAXILLOFACIAL INJURY

What potential injuries are associated with an oral-maxillofacial (OMF) injury?

Cervical spine injury

What is the first consideration when doing the primary survey?

Airway obstruction

What are some considerations in an OMF injury?

Important to consider life-threatening bleeding in the thoracic, abdominal, head, and extremities.

What percentage of OMF injuries does mandibular fractures make-up?

2/3

What is the most common mechanism of injury in mandibular injury?

Blunt trauma from assaults

What parts of the mandible are most susceptible to injury?

Condyle, angle, and symphysis

How can airway obstruction occur in the setting of OMF injury?

Dentures/avulsed teeth and aspiration of blood

What are the most common maxillofacial injuries that occur in blunt trauma?

Nasal and mandibular fractures

What is the most common physical finding of mandibular fractures?

Malocclusion of the teeth

What are some physical findings of a mandibular fracture?

Malocclusion, trismus, pain, ecchymosis of the floor of the mouth, and deviation on opening the mouth.

What is important to remember about mandibular fractures?

Fracture in two or more places greater than 50%

What is the diagnostic test of choice for mandibular fractures?

Dental panoramic view (Panorex), but many often will obtain a CT with facial reconstruction to evaluate for other facial injuries.

What are some considerations in the management of mandibular fractures?

Consultation with ENT for reduction/fixation; open fractures typically require antibiotics; update tetanus status

What are some common causes of mandibular dislocations?

Excessive opening of mouth (ie, laughing) and trauma

What are some signs and symptoms of a mandibular dislocation?

Jaw displaced to unaffected side, difficulty talking/eating, and anterior open bite

What is commonly done for a mandibular dislocation?

Manual reduction

What is the main reason to obtain an x-ray evaluation?

Evaluate for possible associated fractures

What areas of the face define the midface?

Orbital-zygomatic-maxillary complex

What is the typical mechanism of injury to the midface?

Blunt trauma from MVC and assault

What does mobility of the maxillary dentition indicate?

Maxillary fracture

What physical finding is most common in midface fractures?

Malocclusion

What physical maneuver can confirm a suspected midface fracture?

Grab anterior maxillary teeth and check for mobility of the hard palate

What specific exam should be done for any orbital/zygomatic complex?

A thorough ophthalmology exam

What diagnosis is suspected when one finds a firm fixed point of limitation in gaze?	Entrapment of extraocular muscles
Does an anterior or posterior epistaxis bleed more?	Posterior
What fractures are CSF leaks associated with?	Midfacial, frontal sinus, and basilar skull fractures
What is the radiographic test of choice for midface fractures?	CT scan with facial reconstructions
When does osseous healing begin to occur?	7 days
What are the four stability points of the zygoma?	1. Frontal bone 2. Maxilla 3. Temporal bones 4. Frontozygomatic structure
What is the general physical finding in zygomaticomaxillary (ZMC) fractures?	Depression at the site of trauma, pain on mandibular opening, or limited opening.
What is the goal of the treatment of ZMC fractures?	Surgical reduction without internal fixation
What is an orbital blowout fracture?	Fractures of any of the orbital walls secondary to direct impact of the globe.
What is the weakest section of the orbital complex?	The medial wall and floor of the orbit
What are some signs and symptoms of an orbital blowout fracture?	Enophthalmos, upward gaze palsy, diplopia, pain on eye movement, and V_2 paresthesia.
What is the mechanism by which extraocular eye movement dysfunction occurs?	Extraocular muscle entrapment
What is the radiographic test of choice?	Modified—Waters view
What are some considerations in the management of an orbital blowout fracture?	Patients should get ophthalmology follow up; persistent entrapment requires surgery; consider antibiotics if sinus involvement; most often can be managed conservatively
What are maxillary fractures commonly due to?	Direct trauma to the face (large force)

How are maxillary fractures commonly classified?

    LeFort I   Palate-facial

    LeFort II   Pyramidal

    LeFort III   Craniofacial

What are some signs and symptoms of maxillary fractures?

Midface mobility, malocclusion, CSF rhinorrhea, and soft-tissue swelling

What is the preferred imaging modality for maxillary fractures?

CT with facial reconstruction

What are some considerations in the management of maxillary fractures?

ABCs; CT to delineate the extent of fracture; antibiotics if sinus involvement; can often be managed conservatively if non-displaced

SPINAL TRAUMA

Name three common mechanisms of spinal cord injury (SCI):

1. MVC
2. Violence
3. Falls

What is the average age and gender of those who sustain spinal cord injury?

Males with an average age of 30

What is the percentage of patients with SCI who also have other significant injuries?

50%

What fraction of SCI involves the cervical spine?

50%

What is the general treatment for spinal column injury?

Treatment centers on preventing further injury through fixation (internal or external).

Describe the general composition of the spinal column.

7 cervical vertebrae, 12 thoracic vertebrae, 5 lumbar vertebrae, and 5 fused sacral vertebrae

Is the thoracic column flexible?

No—it is relatively stiff due to the orientation of facets and interaction with ribs.

Is the lumbar column flexible?

Yes

Why is this important?

The point where the thoracic column and lumbar column meet creates a point where shear stress occurs making T12-L1 a site of common spinal trauma.

What are the three main spinal cord pathways and what fibers are carried?

1. Dorsal column pathway: position/vibration
2. Spinothalamic pathway: pain/temperature
3. Corticospinal pathway: movement

What is the "three columns of the spine" theory?

A way to visualize the biomechanical stability of the spine.

Name the boundaries of the three columns of the spine:

Anterior column

Anterior 2/3 vertebral body and anterior longitudinal ligament

Middle column

Posterior 1/3 of the vertebral body and posterior longitudinal ligament

Posterior column

Facets and posterior ligaments

How many of the columns must be compromised in order for the spine to be considered unstable?

2 out of 3

What is the consequence of an unstable vertebral column?

Spinal cord injury with possible paralysis

Does spinal column injury equate to spinal cord injury?

Not necessarily

What are some examples of different types of mechanisms that can cause spinal injury?

Axial loading; hyperflexion/extension; rotational injuries

What is complete spinal cord injury?

Irreparable damage with no discernible motor, sensory, or electrical function.

What is incomplete spinal cord injury?

Some preservation of sensory and/or motor function

What are some examples of incomplete spinal cord injury:

Posterior cord injury

Loss of vibration and position

Anterior cord injury

Loss of bilateral motor, temperature, and pain

Central cord injury	Loss of pain and temperature; motor loss (arms > legs)
Brown-séquard injury	Ipsilateral loss of position/vibration/motor; contralateral loss of pain/temperature
What presumption must be made with any tenderness along the spinal column?	There is vertebral fracture and/or ligamentous injury
For which patient populations should one have a higher index of suspicion for spinal injury?	Elderly, children, patients with osteoporosis, and history of cancer with metastatic bone lesions
What is SCIWORA?	Spinal cord injury without radiographic abnormality.
Why is this more common in children?	Elasticity of their ligaments
Why is this more common in the elderly?	Underlying cervical stenosis
When should a cervical spine injury be suspected?	High-speed MVC; fall >15 feet; any injury above the clavicle; diving accidents; electrical injury; in any scenario where trauma may be possible such as found down unresponsive
What are the most commonly missed fractures in the cervical spine?	C1-C2 and C7-T1
What are the NEXUS criteria?	Decision rule that helps to identify those patients with a low probability of injury to the cervical spine.
List the Nexus criteria:	Normal alertness; not intoxicated; no cervical midline tenderness; no focal neurologic deficits; no distracting injuries
What are the three views recommended to assess cervical injury?	1. Lateral 2. AP 3. Open mouth (odontoid view)
Which view is commonly obtained?	Lateral alone is adequate in 90% of cases
True or False: as long as all cervical vertebrae are visualized, the film is adequate.	False. C7-T1 must be visualized

What are the ABCS of assessing lateral films?	Alignment Bone Cartilage Soft tissue
Alignment	Anterior/posterior/spinolaminar lines
Bones	Check vertebral body heights
Cartilage	Intervertebral spaces and facets
Soft tissue	Look for soft tissue swelling, especially at C2-C3
When is a CT of the cervical spine indicated?	Inadequate plain films; fracture on films; unconscious patients; high suspicion of cervical spine injury
When is an MRI indicated?	Any evidence of neurological deficits
What is a flexion-extension film useful for?	A flexion-extension film is typically used to assess ligamentous injury and often not obtained in the acute phase of trauma as it requires movement of the spine.
What is a Jefferson fracture?	Axial loading injury that results in a C1 burst fracture with C2 involvement.
What is an odontoid fracture?	
Type I	Involves the tip of the dens of C2
Type II	Traverses the dens at the junction of the body of C2
Type III	Involves C2 vertebral body
Which odontoid fracture carries the worse prognosis?	Type II
What is a clay shoveler's fracture?	Avulsion of the spinous processes of C6-T3 typically the result of flexion injury or direct trauma (managed conservatively).
What is a hangman's fracture?	Bipeduncular fracture of C2 due to excessive extension.
What is the most common site of injury in the thoracolumbar injury?	T12-L1
When are AP and lateral films indicated?	Patient complains of pain in the region or mechanism of injury is suggestive.

What is a compression fracture?	Anterior vertebral body fracture
What is a burst fracture?	Vertebral body is crushed in all directions.
What is a chance fracture?	Fracture due to excessive flexion such as an MVC where a seatbelt is used.
What are some considerations in the management of spinal injury?	Protect the cord by stabilization; CT scan if plain films are indeterminate or if high suspicion of injury
What is the role of steroids in the setting of spinal injury with evidence of spinal injury?	While there is controversy; advocates often will initiate high-dose steroids.

THORACIC TRAUMA

What fractions of patients who sustain injury to the chest require thoracotomy?	10-25%
What findings are indicative of serious chest injury?	JVD, subcutaneous emphysema, and tracheal deviation
If a patient with penetrating thoracic injury loses vital signs in the ED, what procedure is indicated?	Emergent thoracotomy
If a patient with blunt thoracic injury loses vitals in the ED, would one still do a thoracotomy?	Rarely—the mortality rate approaches 100%
What are some primary indications for urgent thoracotomy or sternotomy?	Massive hemothorax; cardiac tamponade; aortic tear; esophageal disruption or perforation; open pneumothorax
Name the six immediate life-threats associated with thoracic trauma:	1. Airway obstruction 2. Tension pneumothorax 3. Massive hemothorax 4. Open pneumothorax 5. Flail chest 6. Cardiac tamponade
What are the six potential life-threatening injuries to the thoracic region?	1. Blunt cardiac injury 2. Traumatic rupture of the aorta 3. Major tracheobronchial injury 4. Diaphragmatic injury 5. Esophageal perforation 6. Pulmonary contusion

Open Pneumothorax

What is the most common cause?	Penetrating injuries
What size is considered a large defect?	>3 cm
What are some signs and symptoms of an open pneumothorax?	Hypoxia; hypoventilation; tachypnea; chest pain
Should the wound be fully closed with a dressing?	No! It can convert to tension pneumothorax
What is the standard treatment?	Tube thoracostomy on the affected side
What is the proper chest tube size?	16-24 French (F) is adequate for a pneumothorax but a larger one may be required for hemothorax (32-40) where clots may be a concern.

Tension Pneumothorax

What is the pathogenesis of tension pneumothorax?	Air is able to enter, but not leave the pleural space which is essentially a ball-valve effect.
What are some signs and symptoms of tension pneumothorax?	Decreased breath sound on one side; tracheal deviation (late finding); subcutaneous emphysema; hypotension
What immediate action is required for tension pneumothorax?	Needle decompression followed by tube thoracostomy (the latter is the mainstay treatment where the former should only be utilized if a tube is not possible).
Where do you insert the needle for needle decompression?	Second intercostal space mid-clavicular line or fifth intercostal space in anterior axillary line.
What is the consequence of decompression?	Converts tension pneumothorax into simple pneumothorax

Hemothorax

What is a common cause of a hemothorax?	Damage to the primary or secondary pulmonary vessels

How much blood can each hemothorax contain?	Up to 3 L
What will the chest x-ray show?	Total opacity of the affected side "white out"
How much fluid is required before an upright CXR can detect it?	200 mL
What are some signs and symptoms of a hemothorax?	Dullness to percussion, diminished breath sounds, and decreased tactile fremitus.
Does every hemothorax need surgical intervention?	No—most are self-limited
What are some indications for surgical intervention for a hemothorax?	Initial chest tube output is >1500 mL; 50% hemothorax; chest tube output is >200 mL/h over 4 to 6 hours

Flail Chest

What are some signs and symptoms of a flail chest?	Paradoxical movement of the flail segments with spontaneous breathing.
What are some common radiographic findings in a patient with flail chest?	Two or more consecutive rib fractures with pulmonary contusions
What is the patient at high risk for?	Pneumothorax and hemothorax
What is the test of choice?	CXR (CT more accurate)
What are some considerations in the management of a flail chest?	Low threshold for ET intubation; pain control; pulmonary physiotherapy; high-risk for respiratory failure requiring intubation
What are some indications to intubate?	$PaCO_2$ >55 mmHg; respiratory fatigue; PaO_2 <60 mmHg, but clinical picture is more important than numbers

Cardiac Tamponade

What is cardiac tamponade?	Build-up of fluid in the pericardial space that obstructs effective cardiac pumping.

What is the mechanism by which cardiac tamponade commonly occurs?	Penetrating injuries
What is the most common site of perforation that leads to cardiac tamponade?	Right atrium
What is Beck Triad?	Hypotension; muffled heart sounds; jugular venous distension (JVD)
How commonly does Beck triad present?	1/3 of cases
What is a characteristic ECG finding of cardiac tamponade?	Electrical alternans
What are some other physical exam findings that may help make the diagnosis?	Pulsus paradoxus, tachycardia, diastolic collapse with bedside ultrasound
What are some considerations in the management of cardiac tamponade?	Ultrasound can rapidly diagnose tamponade; pericardiocentesis is temporizing until an open thoracotomy can be done in the OR; IV fluids

Traumatic Aortic Rupture

Where is the site where the aorta most commonly tears?	Ligamentum arteriosum
What is the most common mechanism by which aortic rupture occurs?	Sudden deceleration (ie, falls and MVCs)
About how many patients who sustain a traumatic aortic rupture die at the scene?	Up to 90%
What are some signs and symptoms of a traumatic aortic ruptures?	Retrosternal pain; pulse deficits; dyspnea; upper extremity hypertension with decreased femoral pulses
How is the diagnosis of aortic rupture usually made?	History is very important, but an abnormal CXR along with confirmative studies can confirm the diagnosis.
What are some findings on CXR that may be suggestive of aortic rupture?	Superior mediastinum widening, indistinct aortic knob, rib fractures, left hemothorax, and left apical pleural cap.

What are two confirmative tests that can be used to help diagnose aortic rupture?	1. CT 2. Transesophageal echocardiography (TEE)
What are some considerations in the management of aortic ruptures?	Immediate surgical repair with early involvement of CT surgery; regulate BP to minimize tear

Blunt Cardiac Injury

How does a blunt cardiac injury (BCI) commonly occur?	Commonly occurs in a high-speed MVC where the chest strikes the steering wheel.
What is the spectrum of BCIs?	Myocardial concussion; myocardial contusion; tamponade; cardiac rupture
How do myocardial concussions occur?	Typically the heart will strike the chest wall with no permanent cell damage
What are some possible complications of myocardial concussions?	Hypotension; dysrhythmias
What are some considerations in the management of a myocardial concussion?	Most will resolve without treatment; ACLS for dysrhythmias (ie, asystole)
What is a myocardial contusion?	More forcible injury to the myocardium from impaction against the chest wall.
What ventricle is more commonly injured in a myocardial contusion?	Right ventricle
What are some commonly used tests to distinguish low-risk from high-risk patients?	ECG; echocardiography
What are some considerations in the management of a myocardial contusion?	Observation for low-risk patients (normal vitals, asymptomatic, etc); admit patients with conduction abnormalities

Pulmonary Contusion

What is a very common mechanism by which a pulmonary contusion occurs?	Deceleration (MVCs or falls)
What is an important point to know about a pulmonary contusion?	Most common potential lethal chest injury

What are some signs and symptoms of a pulmonary contusion?	Dyspnea, tachycardia, tachypnea with chest wall tenderness
What are some common CXR findings in a pulmonary contusion?	Typically show patchy alveolar infiltrate to consolidation, usually within 6 hours of injury.
What are some potential complications of a pulmonary contusion?	Pneumothorax; pneumonia (most significant)
What are some considerations in the management of a pulmonary contusion?	Adequate ventilation to allow healing; low-threshold for intubation; liberal pain control to allow adequate breathing, coughing, and clearing secretions

Diaphragmatic Injury

Which side of the diaphragm is most injured in blunt trauma?	Left, presumably due to an inherent weakness on that side
Which side of the diaphragm is most injured in penetrating trauma?	Left, since most assailants are right-handed
What is the operative approach for diaphragmatic repair?	Celiotomy
What are some sequelae of a diaphragmatic rupture?	Herniation of viscous that can result in SBO, incarceration, and compression of the heart/lungs (these can present years later).
True or False: most diaphragmatic tears will spontaneously heal.	False: most ruptures will require operative repair

ABDOMINAL TRAUMA

How should any abdominal injury be categorized?	Blunt versus penetrating trauma
What are three common causes of blunt trauma?	1. MCV 2. Falls 3. Assaults
What are two common causes of penetrating trauma:	1. Gunshot wounds 2. Knives

Name three regions of the body to consider in abdominal trauma:	1. Peritoneal cavity 2. Retroperitoneal cavity 3. Pelvis
What is the general management for anyone who is hemodynamically unstable or has peritoneal signs?	Immediate operative intervention, should not attempt further diagnostic tests such as a CT
What are the goals of exploratory laparotomy?	Immediate hemostatic control; control any GI contamination; operative repair→damage control
What are some signs of hypotension?	Tachycardia, obtundation, cool skin, poor capillary refill
What are peritoneal signs caused by?	Irritation to the peritoneal lining caused by leaking of blood, bile, or gastric juices
What are some peritoneal signs?	Guarding, rigid abdomen, or rebound tenderness
What percentage with hemoperitoneum will have acute findings?	80%
What is the most important thing to do in a suspected abdominal injury with an initial benign exam?	Serial abdominal exams
What other factors in a trauma situation are associated with abdominal injury?	Chest injury, pelvic fracture, hypotension, and lap belt contusion.
What is the most commonly injured solid organ?	In blunt trauma: spleen; in penetrating trauma: liver
What is the most commonly injured hollow organ?	Small bowel
What are the three diagnostic tests to consider in any trauma to the abdomen?	1. Diagnostic peritoneal lavage (DPL) 2. Focused abdominal sonography for trauma (FAST exam) 3. CT
Diagnostic peritoneal lavage (DPL):	
What is it	Catheter placement in the peritoneal cavity to see if there is any initial return of fluid. If nothing, place liter of warm saline and drain
Indications	Hemodynamically unstable with questionable abdominal injury

Accuracy	Sensitivity and specificity is 95%
Advantages	Fast, accurate, and inexpensive
Disadvantages	Invasive, nontherapeutic rate of 20%, inability to pick up retroperitoneal and isolated diaphragmatic injuries
Criteria for positive DPL	10 mL of gross blood; >100 k RBC/mm^3; >500 WBC/mm^3; Bacteria, bile, and food particles

FAST exam:

What is it	Use of sonography to rapidly detect hemoperitoneum
Indications	Hemodynamically unstable with questionable abdominal injury
Accuracy	Sensitivity and specificity is between 70 and 90% and poor at detecting solid organ damage
Advantages	Fast, accurate, and inexpensive
Disadvantages	Poor at detecting solid organ damage and small amounts of blood, operator dependent

CT:

What is it	CT is used to evaluate solid organ injury and detect fluid/air in cavity
Indications	Hemodynamically stable patients that require abdominal evaluation
Accuracy	92-98%
Advantages	Noninvasive, evaluates solid organ injury, and retroperitoneal injuries
Disadvantages	Radiation exposure, expensive, time, variable in detecting hollow viscus injury

Blunt Abdominal Injury

What is the first thing to assess in blunt trauma to the abdomen?	ABC! Airway with proper ventilation and hemodynamic stability
What is the most common abdominal organ injured in blunt trauma?	Spleen followed by liver

If the patient is unstable and has obvious peritoneal signs, what is the next step?	Proceed directly to exploratory laparotomy
What is the test of choice in a stable patient with suspected abdomen injury?	CT
What are the major forces involved with blunt trauma?	Crushing, shearing, and stretching

Name the possible organ injury with the following:

Right lower rib fracture	Liver and gallbladder
Left lower rib fracture	Spleen and left kidney
Epigastric contusion	Duodenum, pancreas, and mesentery
Anterior pelvis fracture	Bladder and urethra

Penetrating Abdominal Injury

What percentage of those with GSW require operative repair?	Up to 90%
What proportion of those with knife wounds require operative repair?	1/4
What abdominal organ is most commonly injured in penetrating injuries?	Liver
Is CT useful in GSW?	When the patient is stable it is useful to locate injuries. Exploratory laparotomy is diagnostic and therapeutic.
What proportion of those with anterior stab wounds has peritoneal violation?	2/3
Of those with peritoneal violation, how many require operative management?	1/2
What are some indications for Ex Lap in a knife wound?	Hemodynamically unstable, peritoneal signs, obvious evisceration
What is recommended in a stable patient with a knife wound?	Local wound exploration

GENITOURINARY TRAUMA

What is the cause of most genitourinary (GU) injuries?	Blunt trauma
What is a key marker of GU injury?	Hematuria
What are the possible locations of GU injury?	Upper: kidney and ureter; lower: bladder and urethra
What should be done with macroscopic hematuria?	Further evaluation
What percentage of renal injuries will have no hematuria?	15%
Is initial return of blood on catheter placement concerning?	No—is usually catheter-related
What should be done with microscopic hematuria?	Further imaging if mechanism of injury is suggestive
What are some diagnostic tests utilized?	
Urethrogram	In any suspected urethral injury
Cystogram	Important to fully inflate bladder to detect small injuries and done postvoid
CT	Test of choice for renal trauma
US	Useful for detecting renal parenchyma injury
Intravenous pyelogram	Largely replaced by CT for staging
What percentage of renal injury is from blunt trauma?	80%
What percentage of those with blunt renal trauma will lose a kidney?	5%
What is the general management of renal trauma in patient that is stable?	Nonoperative management
What is the indication of operative management?	Unstable, hilar/pedicle damage, and significant blood in urine
How common is post-injury hypertension?	15%

What is the cause of most bladder injury?	Blunt trauma
What percentage of blunt trauma is extraperitoneal?	80%
What are the indications for a cystogram?	Gross hematuria; seatbelt contusions; pelvic fractures
What are extraperitoneal injuries associated with?	Fractures of superior and inferior pubic rami
What are intraperitoneal injuries associated with?	Seatbelt injuries with a full bladder
What is the general treatment for bladder rupture?	Ex Lap followed by primary repair
How are most extraperitoneal bladder injuries managed?	Bladder drainage alone
What is the cause of most ureteral injuries?	Penetrating trauma
What are the diagnostic tests of choice?	Intravenous pyelogram (IVP) and CT
What is the general treatment?	Primary repair and stenting
What is the cause of most urethral injuries?	Blunt trauma
What are posterior urethral injuries associated with?	Pelvic fracture
What are anterior urethral injuries associated with?	Penetrating trauma
What is the diagnostic test of choice?	Urethrogram

ORTHOPEDIC TRAUMA

What is a dislocation?	Total loss of articulation contact
What is a subluxation?	Partial loss of articular congruity

What is a fracture?	Break (partial or complete) in continuity of the bone
Open fracture	Fracture with skin disruption
Closed fracture	Fracture with intact skin
What are some important descriptions for bone fractures?	Pattern, morphology, location, open versus closed, and neurovascular status
Name the possible nerve injury:	
Anterior shoulder dislocation	Axillary nerve injury
Humeral shaft	Radial nerve injury
Posterior hip dislocation	Sciatic nerve injury
Proximal fibular fracture	Peroneal nerve injury
What percent of fractures are missed in patients with multiple injuries?	10 to 15%
What are important components of the physical exam?	Inspection, palpation, range of motion, and neurovascular status
What is the initial diagnostic test of choice?	Plain films with at least two views, above and below the injury
What is the initial treatment in any fracture?	Reduction; splint; irrigate and update tetanus status if open
Are antibiotics recommended in open fractures?	Yes
What is the purpose of splinting?	Immobilization to help control bleeding, pain, and prevent secondary injuries
Should open fractures be splinted?	Yes—splint as they are
What is important to assess after splinting of all fractures?	Neurovascular status
What is the gold standard of splinting?	Plaster of paris
What is the mangled severity scoring system (MSSS)	A scoring system to help guide whether a severely mangled limb should be salvaged versus amputated.
What are the primary components of the MSSS?	Skeletal/soft tissue injury; limb ischemia; shock; age
What is the most important factor when deciding amputation versus salvage?	Neurologic status

What is the primary issue in any open fracture?	Infection (osteomyelitis)
What is an important management issue in addition to antibiotics?	Adequate debridement
What is the initial treatment for open fractures?	Early irrigation; early splinting
What is a typical antibiotic regiment?	First generation cephalosporin or aminoglycoside; penicillin if the injury is barnyard related; update tetanus
Is operative management indicated for open fractures?	Yes—OR within 6 to 8 hours

Hip dislocations:

Are anterior or posterior dislocations more common?	Posterior
What is a common cause of posterior hip dislocations?	MVC
What percent of hip dislocations result in sciatic nerve injury?	10 to 15%
What is the most concerning complication?	Avascular necrosis (AVN)
What is done to avoid AVN?	Immediate reduction (closed or open)

Femoral neck/shaft fractures:

What is a common cause of a femoral neck fracture in children/adults?	High-energy impacts (ie, MVC)
What is a common cause of a femoral neck fracture in elderly patients?	Low-energy impacts (ie, falls)
What is a particular concern?	AVN
What is the typical treatment?	Open reduction internal fixation (ORIF)
What is important to rule-out in femoral shaft fractures?	Femoral neck fractures
What is the typical treatment for femoral shaft fractures?	Intramedullary nailing

Knee dislocations:

What is a common cause of knee injury?	Any high-force impact
How often is the popliteal artery injured?	20%
What is typically done to assess the popliteal artery?	Arteriography

What nerve injuries are typically associated with knee dislocations?	Tibial and peroneal nerve
What is the initial management in knee dislocations?	Urgent reduction

Tibial shaft fractures:

What is a common cause of tibial shaft fractures?	High-energy impacts (ie, MVC)
What syndrome are tibial fractures associated with?	Compartment syndrome
What is the typical treatment for tibial shaft fractures?	ORIF

Pelvic fractures:

What is the primary concern in any pelvic fracture?	Life-threatening bleeding
How many liters of blood can the pelvis accommodate?	5 L
What do pelvic fractures have a high association with?	Head, thoracic, and abdominal trauma
What is the mortality rate of open pelvic fractures?	50%
What is the mortality rate of major vascular disruption secondary to pelvic fractures?	75% (it is rare)
What is the initial management in suspected pelvic fractures?	External fixation of the pelvis with sheet or other device
What type of physical exam is important to perform in a pelvic fracture?	Detailed lower neurovascular exam

Hand trauma:

What is important to know about hand injuries?	It is the most commonly injured part of the body
What assumption must be made if there is a laceration, swelling, and ecchymosis?	Neurovascular damage
What is the Allen test used for?	To test patency of both the radial and ulnar artery
What is the function of the radial nerve?	Extension of the wrist
What is the function of the median nerve?	Flexion of the wrist and opposition of thumb
What is the function of the ulnar nerve?	Assist in flexion of wrist

What is compartment syndrome? A significant increase in pressure within a confined space (fascia).

What is a common cause of compartment syndrome? Any injury that leads to swelling within a confined space.

What percent of compartment syndromes do fractures account for? 50%

What fractures are highly associated with compartment syndrome? Tibial fractures

What factors are associated with compartment syndrome? Reperfusion after 4 to 6 hours of swelling; significant crush injury; combined arterial and venous injury

What is a common physical finding on exam? Pain out of proportion followed by paresthesias

What are some common signs on exam? Swelling with pain on passive stretching

What is the first sign of compartment syndrome? Loss of function

What is a late finding of compartment syndrome? Loss of pulses

What is the primary treatment for compartment syndrome? Fasciotomy

What is the typical pressure reading for fasciotomy? Greater than 30 mm Hg or 20 to 30 mm Hg with symptoms

What is rhabdomyolysis? It is any type of significant muscle injury that results in release of toxins.

What is the most feared complication of rhabdomyolysis? Kidney failure

What is the most sensitive marker for muscle damage? Serum creatine phosphokinase (CPK)

What is the most common cause of rhabdomyolysis in trauma? Anything that causes muscle death such as crush injuries.

What is the most common cause of rhabdomyolysis in non-trauma situation? Neuroleptic malignant syndrome; malignant hyperthermia; medications (statins)

What is the pathogenesis of rhabdomyolysis?	Fe: forms toxic oxygen metabolites; myoglobin: forms casts to clog renal tubules
What is the primary objective in treatment?	Adequate fluids to ensure renal perfusion
What is another concern in rhabdomyolysis?	Hyperkalemia
What is the standard treatment for hyperkalemia?	Calcium to stabilize the heart; sodium bicarbonate and insulin to drive potassium into cells; kayexalate to bind potassium
What is the prognosis of rhabdomyolysis?	Generally good with most patients returning to baseline kidney function in 3 to 4 weeks
What is the role of alkalization with rhabdo?	Generally adequate volume restoration is sufficient

TRAUMA IN PREGNANCY

What are some important points about trauma in pregnancy?	Most common cause of nonobstetric death; fundamentally treating two patients; management centers around mother; "What is good for the mother is good for the child"
What are some important caveats about the airway management of pregnant trauma patients?	Continuous 100% oxygen (especially fetal Hb); pulse oximetry monitoring; RSI as required with normal medications; thoracostomy at third or fourth ICS
What are some important points in regards to circulatory status in pregnant trauma patients?	Increased HR/low BP may reflect normal pregnancy, not shock; avoid supine position; LR is preferred over NS; blood transfusion if failure to improve after 2 L of crystalloid
What is supine hypotension syndrome?	When the gravid uterus compresses the IVC, decreasing preload and CO when in supine position.
What is the optimal position to lay a pregnant trauma patient?	Left lateral decubitus position

What are some important components of the obstetric evaluation?	Uterine contractions; fetal heart rate (ensure between 120 and 160); fundal height and tenderness; fetal movement; pelvic and rectal examination
When is a fetus considered viable?	Gestational age >24 weeks
What is the most common cause of fetal death following blunt trauma?	Placental abruption
What are some clinical features of placental abruption?	Uterine tenderness, fetal distress, abdominal cramps, and signs of shock
What is the most important preventative measure in MVCs?	*Properly* worn seatbelts

CLINICAL VIGNETTES—MAKE THE DIAGNOSIS

20-year-old man is brought in by his parents due to concern for a head injury after a football game where the patient ran head first into another player, patient mentions he "blacking-out" but otherwise feels fine; PE: no focal neurologic deficits; CT of head: normal

Concussion

20-year-old man who was at a swimming hole is brought in by EMS in cervical precautions. Patient dove from a very high cliff and mentions he could not extend his arms in time; cervical films: C1 ring is fractured in multiple places

Jefferson fracture

71-year-old woman with a history of atrial fibrillation was seen in the ED 3 days ago after falling and hitting her head, had a negative CT of the head at that time, but now is presenting with confusion; PE: unremarkable neuro exam; CT of head: now shows a crescent-shaped lesion

Subdural hematoma

21-year-old man was stabbed in the chest is currently complaining of dyspnea; PE: decreased breath sounds and hyperresonance to percussion on the right chest

Simple pneumothorax

You arrive at a scene involving a car accident. A patient was just extricated and is in obvious respiratory distress with suspected cervical spine injury. Is nasotracheal intubation the procedure of choice?

No—orotracheal intubation, with in-line cervical spine stabilization, is still the procedure of choice

16-year-old man who was involved in a gang fight and hit squarely in the back with a bat is now complaining of back pain; PE: remarkable tenderness of his upper back; thoracic plain film: avulsion fracture of the spinous process of T2

Clay shoveler's fracture

23-year-old woman is emergently brought in by helicopter to the trauma bay to be evaluated for a gunshot wound to the chest, patient is intubated and suddenly becomes hypotensive; PE: jugular venous distension and muffled heart sound

Pericardial tamponade

45-year-old alcoholic man is brought into the ED by EMS after being knocked unconscious in a bar fight, patient was awake and demanding to go home, but now is unconscious; CT of head: biconvex lesion near the temporal bone

Epidural hematoma

67-year-old woman is brought into the ED by paramedics after being extricated from a high-speed car collision, she is unconscious and unresponsive; PE: posturing; CT of head: widely scattered neuronal damage

Diffuse axonal injury (DAI)

21-year-old man is brought in by EMS from a high speed MVC where the patient was extricated and his side passenger was found dead; PE: fractured left femur and multiple scalp lacerations; CXR: fracture of the first rib and 9 cm superior mediastinum along with an indistinct aortic knob

Traumatic aortic dissection

15-year-old woman with no PMH presents to ED with an injury to her left eye. Patient mentions she was hit squarely in her left eye with a softball and now has double vision; PE: inability of the left eye to gaze upward; modified Waters view: air fluid level in maxillary sinus

Orbital floor fracture with entrapment

26-year-old woman is brought in by EMS after being hit by a car and thrown 15-ft across the street, patient is currently hypotensive and unresponsive to fluids; FAST exam: blood in the Morrison pouch

Abdominal injury requiring laparotomy

9-year-old girl is brought into the ED by her mother after being kicked in the chest by a horse at the ranch, the patient is having difficulties breathing and in significant pain; CXR: frank consolidation on the right lung

Pulmonary contusion

22-year-old man is brought into the ED by EMS after a diving accident where the patient dove head first and lost consciousness, patient is now in cervical precautions and is A&O x4; PE: clear fluid is slowly dripping down his left ear

Basilar skull fracture

52-year-old man with no PMH presents after an MVC where his chest hit the steering wheel and has complaints of chest pain; PE: tenderness with palpation of the anterior chest wall; ECG: sinus tachycardia; labs: normal cardiac enzymes

Myocardial concussion

22-year-old man with a gunshot wound to the chest is currently being evaluated in the trauma bay when he suddenly becomes hypotensive and in respiratory distress with distended neck veins

Tension pneumothorax

CHAPTER 16

Environmental Exposures

HIGH-ALTITUDE ILLNESSES

What are some examples of high-altitude illness?

Acute mountain sickness (AMS)
High-altitude pulmonary edema (HAPE)
High-altitude cerebral edema (HACE)

Define various heights of altitude:

High

8,000-10,000 ft (Denver = 5,281)

Very high

10,000-18,000 ft (Highest point in continental US = 14,505)

Extremely high

>18,000 ft (Everest = 29,029)

Name some groups at risk for high-altitude illness:

Mountaineers, military personnel, and aviators

What is acute mountain sickness (AMS)?

It is a syndrome of high-altitude illness that is characterized by a vague set of symptoms similar to carbon monoxide poisoning or influenza caused by acute exposure to low partial pressure of oxygen at high altitude.

Is AMS life-threatening?

No—but it is important to monitor for symptoms of HAPE and HACE which are life-threatening.

What are some risk factors in the development of AMS?

Rate of ascent/altitude acclimatization
History of altitude sickness
Duration of stay at a given altitude

What are some signs and symptoms of AMS?

Most important feature is a headache with other associated symptoms such as fatigue, insomnia, and nausea.

What is the most important step to consider when AMS is suspected?	To immediately stop further ascent to allow acclimatization
What are some indications for immediate descent?	Evidence of developing HAPE or HACE, such as severe pulmonary edema or neurologic symptoms such as confusion or ataxia.
Name some treatment options for moderate AMS:	Acetazolamide Oxygen Dexamethasone for more severe cases
Name some preventative measures to help avoid AMS:	Slow ascent Hydration Avoidance of opioids Acetazolamide may have a role in prevention of AMS
What is the mechanism of action of acetazolamide?	It is a carbonic anhydrase inhibitor that induces a bicarbonate diuresis, causing a metabolic acidosis and increasing ventilation and oxygenation.
What are some contraindications of acetazolamide?	Sulfa allergy and pregnant women
What is the most common fatal form of high-altitude illness?	High-altitude pulmonary edema (HAPE)
What are some important features of HAPE?	Typically more common at higher altitudes (>12,000 ft) Presentation can be sudden Increased risk with children and younger adults
What are some signs and symptoms of HAPE?	Dry cough Fatigue with minimal exercise Dyspnea at rest Cyanosis Tachycardia and tachypnea
What are some important tests to consider if available?	Chest radiograph: typically bilateral patchy infiltrate Electrocardiogram: may show tachycardia, right heart strain, and abnormal P wave morphology

What is the differential diagnosis of HAPE?	Pneumonia Pulmonary embolism Bronchitis
What is the most critical action in the management of HAPE?	Early recognition
Name some treatment options for HAPE:	Rest Oxygen Descent (mandatory if above is not possible) Hyperbaric chambers (stimulate descent if unable to move patient)
Name some preventative measures to help avoid HAPE:	Nifedipine Slow ascent
What is high-altitude cerebral edema (HACE)?	The most severe form of high-altitude illness which typically is associated with AMS or HAPE
What are some signs and symptoms of HACE?	Severe headache Altered mental status Ataxia (most sensitive sign) Seizures Papilledema Retinal hemorrhage
Name some treatment options for HACE:	Oxygen Descent Hyperbaric chambers (stimulate descent if unable to move patient)

DYSBARISM

What is the definition of dysbarism?	They are illnesses that result from exposure to increased ambient pressure that typically affect scuba divers but anyone who works in pressurized environments.

What are some elements to obtain in a diving history?	Activities prior to diving (especially flying) Location (ie, ocean) Equipment used and gases breathed (ie, air only or oxygen enriched mixture) Maximum depth, time spent, and rate of ascent Dive problems
Name three common gases typically used in diving:	Oxygen Nitrogen Helium
What are some complications associated with diving injuries?	Hypothermia Submersion injuries (near-drowning) Decompression sickness Nitrogen narcosis Barotrauma Envenomation
What is nitrogen narcosis?	Also known as "rapture of the deep," is a reversible alternation in consciousness from increased tissue nitrogen concentration.
Is nitrogen narcosis life-threatening?	The effects are reversible on ascent, but morbidity results from impaired judgment that may place the diver at risk.
What is the most common form of diving injury?	Barotrauma
What is barotrauma?	It is an injury caused by pressure changes, due to inability to equalize the pressure within air-filled structures to the ambient pressure of the environment.
Name some examples of barotrauma:	Pulmonary barotraumas Pneumomediastinum Pneumothorax Ear barotrauma
Name a life-threatening complication of diving:	Air gas embolism (AGE)—one of the leading causes of death after drowning in scuba divers when air dissolving in serum at high pressure returns to gaseous state during ascent.

What are two serious sequelae of AGE?	Myocardial infarction and cerebral vascular accident
What are some signs and symptoms of AGE?	Can include dysrhythmia, cardiac arrest, change in mental status, and visual disturbances often sudden and dramatic
What are some critical actions in the management of AGE?	100% oxygen Recompression therapy (hyperbaric oxygen chamber) Ground transport to chamber to avoid low ambient air pressures during flight
What is another complication of diving?	Decompression sickness (DCS)
What is DCS?	It is a spectrum of illness from the release of nitrogen bubbles due to rapid reduction in pressure.
What are two groups of DCS?	Type 1 DCS: muscles and skin Type 2 DCS: any other organ system
What are some signs and symptoms of Type 1 DCS?	Also known as the "bends." Pain to the arms or legs that ranges from mild discomfort to severe pain or may present as pruritus alone.
What are some considerations in the management of Type 1 DCS?	Recompression therapy (hyperbaric oxygen chamber) Monitor for progression to Type 2 DCS
Name three examples of Type 2 DCS:	1. Cerebral DCS (common in aviators) 2. Spinal DCS (common in divers) 3. Pulmonary DCS
What are some signs and symptoms of cerebral DCS?	Seizures Visual disturbances (blurry, diplopia, etc.) Hemiplegia
What are some signs and symptoms of spinal DCS?	Paresthesia Neurogenic bladder Incontinence
What are some signs and symptoms of pulmonary DCS?	Cough Dyspnea Chest pain

What are some important points in the management of Type 2 DCS?	Reduce size of bubbles via recompression
	100% oxygen to wash out nitrogen
	Admission for observation
	Further recompression if new symptoms

HYPOTHERMIA

What are the classifications of hypothermia?	
Mild hypothermia	Core temperature 32-35°C
Moderate hypothermia	Core temperature 28-32°C
Severe hypothermia	Core temperature below 28°C

What are some examples of physiological response to hypothermia?	Shivering
	Increased adrenal activity (hypertension/tachycardia)
	Increased thyroid activity
	Peripheral vasoconstriction

| Is a standard thermometer useful to measure the degree of hypothermia? | No—most cannot measure temperatures below 34-35°C |

| What methods are used to measure temperature in hypothermia? | Rectal probe, tympanic membrane probe, and bladder probe |

What are some predisposing factors for hypothermia?	Typically a combination of impaired regulation, decreased heat production and increased heat loss
	Environmental exposure
	Malnutrition
	Sepsis
	Medications
	Toxicologic
	Hypothyroidism
	Hypopituitarism

What are some signs and symptoms of mild, moderate, and severe hypothermia:	
Mild hypothermia (32-35°C)	Confusion
	Shivering
	Hypertension
	Tachycardia (initially)

Moderate hypothermia (28-32°C)	Decreasing level of consciousness
	Dilated pupils
	Loss of shivering mechanism
	Bradycardia
	Atrial fibrillation
	Cold diuresis
Severe hypothermia (below 28°C)	Coma
	Asystole at <20°C
	Oliguria
	Pulmonary edema
What are some complications of hypothermia?	Lactic acidosis
	Bleeding diathesis
	Rhabdomyolysis
	Bladder atony
	Frostbite
What are the characteristic ECG findings of hypothermia?	Initial tachycardia followed by bradycardia
	Prolongation of all intervals
	Osborne wave (J-point elevation)
What is paradoxical undressing?	Considered a preterminal event where clothes may be discarded due to maladaptive response to severe hypothermia, often mistaken as a victim of sexual assault.
List the important changes that occur in the following laboratory values in hypothermic patients:	Arterial blood gas: falsely show higher oxygen and carbon dioxide levels and lower pH than actual value
	Complete blood count: hematocrit falsely increases 2% for every 1°C drop in temperature
	Coagulation studies: may see prolonged Pt and PTT which corrects with warming of patient (but clotting truly is dysfunctional while patient is cold)
What are some general issues to consider in the management of the hypothermic patients?	Continuous core temperature recording—rectal probe is most practical
	Avoid aggressive handling of the patients (irritable myocardium)
	Critical to address volume status and use of warmed crystalloids (40°-42°C)
	Most medications are temperature dependent

What are two important diagnoses to consider if a patient fails to rewarm?

Myxedema coma

Adrenal insufficiency

Treatment options for hypothermia

Table 16-1 Treatment Options for Hypothermia

Rewarming Modalities	Techniques	Comments
Passive external	Insulate patient	Non-invasive
		Allow gradual rewarming
Active external	Heating pads/blankets Warm fluids	Useful for moderate hypothermia
Active internal	Warm peritoneal dialysis	Invasive
	Extracorporeal rewarming-cardiopulmonary bypass	Consider if patient is in extremis
	Airway rewarming	
	Thoracic lavage	

HEAT ILLNESS

What is hyperthermia?

It is an elevation of core temperature above 37°C usually due to the combination of excessive heat production, inability to dissipate heat, and dysregulation.

Name four ways that heat is dissipated:

1. Convection (heat carried away via bulk flow/currents)
2. Conduction (heat dissipation without flow)
3. Radiation
4. Evaporation

What are some important differential diagnoses of hyperthermia?	Heat stroke
	Malignant hyperthermia (general anesthesia)
	Neuroleptic malignant syndrome (antipsychotic meds)
	Serotonin syndrome (antidepressants, opioids, stimulants, psychedelics, other drugs)
	Drugs (ie, cocaine)
	Metabolic (ie, DKA)
What are some risk factors for hyperthermia?	Poor physical fitness
	Obesity
	Drug use
	Dehydration
What are heat cramps?	They are brief and intermittent muscle cramps that appear to be related to a salt deficiency often from copious sweating and hydration with hypotonic fluids.
What is the management of heat cramps?	The typical response to salt solutions
What is the definition of heat exhaustion?	It is a form of heat illness characterized by either volume depletion (more common) or salt loss in the setting of heat stress.
What are some signs and symptoms of heat exhaustion?	Fatigue and headache
	Often have normal core temperature ($<40°C$)
	Orthostatic hypotension
	Tachycardia
	Intact mental status (primary distinction between heat stroke)
What does the management of heat exhaustion consist of?	Assess volume status and replete fluid
	Evaluate for electrolyte disturbances as indicated
What is the definition of heat stroke?	It is a life-threatening form of heat illness characterized by global dysfunction often associated with temperatures greater than 40.5°C.

What is the clinical hallmark of heat stroke?	Central nervous system dysfunction
List other common features of heat stroke:	Elevation of hepatic transaminases Can either be sweating or dry (dry due to compromised thermoregulatory response)
What are some characteristic features of classic and exertional heat stroke:	
Classic heat stroke	Occurs commonly in elderly and the sick Compromised thermoregulation Often with elevated ambient temperatures Anhidrosis
Exertional heat stroke	Common in young athletes Typically massive exogenous heat Exertional heat production Rhabdomyolysis Diaphoresis
When is the optimal time to begin cooling?	Immediately! Delay to immediate cooling increases mortality substantially
What are some modalities utilized in cooling?	Immersion therapy Cold pack to axillary areas and groin Mist and fan (limited success) Cooling blanket Gastric lavage (invasive and only if in extremis)

BURNS

What are some common causes of burns?	Thermal Chemical Radiation Electricity
Why are infants and elderly more susceptible to deeper burns?	Thinner skin
What is the "rule of nine"?	An estimation of total body surface area (BSA) affected

Table 16-2

Head and neck	9%
Each arm	9%
Anterior trunk	18%
Posterior trunk	18%
Each leg	18%
Perineum	1%

Can this be applied to infants and young children?	No—they have proportionally larger heads
What are some clinical features to know for each of the following types of burns:	
Superficial (First degree)	Confined to superficial layer of skin; erythema and pain, but no blisters; sunburn most common cause; heals in a week (does not scar)
Partial thickness (Second degree)	Epidermal and top dermis involved; blister formation is the hallmark; thermal liquids most common cause; heals in 2 weeks (some scarring)
Full thickness (Third degree)	Epidermal and full dermis involvement; charred with leather appearance; full skin and nerve permanently destroyed; healing will only occur with grafting/surgery
Musculoskeletal (Fourth degree)	Involvement of muscle/fascia/bone; necrosis is common; melted metal is common cause; debridement/amputation is common
What are some risk factors that make a burn patient more predisposed to complications?	Immunocompromised Extremes of ages Associated head injury Concomitant inhalation injury

Name some criteria of severe burns:

Greater than 5% BSA full thickness burn

Particular areas of the body such as face, joints, and perineum

Associated with trauma

Co-morbid conditions

What are some signs of an endangered airway in patient with thermal burn?

Respiratory problems (ie, stridor)

Carbonaceous sputum

Singed hair

Oropharyngeal swelling

What is involved in the initial management of burn patients?

Very close monitoring of airway, breathing, circulation (ABCs)

Low threshold for intubation

Aggressive fluid resuscitation in all but the most superficial of burns (per Parkland formula)

List some indications for endotracheal intubation of burn patients:

Significant orofacial burns

Hypoxia despite high-flow oxygen

Any upper airway obstruction

What total body surface area (TBSA) will typically require aggressive fluid resuscitation?

TSBA >20%

What is the Parkland formula?

Used to calculate the amount of fluid to give in the first 24 hours for moderate to severe burns.

How is the Parkland formula used in the first 24 hours?

LR at 4 mL × kg × BSA burn with the half given over the first 8 hours and the rest given over 16 hours.

What are some ways to measure response to fluid resuscitation?

Heart rate (<100 beats/min)

Urinary output (0.5-1 mL/kg/h)

Mentation

What are some other management guidelines to remember with burns?

Opioids are commonly used for pain control

Prophylactic antibiotics for select patients

Tetanus prophylaxis

Contact burn centers for major burns

Low threshold for performing an escharotomy with circumferential burns, as perfusion may be compromised

Where are circumferential burns most dangerous?

Thoracic chest (compromise breathing)

Extremities (compartment syndrome)

List some important burn-care guidelines for minor burns:

Debride any lost tissue or broken blisters

Blisters on sole or palms can be left intact

Cool compresses for burn area

Remove all jewelry

Topical antibacterial agent

Discharge with proper analgesia and follow-up

What are some commonly used topical antibacterial agents for minor burns?

Bacitracin

Polymyxin B

Silver sulfadiazine

ELECTRICAL, LIGHTNING, AND CHEMICAL INJURIES

What are some important facts about electrical injuries?

Leading cause of occupation-related death

It is more frequent in males between ages 20 and 40 years

Up to 45% of severe electrical injuries are fatal

What types of electrical injuries are there?

Low voltage (<1000 volts)

High voltage (>1000 volts)

Lightning

What tissues of the body have the highest resistance to electricity?

Bone

Fat

Tendon

Why is alternating current (AC) considered more dangerous than direct current (DC)?

Continuous muscle contraction which may cause the hand to grab the source of current closer to the body.

What are some factors that contribute to the severity of electrical injuries?

Current

Voltage

Resistance

Type of current (AC/DC)

Duration of contact

What are some features of exposure to AC currents?

Repetitive stimulation of muscles (spasms)

Prolonged contact with electricity

AC current prevents self-release from source

Vfib most common dysrhythmia

What are some features of exposure to DC currents?

Single muscle spasms (typically thrown)

Increased risk of trauma due to being thrown

Asystole most common dysrhythmia

What is the most common electrical injury seen in children younger than 4 years of age?

Mouth burns

What is potential complication of the above injury?

Delayed bleeding from the labial artery

What is the most common mechanism of injury in the following:

    Low voltage

Working on electrical circuits or appliances; biting into cords (infants); electrical weapons (taser)

    High voltage

Conductive object contact with high voltage overhead lines

    Lightning

In open field or near a tall object

What is a common cause of death in electrical injuries?

Cardiac arrhythmias

What are some important baseline studies to consider?

Complete blood count

Chemistry panel

Coagulation studies

ECG

Creatine kinase

Radiographic studies if suspect trauma

What are some other complications associated with electrical injuries?

Burns

Rhabdomyolysis

Myoglobinuria

Autonomic dysfunction

Vascular injuries

Cataracts

What are some critical actions in the management of electrical burns?

Aggressive fluid replacement for significant body surface area involvement

Cardiac monitoring in severe injuries

Monitor for compartment syndrome

Also monitor for rhabdomyolysis

Tetanus prophylaxis

Do all patients with electrical injuries require admission?

No—asymptomatic patients with normal ECG from low-voltage exposure typically can be discharged.

What are some important points to know about lightning injuries?

Leading cause of weather-related death

High-intensity bursts of short duration

Direct current (up to 1.5-2 billion volts)

Rarely causes deep tissue burns

Fluid loss is rarely an issue

What are some common mechanisms by which lighting can cause injury?

Thermal burns

Blunt trauma from blast impact

Direct lightning strike

Lightning strikes nearby object

What are some signs and symptoms of a lightning strike?

Missing clothes/shoes

Stunned

Evidence of burns (not always)

Unconsciousness

Headache

Vision/hearing problems

Tachycardia/hypertension

What is a feathering burn?

They are not true burns; it is a fern pattern on the skin due to electron showering from lightning.

What are some ECG findings in lightning injuries?

Sinus tachycardia

Transient ST segment elevation

Premature ventricular contractions

Atrial fibrillation

Asystole and ventricular fibrillation can also occur

What are important lightening-induced injuries to consider in the following organ systems:

Central nervous system

Seizures; loss of consciousness with amnesia; peripheral nerve damage

Cardiovascular system

Dysrhythmias pericardial tamponade; respiratory arrest

Ocular and auditory

Ruptured tympanic membrane is common; corneal damage; cataract formation

What are some critical actions in the management of lightning injuries?

Crucial to exclude traumatic injuries

Treat lightning burns like regular burns

Tetanus prophylaxis

Patients should be admitted with cardiac monitoring

Do all patients with lightning injuries require admission?

Most patients require observation

What are some points for the following types of chemical burns:

Acids

Acids are proton donors; coagulation necrosis by denaturing proteins; acid burns are typically more superficial

Bases

Bases are proton acceptors; severe injury (ie, liquefaction necrosis); bases tend to penetrate deeper into the tissue

What are some factors that determine the severity of a chemical burn?

Length of contact

pH of the agent

Concentration of the agent

Volume of the agent

What are some commonly encountered acids?

Hydrochloric acid

Sulfuric acid

Hydrofluoric acid

What are some commonly encountered bases?

Sodium hydroxide

Sodium hypochlorite

What route of exposure is associated with substantial morbidity and mortality?

Oral ingestion

What is the critical management with an ocular exposure to chemicals?

Immediate irrigation for the eyes should take place

What are some diagnostic tests to consider in chemical burns?

Usually none in minor chemical burns

Complete blood, chemistry panel, coagulation panel, and acid-base status in severe burns

Endoscopy for significant ingestions

DROWNING

Define the following:

Drowning

Death within 24 hours following submersion in a liquid medium

Near-drowning

Survival after suffocation in a liquid medium for at least 24 hours

What are some epidemiologic information to know about drowning and near-drowning?

Leading cause of unintentional death

Incidence highest in young male children

Drowning is much more common during the summer months

What are some medical problems associated with an increased risk of drowning:

Seizure disorder

Prolonged Q-T syndrome

Developmental delay

What are some risk factors of near-drowning?

Inability to swim

Use of illicit drugs or ethanol

Poor adult supervision

Risk-taking behavior

What are some complications of near-drowning?

Hypothermia

Acute lung injury

Bradycardia

Hypoxia

Disseminated intravascular coagulation

What is important to note about hypothermia in the setting of near-drowning?

It has a neuroprotective effect which may allow prolonged resuscitation without permanent sequelae (ie, do not stop CPR unless rewarming has taken place as patient is still not responding)

What are some neurologic complications of near-drowning?

Cerebral edema

Seizure

What are some poor prognostic factors in near-drowning?

Submersion >10 min

Time to CPR >10 min

Water temp >10°C; GCS <8

Resuscitation >25 min

What are some pre-hospital management issues in near-drowning?

CPR

Possible cervical injury should be suspected

Pulses are difficult to palpate in hypothermia

Remove wet clothing

Consider various rewarming techniques (see hypothermia section)

What are some diagnostic tests to consider in near-drowning?

Cardiac monitoring and an electrocardiogram

Arterial blood gases submersion victims

Chest radiograph

Computed tomography of the head is rarely indicated unless trauma is suspected

What are some critical management issues concerning near-drowning?

Pulmonary support is essential to optimize a favorable neurologic outcome

Supportive care is the mainstay

RADIATION

What are some potential sources of injuries following nuclear weapons?

Thermal injuries

Mechanical injuries from the blast

Ionizing radiation

Name a major source of radiation exposure to the public:

Radon gas

Define the following terms:

  Radioactivity:

It is an unstable atom (spontaneously decaying) which releases particles or energy.

  Nonionizing radiation:

All forms of the electromagnetic spectrum with frequencies equal to or less than UV light. Often produce local heat, but do not induce molecular damage.

Ionizing radiation:	Higher frequency electromagnetic energy, including x-rays and gamma rays which are sufficient energy waves to induce molecular damage.
Alpha particles:	They are composed of two protons and two neutrons that dissipate their energy quickly and have poor penetration.
Beta particles:	Smaller mass and charge than alpha particles, and have tissue penetration of up to 9 mm.
Gamma rays:	Have no mass and no charge and capable of penetrating tissue deeply.
What is the best indicator of significant radiation exposure?	Absolute lymphocyte count at 48 hours
Name some tissues that are sensitive to radiation injury:	Tissues with a rapid turnover are most susceptible such as gastrointestinal tract and bone marrow.
What are some methods health care providers can utilize to minimize radiation exposure?	Universal precautions Undress the patient immediately, and all clothing should be placed in radioactive waste sealed containers

CLINICAL VIGNETTES—MAKE THE DIAGNOSIS

21-year-old male presents with complaints of pain on the back of his skin, he mentions he was on the beach the day before; PE: skin on the back is red and tender to touch, but does not have blisters

First degree burn

Serving as the team physician on a mountain expedition, what is the most likely diagnosis based on the symptoms for each of the following members:

A few days into the ascent to 9,000 ft, a member is complaining of a bad headache, which is worse in the morning and has had trouble sleeping. Her neurologic exam is normal:

Acute-mountain sickness (AMS)

Four days into the ascent to 10,000 ft, a member complains of increasing dyspnea at rest, fatigue, headache, cough; PE: rales and cyanosis:

High-altitude pulmonary edema (HAPE)

A member is beginning to display odd behavior, seeing things that are not there and often acting confused. Neurologic exam shows ataxia:

High-altitude cerebral edema (HACE)

35-year-old male is brought into the ED via EMS for profuse sweating along with nausea while he was jogging at the beach several hours ago; PE: tachycardia, hypotension, normal temperature

Heat exhaustion

21-year-old female presents with severe muscle cramps in her calves after running 3 miles in hot and humid weather; PE: normal vitals

Heat cramps

CHAPTER 17

Toxicological Emergencies

TOXICOLOGY SUPPLEMENT

Table 17-1

Toxin	Antidote
Acetaminophen	N-Acetylcysteine (NAC)
Anticholinergics	Physostigmine
Arsenic	D-penicillamine/Dimercaprol
Benzodiazepines	Flumazenil
Beta-blockers	Glucagon
Black widow spider	*Latrodectus* antivenin
Botulism	*Botulinum* antitoxin
Brown recluse spider	*Loxosceles* antivenin
Calcium channel blockers	Calcium and high-insulin/euglycemic therapy
Cholinergics	Atropine
Coral snake bite	Elapid antivenin
Cyanide	Amyl nitrite, sodium nitrite, sodium thiosulfate, and hydroxocobalamin (B12a)
Cardioactive steroids (digoxin)	Digoxin-specific antibodies
Ethylene glycol	Ethanol or fomepizole (4-MP)
Heparin	Protamine sulfate
Hydrogen sulfide	Sodium nitrite, hyperbaric oxygen
Hypoglycemic agents	Dextrose
Iron	Deferoxamine
Isoniazid	Pyridoxine (B6)
Lead	Dimercaprol

(Continued)

Table 17-1 (*Continued*)

Toxin	Antidote
Methanol	Ethanol or fomepizole
Methemoglobin	Methylene blue
Methotrexate	Leucovorin
Opiates	Naloxone
Organophosphorus compounds	Atropine and pralidoxime
Crotalid (pit viper) bites	*Crotalidae* antivenin (CroFab)
Tricyclic antidepressants	Sodium bicarbonate
Warfarin	Vitamin K, FFP, PTC, or Factor VIIa

Table 17-2

Toxidromes	Temp	HR	RR	BP	Pupil	Diaphoresis	MS
Anticholinergic	↑	↑	+/–	–	↑	↓	Delirium
Cholinergic	–	–	+/–	+/–	+/–	↑	Normal
Sympathomimetic	↑	↑	↑	↑	↑	↑	Agitated
Sedative-hypnotics or ethanol	↓	↓	↓	↓	+/–	–	Depressed
Opioids	↓	↓	↓↓	+/–	↓	–	Depressed
Withdrawal from opioids	–	↑	–	↑	↑	↑	Normal-anxious
Withdrawal from sedative-hypnotics or ethanol	↑	↑	↑	↑	↑	↑	Agitated confused

GENERAL APPROACH

What is the first course of action for any patient who presents with a suspected ingestion?	Airway, breathing, circulation (ABC)
What are some other actions to take once ABC's have been established?	O$_2$ saturation for hypoxia; finger stick for glucose; assess vitals; accurate history
What two organ systems should be strongly considered?	1. Cardiovascular system (CVS) 2. Central nervous system (CNS)

Why concentrate on the CNS and CVS during the exam?

The most lethal adverse affects of an acute toxicological ingestion will involve the CVS and CNS.

What are some actions to consider for any poisoned patient?

Treatment is primarily supportive; always consider co-ingestions; call poison center for recommendations

What is gastric decontamination?

The use of various techniques to either remove the toxin or expedite passage through the GI tract to limit absorption.

Name five methods of gastric decontamination:

1. Ipecac
2. Activated charcoal (AC)
3. Whole bowel irrigation
4. Intestinal evacuants
5. Orogastric lavage

Are gastric decontamination methods routinely used in acute poisonings?

No—while historically commonly used, gastric decontamination is now used in select cases.

What are important things to know about ipecac?

Derived from plant alkaloids; single dose produces emesis in over 90% of patients; emesis typically occurs around 30 min

What are some indications for the use of ipecac?

Considered where AC binds poorly to toxins; in acute ingestions (<1 h); if removal of small amount has significant impact on outcome; patient should have intact gag reflex

What are some contraindications of ipecac?

Prior significant emesis; avoid if unconsciousness/altered mental state; nontoxic ingestions; avoid if ingested caustic substances

What are some complications with the use of ipecac?

Aspiration; lethargy; Mallory-Weiss tear; intractable emesis

What is gastric lavage?

Orogastric lavage with a large-bore tube to lavage with adequate volumes until clear while removing any remaining toxins.

What are some indications for the use of gastric lavage?

Consider if ingestion occurs within an hour; preferred for patients who have no gag; consider where a rapid deterioration is expected (ie, TCAs); also may consider if patient is intubated, an awake lavage is exceedingly difficult to perform

What are some contraindications for the use of gastric lavage?

Any caustic ingestions; if drug is most likely not in the stomach; any large foreign bodies or sharp objects

What are some complications of gastric lavage?

Aspiration; esophageal/gastric perforation; tension pneumothorax (should not be routinely performed)

What is activated charcoal (AC)?

Fine black powder produced by burning carbonaceous material that will result in a substance in a huge surface area to bind many substances.

While AC will bind many substances, what are some substances that AC does not bind well?

Strong acids and bases; metals (ie, iron and lithium); alcohols

What substances does multiple-dose activated charcoal (MDAC) prove effective in?

Theophylline; digoxin; phenytoin; carbamazepine

What are some contraindications of AC?

Any perforation; loss of airway reflex

What are some complications of AC?

Small bowel obstruction (very rare); aspiration

What is whole bowel irrigation?

Use of large volumes of fluid to cleanse the entire GI tract that will clear most matter (ie, toxin) within a few hours.

What substance is commonly used in whole bowel irrigation?

Polyethylene glycol (PEG)

What are some indications for whole bowel irrigation?

Toxic substance not well absorbed by AC; toxins with prolonged absorption; GI drug concealment ("body packing")

What are some contraindications of whole bowel irrigation?

Bowel obstruction and perforation; hemodynamic instability; evidence of no bowel activity

What are some toxins where hemodialysis (HD) is commonly indicated in severe cases?

MEAL
Methanol; Ethylene glycol;
Aspirin; Lithium

What are some indications where HD should be considered?

Sign of end-organ damage; failure of standard therapy; contraindication of standard therapy; predetermined drug concentration

What are some complications of HD?	Blood loss; hypotension; coagulopathy from heparin; decrease in platelets
What is urinary alkalinization?	A method of enhanced elimination by alkalinization of urine (via bicarb) to enhance ion trapping and elimination via urine.
What are some substances where urine alkalinization is indicated?	Aspirin; chlorpropamide; methotrexate; phenobarbital

OVER-THE-COUNTER DRUGS

Acetaminophen

What are some important things to know about acetaminophen (APAP)?	APAP is found in over 100 drug preparations; leading cause of liver failure requiring transplantation; leading drug involved in ingestion
What is the normal metabolism of APAP?	>90% conjugated to glucuronide/sulfate conjugates (eliminated by kidney after); 2% excreted by kidney unchanged; 5% oxidized to N-acetyl-*para*-benzoquinone imine (NAPQI)
What is the primary toxic metabolite of APAP that is responsible for liver necrosis?	NAPQI
What is the body's method to detoxify NAPQI under normal circumstances?	Glutathione binds to NAPQI preventing hepatocyte necrosis
What happens when there is an APAP overdose?	Conjugation and sulfation pathways are saturated which means more NAPQI is produced and overwhelms glutathione stores.
What is the toxic dose of APAP in an acute setting?	150 mg/kg (7.5 g) in an adult (24 h) lowest dose capable of causing hepatotoxicity
What is the time course of APAP toxicity:	
Phase 1 (0-24 h)	Anorexia, nausea, emesis, and elevated transaminases
Phase 2 (24-72 h)	Right upper quadrant (RUQ) pain, bilirubin and PT elevate, and transaminases begin to peak

Phase 3 (72-96 h)	Maximal hepatotoxicity (may get encephalopathy, jaundice, and death)
Phase 4 (96 h-2 weeks)	If patient survives fulminant hepatic failure total recovery of liver
What is the Rumack-Matthew nomogram?	Predicts the risk of toxicity assuming a one time ingestion with complete absorption
Based on the nomogram, what is the cut-off level in deciding to treat or not?	150 mg/mL (in the United States) at 4 hours
What are some limitations of applying the nomogram to an APAP overdose?	Does not apply to multiple ingestions; not applicable to chronic ingestions; also cannot apply the nomogram with ingestions past 24 hours
What is the antidote for APAP toxicity?	N-acetylcysteine (NAC)
What is the mechanism by which NAC works?	Precursor to cysteine then to glutathione; enhance sulfation of APAP; can act as free radical scavenger; glutathione substitute
When is the optimal time to give NAC following APAP overdose?	Within 8 hours (nearly 100% protective)
How is NAC administered?	Oral; IV (Both are equally effective if given within 8 h)
What are adverse reactions to IV NAC?	Anaphylactoid reaction; hypotension and death (very rare); artificial elevation of PT
What are some poor prognostic factors after APAP overdose?	pH <7.30; creatinine >3.3; grade III/IV encephalopathy (King College Criteria)

Salicylates

What are some of the therapeutic properties of aspirin (ASA)?	Antipyretic; analgesic; anti-inflammatory
What are some important things to know about ASA?	A significant source of poisoning; ASA can produce substantial toxicity/death; there are more than 200 products with ASA
What are some sources of salicylates?	Oil of wintergreen (methyl salicylate); arthritis/decongestants/cold preparations; keratolytics; Pepto-Bismol

What is the toxic level of ingestion for acute ASA poisoning?

300-400 mg/kg produces serious toxicity; 100 mg/kg/day for over 2 days will produce chronic toxicity

Table 17-3

Serum Salicylate Level	
50 mg/dL	Moderate toxicity
75 mg/dL	Severe toxicity
100 mg/dL	Potentially lethal (also indication for extracorporeal removal)

Do symptoms correlate well with serum concentrations?

Symptoms correlate better with CSF levels, treatment should be based on clinical picture

What are the two primary acid-base disturbances of ASA toxicity?

1. Respiratory alkalosis
2. Metabolic acidosis

What is the mechanism by which ASA toxicity occurs?

Uncouples ox-phos to produce fever; stimulates respiratory drive causing tachypnea; directly causes metabolic acidosis; acidosis will increase the V_d

What are some signs and symptoms of acute ASA toxicity?

Nausea, vomiting, tinnitus, agitation, delirium, seizure, and coma. It is a neurotoxin

What are some signs and symptoms of chronic ASA toxicity?

Nonspecific: altered mental status, lethargy, dehydration, and metabolic acidosis

What is the primary way in which death occurs in ASA overdose?

CNS overstimulation (seizure/hyperthermia); cardiovascular collapse; pulmonary edema

What are some important diagnostic tests to consider in ASA overdose?

Serum ASA concentration (serial levels more useful); ABG (for acid-base disturbances); potassium; renal function

Is there any use for AC in ASA overdose?

Yes—AC binds ASA well

What are some considerations in the management of ASA overdose?

ABCs is the first priority; care is primarily supportive; aggressive rehydration; sodium bicarbonate for acidosis

What is the treatment for moderate-severe ASA toxicity?	Sodium bicarbonate
What are indications for the use of sodium bicarbonate with ASA toxicity?	Concentration of 40-50 mg/dL and/or symptoms
What is a known complication of alkalization?	Hypokalemia
Why is hypokalemia problematic concerning ASA toxicity?	Hypokalemia will cause the kidneys to exchange hydrogen ions in the kidney filtrate in exchange for potassium→this will acidify the urine prolonging elimination of ASA
What is the function of sodium bicarbonate in ASA toxicity?	Alkalinize the urine (enhance elimination); essentially traps salicylic acid to be excreted; treats severe acidosis; alkalinize serum to decrease V_d
What is the role of hemodialysis in ASA overdose?	Used in severely ill patients where immediate removal of salicylic acid is needed as well as correcting metabolic and fluid derangements.
List some indications for hemodialysis in ASA overdose:	Acute ASA level of >100 mg/dL; chronic ASA level >60 mg/dL; renal insufficiency; severe metabolic acidosis (pH <7.1); failure to tolerate sodium bicarbonate

Iron

What are some important things to know about iron overdose?	Unintentional ingestion mostly from children; iron is potentially very toxic; most sources from vitamins and iron pills
What are the three most common preparations of iron and their elemental iron content?	1. Ferrous gluconate 12% 2. Ferrous sulfate 20% 3. Ferrous fumarate 33%
What are some points in the pharmacokinetics of iron absorption?	10-35% is absorbed; iron crosses absorbed in the ferrous state; iron is rapidly cleared and taken up by cells
What is the general toxic dose of iron overdose?	Toxic overdose >60 mg/kg of elemental iron; generally asymptomatic <20 mg/dL

What are some of the toxic effects of iron?

Inhibition of the Krebs cycle; uncoupling of oxidative phosphorylation; mucosal cell necrosis; free radical production

What three organ systems are most affected by iron overdose (primarily from free-radical production)?

1. GI epithelium
2. Heart
3. Liver

What is the most common cause of death in iron overdose?

Circulatory shock

What are the four phases of iron toxicity:

Clinical picture is more important than trying to categorize patients

Phase 1: GI (0-12 h)

Direct injury to the GI mucosa: abdominal pain, diarrhea, emesis, hematemesis, etc; severity ranges from mild to shock

Phase 2: Latent (6-24 h)

Period of apparent recovery. Patients in this phase are usually stable, but they are not asymptomatic. Risk of developing life-threatening hypovolemia and acidosis

Phase 3: Metabolic phase (24 h to 4 days)

Clinical manifestations of the metabolic phase include fever, pallor, cyanosis, jaundice, renal failure, lethargy, coma, shock, and bleeding. Potential for death is highest here

Phase 4: Delayed phase (2-8 weeks)

Characterized by late complications, usually intestinal scarring with GI obstruction

What are important serum iron concentrations to be aware of?

50-150 μg/dL — Normal levels

350 μg/dL — Often significant GI symptoms

500 μg/dL — Significant toxicity likely

>1000 μg/dL — Considerable morbidity

What are some laboratory tests to consider?

CBC/Chem-7/Coags; ABG for moderate-severe cases; lactate; iron studies (ie, TIBC, Fe, etc)

What role does an abdominal radiograph (KUB) play in iron toxicity?

While a KUB may be able to detect opacities (Fe) on film, its absence does not rule out ingestion.

Is gastric decontamination effective with iron overdose?

No—gastric lavage, ipecac, and AC are relatively ineffective with iron ingestion.

What is the antidote commonly used for iron toxicity?	Deferoxamine (DFO)
What is the dose of DFO?	Begin at 5 mg/kg/h and titrate to 15 mg/kg/h. Total dose should not exceed 6-8 g/day
What are some functions of DFO?	Chelation of iron; DFO can remove iron bound to transferrin; DFO can also remove iron from cells
When is the general serum iron level in which to administer DFO?	Generally 500 ug/mL or greater, also consider with significant symptoms such as severe vomiting and hypotension.
What are some adverse reactions with administration of DFO?	Acute renal failure; septicemia from *Y enterocolitica*; acute lung injury; hypotension

PRESCRIPTION MEDICATIONS

Anticoagulants

What are the two main categories of anticoagulants and some examples of each:	
Indanedione anticoagulants	Pindone; diphacinone; valone
Hydroxycoumarin anticoagulants	Brodifacoum; warfarin; fumarin
What are some scenarios where overdose of anticoagulants can occur?	Unintentional ingestion by children; drug interactions; suicidal ingestion; homicidal attempts (ie, rat poison)
What is the mechanism of action of warfarin?	Inhibits the synthesis of vitamin K-dependent factors (II, VII, IX, X, and protein C and S), so that once the existing factors degrade, no more is made by inhibiting both vitamin K 2,3-epoxide reductase and vitamin K quinone reductase.
What are common sites of bleeding with an anticoagulant overdose?	GI tract and genitourinary tract; epistaxis and hemoptysis can be common
What is the most feared complication of an anticoagulant overdose?	Intracranial bleeding

What are the typical abnormal labs with anticoagulants overdose?

Elevated PT/PTT time; platelets and LFT are usually normal

What drug interactions typically lead to excessive anticoagulation?

Cimetidine, erythromycin, metronidazole, and ciprofloxacin typically lead to excess anticoagulation.

What are some distinguishing features of superwarfarins?

Very long-acting anticoagulants; half-life that exceed 3 to 4 months; vitamin K therapy may require months; typically only found in rat poison

What are some key points in the management of accidental ingestion?

If asymptomatic, typically observe; coags/GI decontamination not needed; advise to watch for any signs of bleeding

What are some considerations in the management of intentional ingestion?

Careful monitoring, especially if active bleeding; ABCs—active bleeding can obstruct airway; CBC and coags should be done serially

What are some treatment options for a patient who is actively bleeding from anticoagulants?

For severe bleeding: FFP or whole blood; most other cases: vitamin K

How often should PT be monitored?

Initially every 6 to 8 hours, PT takes days to normalize

What are some routes of vitamin K administration?

Oral, IM, or IV

What are adverse reactions of giving IV vitamin K?

Anaphylactoid reaction (rare); cerebral thrombosis

What is the mechanism of action for unfractionated heparin (UFH)?

Inhibits Antithrombin III that results in prolonged PTT

What are some adverse reactions of UFH?

Heparin-induced thrombocytopenia (HIT); hyperkalemia (inhibits aldosterone)

What are low-molecular weight heparins (LMWH)?

Derivatives of commercial heparin, LMWH inactivate factor Xa, but have a lesser effect on thrombin

What are the three LMWH approved for use in the United States?

1. Enoxaparin
2. Ardeparin
3. Dalteparin

What are some advantages of LMWH over UFH?	Longer duration of action; laboratory monitoring is not necessary; they are much less likely to induce HIT; LMWH can be given to outpatient
What is the treatment of choice for heparin overdose?	Discontinue heparin as it has a very short half-life. Protamine sulfate can be given for serious bleeding as a result of heparin or LMWH.
What are some potential complications with the use of protamine?	Anaphylactic reaction, rate-related hypotension, and it has weak anticoagulation.
What is the dose of protamine?	Typically 1 mg will neutralize 100 units of heparin (max dose is typically 50-60 mg)

Oral Hypoglycemics

What are some important points regarding maintenance of plasma glucose concentrations?	Normally maintained between 70 and 150 mg/dL; glycogenolysis/ gluconeogenesis help maintain normal levels; adult liver has 70 grams of glycogen
What is the relationship of the brain and glucose?	Highly dependent on glucose; first organ to be affected by hypoglycemia; hypoglycemia will activate sympathetic axis resulting in release of catecholamines
What are signs and symptoms of hypoglycemia?	Diaphoresis, tachycardia, tremor, altered mental status, seizure, coma, and rarely focal neurologic deficits that may mimic a stroke.
What is the general principle for initial treatment for all hypoglycemic agents?	Give dextrose then feed the patient
Name some commonly used oral agents in the treatment of non-insulin-dependent diabetes mellitus (NIDDM):	Sulfonylurea; alpha-glucosidase inhibitors; thiazolidinediones; biguanides
What are some examples of a sulfonylurea?	Glyburide; glipizide; tolazamide
What is the mechanism of action of all sulfonylureas?	They cause insulin release from remaining pancreatic cells via cell depolarization (potassium channel) and also improve sensitivity to insulin.

How soon can hypoglycemia occur after the ingestion of a sulfonylurea?

Can vary anywhere from 30 min to many hours after ingestion. Administration of dextrose can mask hypoglycemia.

What are some considerations in the management of hypoglycemia secondary to sulfonylureas?

Carbohydrate-rich meal for awake patients; 50% dextrose for patients with altered MS; glucagon is not effective in hypoglycemia; observe for at least 8 to 12 hours with frequent accuchecks

What are two agents available for refractory hypoglycemia secondary to sulfonylureas?

1. Diazoxide
2. Octreotide (main treatment)

What are some considerations with the use of diazoxide?

Inhibits insulin secretion; causes hypotension and hyponatremia; can cause sodium and fluid retention

What are some considerations with the use of octreotide?

Somatostatin analogue; more effective then diazoxide; inhibits secretion of insulin; generally very well tolerated

What are some considerations in the management of hypoglycemia from sulfonylureas?

A single ingestion by child = admission for potentially delayed hypoglycemia; interactions may enhance toxicity; any patients who present hypoglycemic = admission for observation

What are some other techniques to prevent absorption and enhance elimination?

Activated charcoal

What is the mechanism of action of biguanides (ie, metformin)?

Decreases hepatic gluconeogenesis; increases uptake of glucose; increases utilization of glucose into lactate

What adverse effect is particularly important to monitor with metformin?

Metformin-associated lactic acidosis (MALA)

Who are at increased risk of lactic acidosis secondary to metformin use?

Patients with impaired renal clearance

What is the treatment of MALA?

Treatment is supportive with correction of acid-base disturbance and rehydration—often require dialysis.

Does metformin cause hypoglycemia?

Rarely

Cardiac Glycosides

Table 17-4

	Onset	Time to Peak Effect
Oral	1.5-6 h	4-6 h
IV	5-20 min	1-3 h

What are cardiac glycosides, AKA cardioactive steroids?	Drugs with a steroid ring, with one to four sugars attached to it, and an unsaturated lactone ring.
What are the primary indications for digoxin?	CHF; control of rapid ventricular response from a-fib and a-flutter
What are some sources of cardiac glycosides?	Foxglove; *Bufo* toad venom; milkweeds; oleander
What is the mechanism of action of cardiac glycosides?	Inhibit sodium-potassium exchange pump that will increase intracellular calcium
What are some effects of cardiac glycosides?	Increased vagal tone; increased automaticity; increased contractility
What is the time course for toxicity to develop after an overdose?	Drugs must first move into cells, symptoms generally do not occur for several hours
What are some signs and symptoms of an acute overdose?	Nausea and emesis are almost first symptoms with confusion and weakness, can also develop heart block/bradycardia.
What are other drug classes to consider with bradycardia?	Beta-blocker and calcium channel blockers (will often cause hypotension as opposed to cardiac glycosides, which typically do not)
What are some signs and symptoms of chronic overdose?	Anorexia, nausea, and emesis common with headaches, confusion, and lethargy.
Which patients commonly present with chronic cardiac glycoside toxicity?	Commonly an elderly person with underlying heart disease who presents with nonspecific GI/neuro complaints (usually with precipitating factor such as dehydration).

How does chronic toxicity commonly develop?	Drug interactions that increase levels; worsening renal function; diuretics or infection that lead to dehydration
What are some possible ECG findings in digoxin overdose?	Prolonged PR interval; short Q-T; ST scooping and depression (especially laterally); decreased T-waves
What is an important electrolyte to obtain in an acute overdose?	Potassium
What is the significance of hyperkalemia with an acute overdose?	It is prognostic; patients with a potassium of greater than 5.5 mEq/L often have near 100% mortality in an ACUTE overdose (does not apply to chronic setting).
Should patients with an acute overdose of a cardioactive steroid with hyperkalemia be given calcium?	While most interventions for hyperkalemia should be considered, calcium in this setting may be detrimental.
What are some consideration in the management of acute digoxin overdose?	AC may be considered; HD is not effective; follow potassium closely—treat accordingly; avoid the use of calcium—greater arrhythmias; treat any dysrhythmias accordingly, but avoid type IA/IC antiarrhythmics
What is the standard treatment for cardiac glycoside toxicity?	Digoxin-specific Fab antibody fragment (Digibind or DigiFab)
What are some indications for the use of Digibind?	Serious dysthymias; bradycardia refractory to atrophine; hyperkalemia (>5.5)

Beta-Blockers

What are some indications for the use of beta-blockers?	Hypertension; prevent reinfarction and s/p MI; dysrhythmias; glaucoma; migraine headaches
What are some considerations with beta-blockers?	There are many preparations; agents may be selective or nonselective; with overdose, selectivity is loss
What are some commonly used beta-blockers?	Metoprolol; carvedilol; labetalol; timolol

What is the function of B_1 receptors?	Heart (increase HR/inotrophy/automaticity); eye (increase aqueous humor production); kidney (increase renin production)
What is the function of B_2 receptors?	Liver (gluconeogenesis); smooth muscle relaxation; skeletal muscle (glycogenolysis)
What is the function of B_3 receptors?	Adipose tissue (lipolysis)
How soon after ingestion of beta-blockers do patients manifest symptoms?	Usually within 6 hours (does not apply to extended-release formulations/sotalol)

What are some important clinical manifestations based on systems:

Cardiovascular system	Bradycardia, hypotension, CHF, QRS/QT prolongation (rare)
Respiratory system	Apnea, respiratory depression, and bronchospasms
CNS	Seizure, delirium, and coma (mostly associated with propranolol)
Endocrine system	Children are particularly susceptible to hypoglycemia
What type of beta-blockers are considered the most dangerous?	Ones that are lipophilic, have sodium channel activity, and have potassium channel activity
Which beta-blocker causes a disproportionate amount of deaths?	Propranolol
What are some basic therapeutic measures for overdose with mild symptoms?	Supportive care with fluids; cardiac monitoring
What are some key points in the management of beta-blocker overdose for moderate-severe sick patients?	ABCs; cardiac monitoring/fluids/atropine; catecholamines in severe cases
What is the antidote of choice for beta-blocker overdoses?	Glucagon
What is the mechanism of action for glucagon in the setting of beta-blocker overdose?	Directly increase cAMP concentrations through an alternative receptor pathway not involving the blocked beta-receptor
What are indications for admission?	History of sustained-release overdose; any symptoms/ECG changes within 6 hours

Calcium Channel Blockers

What are some important features of calcium channel blockers (CCB)?	Block L-type calcium channels in myocardium and vascular smooth muscle; decrease myocardial inotropy/ conduction; vasodilation in peripheral vasculature
What are some indications for the use of calcium channel blockers?	Hypertension; angina; dysrhythmias; migraines
What are the three most commonly used CCBs?	1. Diltiazem (benzodiazepine) 2. Verapamil (phenylalkylamine) 3. Nifedipine (dihydropyridine)
How soon after ingestion do symptoms of CCBs overdose appear?	Depending on the formulation, can range from the first hour to 24 hours
What is the mechanism of death in CCB overdose?	Profound cardiogenic and distributive shock, due to decreased inotropy and peripheral vasodilation
What are some important clinical manifestation based on:	
CVS	Hypotension, dysrhythmias, bradycardia, and cardiogenic shock
Respiratory system	ARDS
CNS	Dizziness, seizures, altered MS, and stroke
Endocrine system	Hyperglycemia
What are some key points in the management of CCB overdose?	Prevent and correct hypotension; ABCs; AC; bradydysrhythmias treated with advanced life support (ACLS)
What are important therapeutic maneuvers to reverse hypotension?	IVF bolus; calcium; glucagon and catecholamines; high insulin therapy
What is high-insulin euglycemic therapy (HIE)?	The use of high-dose insulin (1-2 unit/kg of regular insulin!) which may increase contractility as well as improve energy use of the myocardium
What are two complications of HIE therapy?	Hypokalemia and hypoglycemia
Which patients can safely be discharged after CCB overdose?	Typically those who show no symptoms or ECG changes after 6 hours and did not ingest any sustained-release formulation. (verapamil and diltiazem ingestions should be admitted)

PSYCHIATRIC MEDICATIONS

Selective Serotonin Reuptake Inhibitors

Table 17-5

Generic Name	Brand Name
Citalopram	Celexa
Fluoxetine	Prozac
Fluvoxamine	Luvox
Paroxetine	Paxil
Sertraline	Zoloft
Venlafaxine	Effexor

What are some important things to know about selective serotonin reuptake inhibitors (SSRIs)?

SSRIs are generally safe; designed to answer TCA's side effect profile

What is the mechanism of action of SSRIs?

They inhibit presynaptic neuronal reuptake of serotonin

What are some signs and symptoms of SSRIs overdose?

Nausea, emesis, sedation, lethargy, and rarely seizures

What is important to know about citalopram?

Large overdoses can cause seizure and QT prolongation in a delayed manner due to the metabolite which is responsible for these effects.

What are some considerations in the management of SSRI overdose?

Treatment is primarily supportive; important to rule out other overdose such as acetaminophen

What are some general indications to medically clear a patient following SSRI overdose?

Monitor for 6 hours and if no changes, can medically clear with exception of citalopram/escitalopram and extended-release bupropion.

What is serotonin syndrome?

Excessive stimulation of serotonin receptors typically due to ingestion of serotonergic medication ($5\text{-}HT_{1A}$ and $_{2A}$)

What are some mechanisms by which excessive serotonin can occur?

Prevent breakdown of 5-HT; enhance 5-HT release (ie, ecstasy); block reuptake (ie, cocaine)

What are some signs and symptoms of serotonin syndrome?	Mental status change, hyperreflexia, hyperthermia, agitation, myoclonus, and seizure.
What are some considerations in the management of serotonin syndrome?	Benzodiazepines, cooling, and hydration; sedation/intubation in refractory cases
What is another possible treatment option for serotonin syndrome?	Cyproheptadine
What is the mechanism of action for cyproheptadine?	It is an antihistamine that also is a 5-HT antagonist that is available only in oral form.

Other Antidepressants

What are key points of drug overdose for the following antidepressants:

Trazodone and Nefazodone	Inhibits reuptake of 5-HT; overdose may cause sedation; associated with priapism
Amoxapine	Cyclic antidepressant; works on dopaminergic (DA) and norepinephrinergic (NE) receptors; high incidence of seizures; not associated with ECG abnormalities
Bupropion	Prevents reuptake of DA and NE; indicated for smoking cessation; can cause seizures as well as sodium channel blockade

Tricyclic Antidepressants

Table 17-6

Tricyclic Antidepressants

Imipramine

Amitriptyline

Desipramine

Nortriptyline

What are some important things to know about tricyclic antidepressants (TCAs)?	Higher frequency of adverse effects; have low therapeutic index; significant sedative/anticholinergic effect

Why are TCAs fairly toxic in overdose? Primarily due to their nonspecific blockage of reuptake of various neurotransmitters.

What are some of the adverse effects when taken in overdose:

    Anticholinergic Dry skin, hallucinations, delirium, hyperthermia, tachycardia, and mydriasis

    Alpha-adrenergic blockage Peripheral vasodilation with hypotension

    Sodium channel blockage Inhibit fast sodium channels (quinidine-like effect) with widened QRS complex

What is a useful diagnostic test to obtain to further evaluate TCA toxicity? ECG

What is the most sensitive indicator of toxicity on ECG? QRS width

What is the QRS width where seizures and dysrhythmias may occur? QRS width >100 ms

What is the time period in which virtually all patients develop cardiotoxicity? 6 hours (most will develop in the first 2-3 h)

What are some considerations in the management of TCA overdose? ABCs with cardiac monitoring is crucial; AC should also be given <1 hour (assuming no contraindication)

What is the treatment of cardiotoxicity from a TCA overdose? Sodium bicarbonate

How much sodium bicarbonate should be administrated? Typically bolus 1 mEq/kg with the purpose of narrowing the QRS complex

Once the QRS has narrowed in response to bicarb, what is the next action? Place the patient on a bicarb drip

How is a sodium bicarbonate drip prepared? Place 3 amps of sodium bicarbonate into a 1 L of D5NS with a rate of 1.5-2x maintenance

When is it generally safe to discharge patients from the ED after a TCA overdose? No signs of toxicity and continuous monitoring for 6 hours

Monoamine Oxidase Inhibitors

Table 17-7

Generic Name	Brand Name
Isocarboxazid	Marplan
Phenelzine	Nardil
Selegiline	Deprenyl
Tranylcypromine	Parnate

What are some important things to know about monoamine oxidase inhibitors (MAOIs)?	Were among the first class used for depression; were later largely replaced by TCAs; they now have limited indications for use
What is the mechanism of action of MAOIs?	MAOI is an enzyme that breaks down monoamines, so its inhibition will increase the concentration of NE, DA, and 5-HT.
What are some signs and symptoms of an MAOI overdose?	Tachycardia, hypertension, agitation, and diaphoresis; may get cardiovascular as well as neurological collapse in severe overdose
How late can symptoms appear following an MAOI overdose?	Effects can be delayed for over 24 hours
What are some late complications of MAOI overdose?	DIC, rhabdomyolysis, and pulmonary edema
What are some considerations in the management of MAOI overdose?	ABCs; Promptly treat severe hypertension; ACLS for dysrhythmias which may occur; aggressive fluid bolus for hypotension
Can patients be safely discharged after being asymptomatic for 6 hours?	MAOIs are the exception to the "6 hour rule" and should be monitored for at least 24 hours.
What other drugs can interact with MAOIs to produce toxicity?	Any sympathomimetic such as cocaine or dopamine can produce toxicity.
MAOIs are well-known to produce toxicity when ingested with "wine and cheese," why?	These foods contain tyramine, which acts as an indirect sympathomimetic to precipitate toxicity.
What are some other foods that produce toxicity when ingested with MAOIs?	Aged meat; soy sauce; sauerkraut

NEUROLEPTICS

What are neuroleptics?	Originally known as antipsychotics and tranquilizers, these classes of drugs are commonly used for a variety of anxiety and psychotic states.
What are some indications for the use of neuroleptics?	Psychosis; delirium; agitation; nausea
What are some examples of positive symptoms and the receptor that mediates them?	Mediated primarily by central D_2 receptor: delusions; thought disorders; hallucinations
What are some examples of negative symptoms and the receptor that mediates them?	Mediated primarily by $5\text{-}HT_{2A}$ receptor: apathy; social withdrawal; blunted effect
What are some adverse effects from normal use of neuroleptics?	More common with typical neuroleptics: acute dystonia; neuroleptic malignant syndrome; glucose dysregulation
What are some common extrapyramidal symptoms seen with neuroleptics?	Akathisia; parkinsonism; dystonic reactions
What are some adverse reactions when taken in acute overdose?	Reduced seizure threshold; hypotension/reflex tachycardia; hyper- or hypothermia; CNS depression or coma (large doses); quinidine-like effect
What are some key points in the management of neuroleptic overdose?	ABCs with IV access; treat dystonia (ie, diphenhydramine); treat hypotension (ie, fluids); treat cardiotoxicity like TCAs (ie, bicarb)
What are some commonly used medications to treat acute dystonic reactions?	Benzatropine; diphenhydramine; diazepam
When can a patient be medically clear after a neuroleptic ingestion?	No signs and symptoms for 6 hours
What idiosyncratic reaction affects a small percentage of patients on neuroleptics that is potentially fatal?	Neuroleptic malignant syndrome (NMS)
What are some signs and symptoms of NMS?	Autonomic instability (ie, change in HR and BP), profound hyperthermia, mental status change, and rigidity

| What are some clinical features that may help to distinguish NMS from SS? | Often slower in onset and slow to resolve; often rigid extremity as opposed to hyperreflexia and clonus |
| What are some considerations in the management of NMS? | Rapid cooling (ie, spray mist/ice); use of benzodiazepines (paralytics if severe); discontinue the offending agent *bromocriptine have been used since it is a dopamine agonist |

Lithium

Table 17-8

Therapeutic Level	
Maintenance	0.5-0.8 mEq/L
Acute mania	0.7-1.2 mEq/L

What are some facts about lithium?	Alkali metal with a long history of use; used in the past for gout and CHF; up to 90% will have some sign of toxicity
While the exact mechanism of lithium's effects is not fully understood, what are some of its proposed mechanisms?	May substitute for sodium in neurons; increase GABA transmission; affect protein kinases (ie, C and G)
What are some common preparations available?	Immediate release: 300 mg tiq or qid; sustained release: 300 mg bid; controlled release: 450 mg bid
What are some important pharmacokinetic properties of lithium?	95% of lithium is renally cleared; lithium is absorbed preferentially to sodium; any volume-depleted state will result in increased reabsorption of lithium
What are some side effects of lithium at therapeutic doses?	Fine tremors, polyuria, diabetes insipidus, weight gain, leukocytosis, and cog-wheeling rigidity
What are some signs and symptoms of acute lithium toxicity?	Initial symptoms will be GI-related: nausea, emesis, and diarrhea followed by neurologic symptoms such as tremors, lethargy, and seizure, or coma as the lithium moves into the brain.
Is acute lithium overdose directly cardiotoxic?	While ECG may show nonspecific T-wave changes, it is not directly cardiotoxic

What are some signs and symptoms of chronic lithium toxicity?	Primarily neurologic: tremors, nystagmus, seizure, lethargy, and coma as there is already a lithium burden within the CNS.
What are some common causes of chronic toxicity?	Dehydration; Incorrect dosing; renal insufficiency; interaction with other drugs (ie, NSAIDs)
What are some long-term sequelae of lithium use?	Personality changes; memory deficits; diabetes insipidus; cerebellar dysfunction (ie, ataxia)
What is the treatment of choice with lithium toxicity?	Volume restoration through normal saline.
What is the next treatment option for patients who are symptomatic despite use of normal saline?	Extracorporeal removal such as hemodialysis (HD)
What is the absolute lithium concentration where dialysis would be indicated?	4 mEq/L in an acute setting and 2.5 mEq/L in a chronic setting
Why is it important to check lithium levels 6 hours after HD?	Patients will get rebound lithium level as lithium redistributes from tissues.

DRUGS OF ABUSE

Opioids

What is the definition of opioids?	Natural and synthetic substances with morphine-like activity, opioids have analgesic and central nervous system depressant effects, as well as the potential to cause euphoria.
What are endorphins?	Endogenous peptides that produce pain relief (ie, dynorphins/beta-endorphins)
What are some major opioid receptors found in the human body?	Kappa, delta, and Mu
What is the primary opioid receptor that mediates euphoria/analgesia/respiratory depression?	Mu

What are some other signs and symptoms of an opioid overdose?

Most classic finding is miosis, altered mental status that can range from lethargy to coma, and respiratory depression.

What is the most important adverse reaction to monitor with an opioid overdose?

Respiratory depression

Which opioids are associated with seizures?

Meperidine, tramadol, and propoxyphene

Which opioid is found in an anti-diarrheal medication that was once associated with serious toxicity in children?

Diphenoxylate found in Lomotil

Name two opioids used for their antitussive properties:

Codeine and dextromethorphan (no analgesic property)

Are all opioids picked up by the urine tox screen?

No—only opioids that are similar in structure to morphine will trigger a positive test.

Will heroin trigger a positive test opioid screen?

Yes—metabolized to morphine

What are some examples of synthetic opioids?

Methadone, fentanyl, and propoxyphene

What is the mechanism of acute lung injury which is seen with an acute opioid overdose?

Acute lung injury may involve a catecholamine surge with sudden reversal due to high-dose naloxone

What is the agent of choice to reverse opioid overdose?

Naloxone (Narcan)

What is the goal with the use of naloxone?

To reverse respiratory depression (not to wake them up!)

What is the proper dose of naloxone?

Start low! 0.04 to 0.05 mg IV

What is the duration of action of naloxone?

30 to 45 min

What is the concern with the use of naloxone who present with an opioid overdose from a long-acting opioid?

Relapse

What is a treatment option for long-acting opioid toxicity such as methadone?

Can use a naloxone drip, typically 2/3 the dose used to reverse their respiratory depression

What are some indications for admission following opioid overdose?	Anyone who requires a naloxone drip; evidence of NCPE; little improvement after naloxone; life-threatening co-ingestion

Sedatives-Hypnotics

What is the definition of a sedative?	Medication that reduces anxiety and induces relaxation.
What is the definition of a hypnotic?	Medication that induces sleep
Is there really a difference between the two?	Not really, the two terms are used interchangeably
What are some examples of sedative-hypnotics?	Benzodiazepines; barbiturates; buspirone; zolpidem, ethanol
What are some common indications for sedative-hypnotics?	Anxiety; seizures; muscle spasms; insomnia; alcohol withdrawal
What is the mechanism of action of barbiturates?	They enhance the activity of GABA receptors by increasing the duration by which chloride channels open as opposed to benzodiazepines, which increase the frequency of chloride channel opening.
Are barbiturates generally safer than benzodiazepines?	No—benzodiazepines are generally safer as they produce less respiratory depression and minimal cardiac side effects.
What is the "classic toxidrome" of a benzodiazepine overdose?	"Coma with normal vital signs"
What is the antidote of choice for benzodiazepine overdose?	Flumazenil (use with extreme caution if ever)
What are some examples of hypnotic agents which have supplanted the use of benzodiazepines?	Zaleplon (Sonata), Zolpidem (Ambien), and Eszopiclone (Lunesta)
Are these drugs considered dangerous?	Generally safe with a wide safety margin, withdrawal is typically mild
What is the mechanism of action of flumazenil?	Nonspecific competitive benzodiazepine receptor antagonist

Is it always safe to give flumazenil in a suspected benzodiazepine overdose?	No—particularly in multiple drug ingestions where benzodiazepines can have a seizure protective effect with drugs such as TCA or if the patient is on chronic use, as it may induce withdrawal.
Is benzodiazepine withdrawal dangerous?	Yes—it is similar to alcohol withdrawal (ie, hyperthermia, hypertension, seizure, etc) and can be potentially fatal.

Toxic Alcohols

Name the three common toxic alcohols:	1. Methanol 2. Ethylene glycol 3. Isopropyl alcohol
What are some considerations with toxic alcohols?	All can increase the osmol gap; methanol and ethylene glycol will eventual cause a high anion gap metabolic acidosis
Are the parent compounds responsible for the acidosis observed with toxic alcohol ingestions?	No
What are some characteristics of methanol?	Colorless clear flammable liquid that has a slight alcohol odor.
What are some common sources of methanol?	De-icing solutions; shellac; varnish; windshield washer fluid
What is the toxic dose of methanol?	Less than 1 mL/kg can lead to blindness or severe toxicity

Table 17-9

Methanol Levels	
<20 mg/dL	Generally asymptomatic; often threshold to treat
>50 mg/dL	Acidosis
>100 mg/dL	Visual symptoms
>150 mg/dL	Generally fatal

What is the major toxic metabolite of methanol?	Alcohol dehydrogenase (ADH) metabolism to formaldehyde (causes metabolic acidosis) and formic acid (a mitochondrial toxin)

What are some signs and symptoms of methanol toxicity?

Inebriation, nausea, abdominal pain, gastritis, and early visual disturbance such as blurriness and photophobia.

What are some severe symptoms of methanol toxicity?

Coma, seizure, blindness, hypotension, cardiac failure, and pulmonary edema

What are important laboratory tests to obtain?

Chemistry panel; lactate; toxic alcohol panel (often takes time to return), ketones, measure osmolality, ethanol concentration

What are two reasons to obtain an ethanol concentration?

1. It is protective if co-ingested with a toxic alcohol as ADH will bind preferentially with ethanol
2. Important to account for with the calculated osmolarity

What is the mechanism of action of 4-methylpyrazole (4-MP)?

Inhibits alcohol dehydrogenase preventing the formation of toxic metabolites

When should hemodialysis be started?

High (methanol) >20 mg/dL; presence of metabolic acidosis; severe symptoms such as visual changes

What are some common sources of isopropyl alcohol?

Nail-polish remover; glues; rubbing alcohol

What is the metabolism of isopropyl alcohol?

About 50% excreted in urine unchanged; the rest is converted to acetone

Is acetone dangerous?

It is not toxic, but can lead to a ketosis with no acidosis (hallmark of isopropyl alcohol).

How is acetone excreted?

Primarily through the kidney and lung

What is the typical lab finding in isopropyl alcohol?

Increased osmolal gap with no acidosis

What is the treatment for isopropyl alcohol toxicity?

Supportive care; respiratory care

What are some common sources of ethylene glycol?

Brake fluid; automobile coolant systems (antifreeze)

What is the toxic dose of ethylene glycol?

>15 mL/kg

What are some toxic metabolites of ethylene glycol?	Glycoaldehyde; glycolic acid; oxalate
What are some effects of oxalate?	Combines with calcium (calcium oxalate crystals) that damages the kidney and can also damage organs such as liver and brain, in addition, can cause hypocalcemia.
What are some ECG findings associated with ethylene glycol?	ECG can show findings of hypocalcemia such as a prolonged QT or manifestations of hyperkalemia due to acute renal failure.
What are some typical lab findings in ethylene glycol toxicity?	Elevated osmolar gap; elevated anion gap acidosis, renal failure
What is the relationship between an elevated lactate concentration with ethylene glycol?	Some ABG machines will often misinterpret glycolic acid for lactate causing a false elevation.
What are common urinary findings in ethylene glycol toxicity?	Hematuria, proteinuria, and crystalluria
Is gastric decontamination effective?	No—ipecac, cathartics, and gastric aspiration have little role and AC poorly absorbs ethylene glycol.
What are some considerations in the management of ethylene glycol?	Aggressive early therapy is key; correct any acidosis immediately; while ethanol can be given (and is effective); fomepizole is the standard of care now; hemodialysis in severe cases
What are some indications of HD in ethylene glycol toxicity?	Severe metabolic acidosis; renal dysfunction (ie, acute renal injury); levels >20 mg/dL

Cocaine

What is the mechanism of action of cocaine?	Cocaine enhances monoamine neurotransmitter activity in the central and peripheral nervous systems by blocking the presynaptic reuptake pumps for these neurotransmitters.
What is a secondary effect of cocaine that is unique among other stimulants?	Blocks voltage-gated membrane sodium ion channels: Local anesthetic effects; dysrhythmias

| What are two forms of cocaine? | 1. Base (form that can be smoked) |
| | 2. Salt (form that can be insufflated (snorted), ingested or injected) |

Table 17-10

Pharmacokinetics	Onset	Duration
Intravenous	Fast	15-30 min
Inhalation	Fast	15-30 min
Intranasal	20 min	1 h
Gastrointestinal	90 min	3 h

What are some signs and symptoms of acute intoxication?	Euphoria, increased energy, alertness; decreased appetite, need for sleep, and fatigue
What are some adverse effects of cocaine intoxication?	Panic attacks, paranoia, cocaine-induced psychosis, impaired judgment, and dysphoric mood.
What are the effects of cocaine on the following organ system:	
CVS	Increases heart rate, blood pressure, and systemic vascular resistance; cardiac arrhythmias, sudden death, and AMI; cardiomyopathy and myocarditis with chronic use
CNS	Seizures, cerebral vasoconstriction, cerebrovascular disease, and stroke; acute dystonic reactions (ie, akathisia)
Respiratory system	Perforation of the nasal septum and chronic rhinitis from snorting; SOB, wheezing, pneumothorax, and pulmonary edema from smoking
What are some important causes of chest pain to consider in a patient who presents shortly after cocaine use?	Coronary vasospasm (rate of MI is actually low); pneumothorax; aortic dissection; pulmonary infarction
What is the drug of choice for acute cocaine toxicity?	Benzodiazepines
What is the most important vital to be aware of?	Temperature

What is the treatment of choice for severe hyperthermia related to cocaine?	Aggressive cooling through the use of ice baths (mist and fan is actually not very effective)
What is the metabolite that is detected in the urine drug screen for cocaine?	Benzoylecgonine
What is particularly worrisome about intubating a patient with acute cocaine intoxication (ie, having intractable seizures)?	Can still have continued seizures that can lead to permanent brain damage (must have EEG monitoring in place).
What are some signs and symptoms of cocaine withdrawal?	Anhedonia, cocaine craving, anxiety, and depression (it is not life-threatening)—sometimes referred to as cocaine wash-out.
What is the difference between a body-stuffer and a body-packer?	
Body-stuffer	Swallow small packs to avoid police capture; typically mild and transient adverse affects; Tx is observation and AC administration
Body-packer	Smuggle large quantities of drugs (cocaine); often swallow 100+ pre-packed drugs; potentially fatal if they rupture; surgical intervention if bags rupture/obstruct
What are some treatment options for a suspect body-packer?	1. Whole-bowel irrigation 2. Activated charcoal 3. Any evidence of package leakage is an indication for surgery 4. Opioid packages can sometimes be managed with a naloxone drip

Phencyclidine

What are some common street names for phencyclidine (PCP)?	Angel dust, crystal, peep, hog, and PCP
What are some available forms of PCP?	Powder, tablet, crystal, liquid, and capsule
What are some facts about PCP?	Frequently found as mixture in other drugs; often produce brief dissociative reactions; effects are often unpredictable (part of the appeal for many)
What is particularly important about the pharmacokinetics of PCP?	Well absorbed by any route

What is the mechanism of action of PCP?	NMDA receptor antagonist which is responsible for dissociative effect
What is the clinical hallmark of PCP intoxication that allows it to be distinguished from other street drugs?	Vertical nystagmus is characteristic
What are some signs and symptoms of low to moderate PCP intake?	Confusion, ataxia, dysphoria, catatonic behavior, dystonia, violent behavior, and frank psychosis in rare cases.
What are some adverse effects of high dose PCP intake?	Hypertension, seizure, and hyperthermia
What are some considerations in the management of PCP?	Care is supportive (ie, ABCs); benzos for seizure and agitation; reduce external stimuli; physical/chemical restraint if violent; severe HTN should be treated to avoid CVA; prevent/ treat rhabdomyolysis and hyperthermia
What is the morbidity of phencyclidine primarily due to?	Trauma
Name another agent that is similar to PCP commonly used in the emergency department:	Ketamine (known as Special K on the street)
What is another medication commonly abused by adolescents for its dissociative effect?	Dextromethorphan (also known as Robotripping)
Where is dextromethorphan found in?	Robotussin cough syrup
What is the first question that one should ask if a kid triggers a positive PCP screen?	Did they use cough syrup?

Amphetamines

What are amphetamines?	Stimulant agents with sympath-omimetic properties (like cocaine) that act on the CNS and PNS that stimulate both beta- and alpha-receptors.
What are some common amphetamine derivatives?	Methamphetamine (ie, Desoxyn, crank, meth, glass); methylphenidate (ie, Ritalin); 3,4-methylenedioxyamphetamine (ie, ecstasy)

What are some major routes of amphetamine administration?

Oral, intravenous, and inhalation

What are the two organ systems of concern with amphetamine intoxication?

1. CNS
2. CVS

What are some neurologic symptoms of amphetamine toxicity?

Anxiety, aggression, seizure, delirium, euphoria, stroke, and cerebral edema.

What are some cardiovascular symptoms of amphetamine toxicity?

Tachycardia, hypertension, chest pain, dysrhythmias, AMI, and sudden death.

What are some other complications of amphetamine intoxication?

Renal failure, rhabdomyolysis, hyperthermia, anorexia, and complications associated with IVDA

What should be a consideration of a patient who presents with altered sensorium and suspected MDMA usage?

Hyponatremia

What is a frequent and fatal manifestation in patients with drug-induced delirium?

Hyperthermia

What are some considerations in the management of amphetamine intoxication?

Primarily supportive (ie, ABCs); prevent/treat rhabdomyolysis and hyperthermia; benzodiazepines for seizure and agitation

Lysergic Acid Diethylamide (LSD)

What are some commonly used hallucinogens?

Lysergic acid diethylamide (LSD); psilocybin; ketamine; mushrooms; mescaline

What is the mechanism of action of hallucinogens?

Drugs that induce hallucinations, where a user perceives a sensory experience that is not actually there, although in many cases many drugs just distort sensory input (ie, illusions).

Give some examples of common illusions produced by LSD?

Trail: objects in visual field "leave a trail"; feelings of depersonalization; synesthesia: "see sound" or "hear colors"

What are some signs and symptoms of LSD intoxication?

Altered perception is the hallmark along with hypertension, pupillary dilation, sweating, palpitations, blurred vision, in-coordination, and tremors.

What is the hallmark of acute LSD intoxication?	"Bad trip" where the user experiences fear, paranoia, feelings of depersonalization
What is the optimal way to handle a patient with a bad trip?	Reassurance and "talking the patient down" until the drug wears off and consider use of benzos.
What are some long-term complications of LSD use?	Primarily psychiatric: flashbacks (reliving the perceptual distortions), depression, psychosis, and personality change
Is death from LSD common?	LSD generally does not directly cause death, but may indirectly contribute via self-injury or depression/suicide.

METALS, CHEMICALS, AND GASES

General Information

What is important to know about the acute toxicity of metals?	Most metals bind to sulfhydryl groups of enzymes found throughout the body so they have multisystem effects.

What are some common clinical features of acute toxicity of most metals:

Gastrointestinal system	The hallmark of most acute metal toxicity: nausea, emesis, and diarrhea
Cardiovascular	Can range from symptoms of volume depletion (ie, tachycardia) to frank heart failure or dysrhythmias
Renal system	Loss of protein and amino acids in urine, can also get acute tubular necrosis
Nervous system	Peripheral neuropathy is common as well as altered mental status

What are some signs and symptoms of chronic toxicity of most metals:

Nervous system	CNS and PNS disturbances are more prominent than GI symptoms
Renal system	Varying degrees of renal insufficiency is usually noted
Hematology/Oncology	Anemias and neoplasm can be found
Dermatology	Rashes and colored lines of gums/nails often noted

What are some important aspects of the evaluation to focus on with suspected exposure to metals?	History, occupation, lifestyles, hobbies, use of herbal remedies, and travels
What particular area of the exam should one focus on?	Neurologic exam
What are some appropriate laboratory tests to obtain?	CBC with a peripheral smear; chem-7 (assess renal function); liver function tests; urine studies; abdominal films; 24-hour urine metal collection

Arsenic

What group is more likely to get arsenic (As) exposure?	Industrial workers
What are some important things to know about arsenic?	Over 1 million workers are exposed to As; commonly found in pesticides/herbicides; main route of exposure is inhalation
What are other common sources of As?	Shellfish; combustion of fuel; metal alloys/glass/ceramics; may also be exposed via smelting of ore.
What are some forms of As?	Inorganic, organic (arsine), elemental
Which form is generally more toxic?	The inorganic trivalent forms (ie, arsenite), the organic (arsine) form is generally nontoxic
What makes As particularly attractive as a poison?	Resembles sugar and tasteless
What are two primary routes of As exposure?	1. Inhalation 2. Ingestion
What is the primary mechanism by which As exerts its toxicities?	Uncouples oxidative phosphorylation; inhibits mitochondrial enzymes; binds to globin portion of hemoglobin
What are some signs and symptoms of acute As due to inorganic salts?	Nausea, emesis, diarrhea, ECG changes, dysrhythmias, shock, hematuria, seizure, coma, bone marrow suppression, and peripheral neuropathies.
What are some clinical features of chronic toxicity due to As?	Cirrhosis, hematopoietic malignancies, dermatitis, stocking-glove sensory neuropathy, and cancer.

What are some methods to detect As?	Blood levels (<5 mcg/L normal); difficult to differentiate organic versus inorganic; urine "spot" testing
What are some considerations in the management of acute As toxicity?	Supportive care; appropriate lab testing; consider use of chelating agent in the acute setting; should involve medical toxicologist before considering use of chelation
What are some chelating agents used?	Dimercaprol; D-penicillamine; succimer
What are some functions of chelating agents?	Bind to metal to facilitate excretion; deplete tissues of metals

Lead

Which populations are at the greatest risk of lead poisoning?	Adults through occupational exposures; children through lead-based paints
What are some common sources of lead?	Ammunitions; car radiators; ceramic ware with lead glazes; batteries; paints; moonshine; certain herbal supplements
What are major routes of absorption of lead?	Ingestion; dermal absorption; inhalation
What is the primary site of lead storage in the body?	Bones (>90% in adults compared to 75% in children)
What are the long-term cognitive deficits associated with elevated lead concentrations?	Learning, behavioral disorders, and decreased intelligence
How is lead typically absorbed in the body?	Lead initially attaches to red blood cells and then distributes to various locations such as the brain, kidney, and bones.
What are some signs and symptoms of acute lead toxicity?	Abdominal pain, nausea, emesis, lethargy, fatigue, seizure, and coma
What are some signs and symptoms of chronic lead toxicity?	Nephritis, peripheral neuropathy, myalgias, anemia, and motor weakness
What are some other diagnostic tests to consider?	X-ray fluorescence; nerve conduction velocity testing; neurobehavioral testing
What are the classic laboratory findings of lead poisoning?	Basophilic stippling; anemia; hemolysis

What is a normal lead consideration? | <10 ug/dL

What are some considerations in the management of acute lead poisoning? | The removal of the lead source (ie, striping paint) is perhaps the most important intervention; the use of chelating agents depends on the symptoms

What are some possible chelation options for patients with an elevated lead concentration and asymptomatic? | Succimer, an oral chelator, is the preferred agent

What is a chelation regiments for patients with severe symptoms of lead poisoning? | Parenteral chelation with $CaNa_2EDTA$ and Dimercaprol, AKA (BAL). *The use of BAL should precede the use of EDTA by 4 hours to prevent redistribution into the brain when EDTA is given

Hydrocarbons

What are some facts about hydrocarbons? | Common exposure in children; hydrocarbons are ubiquitous; hydrocarbons commonly ingested/ aspirated

What are some common sources of hydrocarbons? | Gasoline; motor oils; petroleum jelly; laxatives; solvents

What are two primary routes of hydrocarbon toxicity? | 1. Ingestion
2. Inhalation

What are some hydrocarbons with systemic effects? | Aromatic hydrocarbons; halogenated hydrocarbons

What are some signs and symptoms of hydrocarbon ingestions? | Drowsiness, seizures, coma, nausea, emesis, and in cases where there is aspiration of hydrocarbons, patients will exhibit respiratory involvement such as dyspnea, coughing, distress, and even hypoxia/cyanosis.

How do most patients do after hydrocarbon ingestion? | Most are asymptomatic after ingestion

What is an important complication of hydrocarbon ingestion? | Aspiration

What are some physical properties that predict the aspiration potential of hydrocarbons?

Greater volatility; lesser viscosity; surface tension

What are some signs that aspiration may have occurred?

Typically patients will cough, gag, and exhibit dyspnea on exertion.

What are some indications for admission with patients with suspected hydrocarbon aspiration?

Symptomatic after 6 hours; abnormal CXR suggestive of aspiration such as infiltrate

What does "sniffing," "bagging," or "huffing" imply?

Inhalation of volatile hydrocarbons with the intention of getting high

What are some signs and symptoms of inhaling hydrocarbons?

Euphoria, agitation, seizure, stupor, and delusions

What is an important cardiac complication of inhaling halogenated hydrocarbons?

Sudden death (fatal dysrhythmias)

What is the mechanism by which halogenated hydrocarbons can cause fatal dysrhythmias?

Heart is sensitized to circulating catecholamines, so any sudden increase in sympathetic response can cause fatal dysrhythmias.

What are some hydrocarbons that may cause thermal burns?

Asphalt; tar

Name the most likely hydrocarbon involved in the following scenario:

A young woman with a history of inhalant abuse presents with profound weakness with profound hypokalemia and a metabolic acidosis.

Toluene

A farmer was in the barn and knocked over a light-bulb shaped fire extinguisher and later presents with hepatic failure.

Carbon tetrachloride

A young man attempted suicide by ingesting paint stripper and later is found to have CO concentration of 35%.

Methylene chloride

What are some considerations in the management of hydrocarbon toxicity?

Supportive care is the mainstay (ie, ABC); monitor carefully for respiratory involvement; avoid emetic agents (ie, ipecac); AC is not particularly useful; standard ACLS for dysrhythmias

Methemoglobin

What is methemoglobin?

Abnormal hemoglobin (Hg) that is in the ferric state (Fe^{3+}) rather then the ferrous state (Fe^{2+}) that renders it unable to accept oxygen or carbon dioxide.

What are some of the physiologic effects of methemoglobin on oxygen-carrying capacity?

Reduces the oxygen-carrying capacity; left shift of the dissociation curve

What is the normal concentration of methemoglobin in a healthy adult?

<1% of total hemoglobin

What are the two primary mechanisms by which methemoglobin is eliminated?

1. NADH electron donation of ferric to ferrous
2. NADPH (accounts for small portion)

What are two common causes of congenital methemoglobinemia?

1. NADH methemoglobin reductase deficiency
2. Hemoglobin M

What is the most common cause of methemoglobinemia?

Acquired methemoglobinemia

What is the mechanism by which acquired methemoglobinemia occur?

Commonly occurs due to drugs or toxins that oxidize the ferrous iron

List some common causes of acquired methemoglobinemia:

Local anesthetics (most common cause); nitrites; sulfonamide; dapsone

What is the hallmark of methemoglobinemia?

Cyanosis that fails to improve with high-flow oxygen (O2 sat often 85%)

What are some signs and symptoms of methemoglobinemia?

Largely dependent on level of methemoglobin: fatigue, anxiety, dizziness, tachycardia, mental status change, and dysrhythmias/acidosis at higher levels.

What is the methemoglobin concentration at which central cyanosis appears?

Methemoglobin levels of 15%

Aside from persistent cyanosis, what are some other diagnostic clues of methemoglobinemia?

Chocolate brown appearance of blood on filter paper; normal partial pressure of oxygen on ABG; MetHb level determined by cooximetry

What is the treatment of choice for methemoglobinemia?

Methylene blue

What is the mechanism of action of methylene blue?	Increases erythrocyte reduction of methemoglobin to oxyhemoglobin
What are some adverse reactions to methylene blue?	Hemolysis in G6PD deficiency; methemoglobinemia at high doses; false low pulse ox readings

Carbon Monoxide

What are facts about carbon monoxide (CO) poisoning?	Leading cause of poisoning in the United States; majority of cases due to fires; suicide contributes to a good portion of cases; CO is odorless and colorless
List some sources of CO:	Incomplete combustion of carbonaceous material (ie, engine exhaust); degradation of heme; vertical transmission (maternal-to-fetal); halogenated hydrocarbons
What is the pathophysiology of CO poisoning?	CO binds with Hb forming carboxyhemoglobin (COHb that decreases oxygen content of blood and will also shift O_2-Hb dissociation curve to the left (decrease oxygen delivery to tissue).
Are the neurologic sequelae primarily just due to decreased oxygen capacity?	Lipid peroxidation
What two organ systems are most profoundly affected by CO poisoning?	1. CNS 2. CVS

Table 17-11 Acute symptoms associated with CO concentrations

COHb concentrations	Symptoms
10-20%	Flu-like symptoms such as headache and nausea
20-30%	Severe headache, irritability, and impaired judgment
40-50%	Loss of consciousness and confusion
60-70%	Unconsciousness, cardiovascular collapse, seizure
>80%	Rapidly fatal

What are the facts about COHb concentrations?	Smokers can have concentrations as high as 10%; does not predict neurologic sequelae

What are some clinical features of CO poisoning in the following organ systems:

CNS — Headaches, dizziness, blurred vision, ataxia, seizure, coma, and even death

CVS — Signs of demand ischemia (ie, chest pain), hypotension, and dysrhythmias

Respiratory — Pulmonary edema and acute lung injury

Renal — Acute renal failure (2° to rhabdomyolysis)

Dermal — Characteristic cherry-red color (more so after massive exposure and death)

What is an important neurologic complication after CO poisoning? — Delayed neurologic sequelae (DNS)

What is DNS? — Neurologic deterioration after a lucid period of around 2 weeks

What are some signs and symptoms of DNS? — Ataxia, tremor, amnesia, memory impairment, paralysis, and dementia

When do the symptoms of DNS resolve? — Range from 1 month to 1 year depending on severity

What is the concern of the fetus with regards to CO poisoning? — Fetal Hb binds CO more avidly than maternal Hb, which can result in anoxic brain injury and death of the fetus

What are some considerations in the management of CO poisoning? — Remove from source as soon as possible; administer 100% O_2 immediately; check COHb by co-oximetry; ABG/ECG when indicated; hyperbaric oxygen when indicated

Table 17-12

FIO2	COHb $T_{1/2}$
Room air	2-6 h
100% at 1 atm	90 min
100% at 3 atm	30 min

What are some indications for the use of hyperbaric oxygen (HBO) in CO poisoning? — Evidence of end-organ damage (ie, LOC); COHb concentration >25%; COHb >15% for pregnant women/child

Persistent symptoms after 1 atm O_2

Cyanide and Hydrogen Sulfide

What are some important sources of cyanide (CN)?	Combustion of many types of material; smoking; food sources (ie, amygdalin); ingestion of cyanide salts (ie, homicide)
What is the pathophysiology of CN toxicity?	Inhibition of cytochrome oxidase (essential for oxidative phosphorylation) that results in cellular hypoxia leading to increased anaerobic metabolism (lactic acidosis).
Name three routes of exposure for CN:	1. Parental 2. Inhalation 3. Ingestion
What are some signs and symptoms of acute CN toxicity?	Headache, confusion, lethargy, hypotension, abdominal pain, nausea, vomiting, traditional cherry-red skin, and severe metabolic acidosis.
When should one suspect CN toxicity?	A fire victim with a coma and acidosis; bitter almond odor; unexplained coma/acidosis (ie, in laboratory or industrial work)
What role do CN concentrations play in the acute management of cyanide?	They cannot be obtained rapidly, so must use clinical judgment
What is a common laboratory finding in acute CN toxicity?	Severe metabolic acidosis with an elevated lactate
What is the initial management for patients with suspected CN toxicity?	Supportive care (ie, establish airway); sodium bicarbonate for acidosis; treat associated conditions (ie, CO); consider use of antidote
What is the antidote typically given for CN toxicity?	Cyanide antidote kite Sodium nitrite; sodium thiosulfate; amyl nitrite pearls
What is the mechanism by which nitrite administration works?	Induces a methemoglobinemia, for which CN has a greater affinity
What is a contraindication for the use of nitrites with suspected CN poisoning?	Where methemoglobinemia would be a concern such as a fire victim
What is another antidote for CN poisoning?	Hydroxocobalamin (B12a) also known as Cyanokit

What is the mechanism of action of hydroxocobalamin?	It is a large metalloprotein that will chelate CN becoming B12
What are some adverse effects of hydroxocobalamin?	Is an intense red-purple and can interfere with common lab assays; can cause hypertension (scavenges NO); anaphylactoid reaction
What antihypertensive is known to contain CN?	Nitroprusside (will release CN molecules if exposed to sunlight)
What other toxin produces effects similar to CN?	Hydrogen sulfide
What are some sources of hydrogen sulfide?	Natural sources (ie, sulfur springs); industrial sources; decay of sulfur containing products (ie, fish)
What is the pathophysiology of hydrogen sulfide?	Similar to CN, but binds to the same enzyme with greater affinity than CN and also causes mucous membrane irritation.
What are some signs and symptoms of hydrogen sulfide toxicity?	Hypoxia, irritation to areas such as eyes, throat, and nasal passage, and severe metabolic acidosis.
When should the diagnosis of hydrogen sulfide be suspected?	Rapid loss of consciousness; odor of rotten eggs; rescue from an enclosed space; multiple victims
What is a common laboratory finding in hydrogen sulfide poisoning?	Severe metabolic acidosis
What is the initial management in patients with suspected hydrogen sulfide toxicity?	Remove the patient from the source; supportive care; nitrite may be of some use; consider HBO therapy

Pesticides

What is a pesticide?	Agent commonly used to destroy or repel pests such as insects or rodents.
What is the mechanism of organophosphate toxicity?	Bind to cholinesterases, especially acetylcholinesterases, preventing the breakdown of acetylcholine (ACh).
What is the mechanism of toxicity of organophosphates?	Cholinergic poisoning due to excessive accumulation of Ach.

What are the clinical effects primarily due to?

Excessive ACh at the nicotinic receptors (autonomic ganglia and skeletal muscle) and muscarinic receptors.

What is "aging"?

It is the process by which organophosphorus compound exhibit irreversible binding with the enzyme.

What are some factors that determine the clinical effects?

Route of exposure; lipid solubility; dose

What is the difference between a carbamate versus an organophosphorus compound?

Carbamates do not exhibit aging, have poor CNS penetration, and undergo hydrolysis

What is "SLUDGE" syndrome?

Clinical effects due to excessive ACh at the muscarinic receptors

Salivation

Lacrimation

Urination

Diarrhea

GI cramps

Emesis

What are some other signs and symptoms of excessive muscarinic activation?

Bronchoconstriction, bronchorrhea, miosis, and bradycardia

What are some CNS effects of excessive ACh activity?

Agitation, confusion, coma, and seizures

What are the nicotinic effects of excessive ACh activity?

Fasciculations, muscle weakness, and paralysis

What is the initial management of organophosphate toxicity?

Supportive care; decontamination of patient; consider use of an antidote

What are two antidotes that can be used in organophosphate toxicity?

1. Atropine
2. Pralidoxime (2-PAM)

What is the mechanism of atropine?

Competitive inhibition of ACh only at muscarinic receptors

What is the endpoint of atropine therapy?

Drying of secretions

What is the mechanism of pralidoxime?

Regenerates organophosphate-bound acetylcholinesterase complex, regenerating its ability to metabolize Ach.

CLINICAL VIGNETTES—MAKE THE DIAGNOSIS

21-year-old man with no past medical history presents with an overdose of his grandfather's antidepressants. He is initially alert and awake, but during his evaluation the patient becomes unresponsive as well as hypotensive and tachycardiac. ECG: QRS 160 ms. What treatment is required?

Sodium bicarbonate (evidence of sodium-channel blockade)

A family of four all present to the ED complaining of an itchy rash as well as warmth that started soon after a family dinner of tuna. All four members are otherwise awake and alert; PE: upper torso urticarial rash greater than lower extremity. What is the toxin?

Scombroid

35-year-old woman presents with inebriation and admits to drinking a liquid to try and get intoxicated. Patient has an unremarkable physical examination, but laboratory values are significant for a metabolic acidosis with an anion gap of 30, osmol gap of 67, lactate of 12 mmol/L, and urine that reveals oxalate crystals. What antidote should be administered early in the patient's course along with a consult to nephrology?

Fomepizole (load 15 mg/kg)

81-year-old woman with a past medical history of congestive heart failure presents with 2 to 3 days of progressive malaise with decreased oral intake. She otherwise is mildly confused and does not remember her medication list; PE: HR of 40 bpm but normal blood pressure; ECG: frequent PVCs. What is the most likely medication involved with this presentation?

Cardioactive steroid (digoxin)

18-year-old woman presents with an overdose of 100 tablets of baby aspirin. She is mildly confused and is found to be tachypneic on examination. Laboratory evaluation is significant for an anion gap acidosis. Salicylate concentration is pending. Aside from sodium bicarbonate, what other intervention should be considered?

Extracorporeal removal (hemodialysis)

42-year-old man presents with an acetaminophen ingestion of unknown amount 4 hours prior to his presentation to the ED. Patient is otherwise awake and alert. Vitals and ECG is normal. His acetaminophen concentration returns at 140 ug/mL at four hours post-ingestion. Is any further treatment required?

No—N-acetylcysteine is not indicated (150 ug/mL is the treatment line at four hours)

31-year-old man with a history of cocaine use presents to the emergency room complaining of chest pain soon after his last cocaine use. Patient is tachycardiac and hypertensive, but is not hyperthermic. ECG shows inverse t-waves concerning for ongoing ischemia. The ED attending wants to bring down the heart rate and blood pressure. Which antihypertensive class in contraindicated in this setting?

Beta-blockers (may cause unopposed alpha agonism leading to a hypertensive emergency)

51-year-old woman is pulled from a burning building. She is unresponsive and found to be in hypotensive and tachycardia. While carbon monoxide is a consideration what other life-threatening toxin should be considered and what empiric treatment should she receive in the field?

Cyanide poisoning and should be empirically treated with hydroxocobalamin (Cyanokit)

CHAPTER 18

Behavioral Emergencies

MEDICAL EVALUATION AND CLINICAL APPROACH

What are some important things to consider in the clinical approach to patients with psychiatric problems?

Is the patient a danger to self or others?; are physical symptoms a manifestation of a psychiatric disorder?; psychiatric disorders may be exacerbated by a physical condition; patients may present with a medical problem caused by a psychiatric disorder

What are some features for each of the following triage categorization for psychiatric patients (as well as for all other patients):

Emergent

Patient has active suicidal ideation; patient has homicidal ideation; acutely intoxicated; life-threatening injury (ie, myocardial infarction); abnormal vital signs

Urgent

Suicidal ideation; agitation/anxiety; incoherent patient

Nonurgent

Does not meet criteria for the first two; patient requests psychiatric help

What is a very important thing to keep in mind when evaluating a psychiatric patient?

All psychiatric patients should receive both a thorough psychiatric and medical evaluation.

How do you deal with a patient who may have uncontrolled behavioral problems?

Restraints or seclusion

What are some warning signs that a patient with a psychiatric problem may require restraints?

Abrupt changes in behavior; threatening violent behavior; patient verbalizes feelings of a loss of control

What are some characteristics that a seclusion room should have?

Safety foremost; continuous observation; low stimulation (ie, low lights); security staff

What are some considerations for the following types of restraints used:

Verbal restraint

Should be attempted in a calm approach; encourage the patient to talk about any concerns and offer reassurance; physical/chemical restraints may be needed

Physical restraint

Commonly used for intoxicated, demented/delirious, and violent patients; has minimal side effects and immediately reversible; consider using in conjunction with chemical restraint; remove restraints when patient is not a danger to self or others

Chemical restraint

Behavioral control once full evaluation done; haloperidol and lorazepam drug of choice; less intrusive than physical restraint; benzodiazepines may worsen dementia and delirium

What are some characteristics of a patient presenting with a psychiatric disorder?

Patient may regard behavior as normal; history of behavioral problems; often will have normal vitals and laboratory test results; can have hallucinations (ie, auditory)

What are some medical conditions that may present as behavioral emergencies?

Toxicological emergencies; urinary tract infection; sedative-hypnotic withdrawal; myocardial infarction; diabetic ketoacidosis; chronic renal disease; thyroid dysfunction; neurological emergencies (head trauma, mass, encephalitis)

What are some laboratory tests to consider in evaluation of a psychiatric patient?

Glucose; complete blood count (CBC) Urinalysis; lytes (also calcium); toxicology screen; carboxyhemoglobin level; thyroid function test

What are some elements in the medical history to consider when evaluating a patient with a psychiatric problem?

Contact current and past primary doctors; obtain all medical and psychiatric records; list of medications, especially sedatives/psych/pain medications; always ask about alcohol and drug use

What are the key components of the mental status examination (MSE):

Level of consciousness	Alert; fluctuating; somnolent
General appearance	Overall appearance (ie, hygiene); movement: chores, tics, tremors, etc; activity level (ie, agitation)
Orientation	Person, place, time, and event
Memory	Immediate, STM, and LTM; three word recall
Mood	Stability; quality (ie, moody vs. anger)
Speech	Fluency, rate, and rhythm; illogical versus logical
Thought content	Perception (ie, hallucination); bizarre thoughts; delusions
Insight and judgment	History can usually infer this
Cognitive function	Ask to perform task such as spelling a word backward or serial 7s

DEPRESSION AND SUICIDE

What are the symptoms of major depressive disorder?

Five or more of the following symptoms for 2 weeks or greater:

Anhedonia; depressed mood; fatigue; sleep disturbance; weight gain/loss; inability to concentrate; sense of worthlessness; psychomotor agitation or retardation; suicidal thoughts

What are some important considerations in the history when evaluating a patient with depression?

Medications (ie, beta-blockers); history of drug use; neurologic conditions (ie, CNS tumor); endocrine conditions; infectious disease (ie, HIV); any previous psychiatric history; suicidal or homicidal ideation; any recent life changes; evaluation of social structure

What is the primary goal when evaluating a patient with depression?

His/her potential for suicide

How common is major depression?

Affects approximately 1 in 6 Americans per year

What are some factors to consider when deciding to admit a patient with depression?

Previous attempts at suicide; social support; younger or older males are more at risk; plan and means to carry out suicide; excessive use of drugs or alcohol

What are some discharge criteria to consider in a depressed patient?

Agrees to return if depression worsens or is contemplating suicide ("Contract for Safety"); support environment exists; not demented, delirious, or intoxicated; close follow-up

Will antidepressants be immediately helpful for treatment of a patient with depression prior to discharge?

No—antidepressants take up to 4 weeks to work and will not acutely treat depression in the ED.

How many people who attempt suicide are successful?

For every 20 attempts, 1 is successful

When do suicide attempts most commonly occur?

During a crisis marked by an acute personal loss

What are some common psychiatric illnesses associated with completed suicides?

Depression; schizophrenia; personality disorders; panic disorders

What role does gender play in suicide?

Females attempt suicide three times more often; males are successful three times more often

Does drug abuse play a role in suicide?

Yes—one fourth of successful suicides involve drugs and alcohol and up to half in adolescent suicides.

List some risk factors associated with suicide attempts:

Underlying psychiatric illnesses; age (rate highest in elderly); chronic pain (ie, cancer); marital status (marriage is protective); presence of lethal means; family history

What is the most common cause of death in suicide in all age groups?

Firearms

What are some warning signs of suicide?

Recent life changes; depression

Will asking a patient directly about suicide intent put ideas into his/her head?

No—one should always ask

What are key questions to ask a patient who expresses suicidal intention?	Ask if they are suicidal; ask if they have a plan; assess if they have the means
What is "silent suicide?"	Killing oneself slowly via nonviolent means such as not taking medication.
What age group is "silent suicide" most common in?	Elderly
Can a suicidal patient leave against medical advice (AMA)?	If they are found to be incompetent or dangerous, they cannot leave AMA.

ACUTE PSYCHOSIS

What is the definition of acute psychosis?	Break in reality often characterized by delusions, hallucinations, and disorganized speech/movement.
Define the following terms:	
Hallucinations	False perception of a sensory modality that does not exist with auditory stimuli being the most common
Delusions	Fixed falsely held belief that is not accepted by a given cultural group and is held despite an evidence to the contrary
Catatonia	Apparent detachment from the environment typically characterized by frozen rigid posture or violent agitation
What are some examples of negative symptoms?	Poverty of speech; loss of volition; flat affect
What is a major psychiatric disorder that can present as an acute psychotic episode?	Schizophrenia
What is the prevalence of schizophrenia in the general population?	1% regardless of race or gender
When is the onset of schizophrenia?	Commonly by late adolescence to early adulthood
What does the diagnosis of schizophrenia require?	Severe impairment in the level of functioning; duration of >6 months; at least two symptoms of acute psychosis for greater than a month; exclusion of medical conditions as cause of symptoms

What are some features for each of the following psychiatric disorders that may present as acute psychosis:

Schizoaffective disorder

Psychosis that is chronic; it is often associated with mood disorders; psychotic features can occur without mood symptoms

Schizophreniform disorder

Psychosis that lasts <6 months; does not occur during a mood disorder

Brief psychotic disorder

Psychosis that lasts <1 month; does not occur during a mood disorder

Major depression with psychotic features

Psychosis that occurs during a depressive episode

What is the most important thing to do when evaluating a patient who is psychotic?

Establishing safety

What are some things to do to ensure safety when evaluating a patient with acute psychosis?

Search for weapons; use restraints if necessary; avoid having the patient between you and an exit point

Should all patients with acute psychosis be admitted?

No, but patients who are a danger to others or themselves should probably be admitted

MANIA

What defines a manic episode?

Three or more of the following for over 1 week:

Impulsivity; distractibility; pressured speech; grandiosity; decreased need for sleep; agitation; flight of ideas

Can a patient with a manic episode also have acute psychosis?

Yes—often with paranoia or grandiosity

What are some medical conditions that can cause mania?

CNS tumors; hyperthyroidism

What are some medications/drugs that are known to cause mania?

Phencyclidine; steroids; EtOH; psychostimulants

What is Bipolar Affective Disorder?

Psychiatric illness characterized by prolonged periods of depression alternating with periods of mania.

What are some elements of the history to attain when evaluating a patient with mania?

Current medications; history of illicit drug use; any prior psychiatric history; any homicidal or suicidal ideation; any recent life stressors

Are antimanic medications such as lithium or carbamazepine useful for an acute episode of mania?

No—take days to weeks to take effect

What classes of drugs are useful for an acute episode of mania?

Antipsychotic medications (ie, haloperidol)

What are some factors when deciding if a patient with acute mania should be admitted?

Impulsivity leads to danger to self or others; poor support structure; active delusions that are dangerous

PANIC ATTACKS

What are some signs and symptoms of a panic attack?

Tremor; shortness of breath; paresthesias; derealization; chest pain; tachycardia; sense of impending doom

Are patients with panic disorder at increased risk of suicide?

Yes—up to 18 times more than the general population

Are patients who present with a panic attack just overreacting?

No—during a panic attack, the patient truly feels threatened and commonly needs reassurance.

What are some medical conditions that may mimic a panic attack?

Asthma; chronic obstructive pulmonary disease (COPD); metabolic disturbances; dysrhythmias; hypoxia; acute MI

What are some characteristics of a panic attack?

Typically begins suddenly; lasts for about 15 min; can occur without provocation

What are some elements of the history to attain when evaluating a patient with mania?

Current medications; any prior psychiatric history; excessive caffeine use; any recent life stressors

Which class of drugs is useful for the short-term management of a panic attack?

Benzodiazepines

What is the most useful intervention for patients with a panic attack?

Reassurance and communication

EATING DISORDERS

What are two eating disorders commonly seen in the emergency department?	1. Bulimia Nervosa 2. Anorexia Nervosa
What is bulimia nervosa?	Chronic eating disorder that often waxes wanes, typically exacerbates during times of stress characterized by "binge and purge."
Describe the typical bulimic patient.	A normal-appearing female around the age of 18 to 24
How prevalent is bulimia?	5% of young adult females
What are some characteristic features of a binge?	Most patients with bulimia binge, that is characterized by excessive consumption of calories (up to 14,000 Kcal!), concealing from friends and family.
Are bulimics typically underweight?	No—often have normal weight
Is binge eating typically from hunger?	Not necessarily—commonly described as a feeling of loss of control
What is purging?	Inappropriate compensatory response to binging often characterized by self-induced emesis.
What are some medical complications of bulimia:	
Ipecac use	Dermatomyositis; cardiomyopathy
Diuretic use	Electrolyte imbalance (ie, hypokalemia); dehydration
Laxative use	Constipation; hypokalemia; dehydration
Self-induced emesis	Electrolyte imbalance; dental problems (ie, erosions); submandibular/parotid gland enlargement; may get esophageal tear or rupture
What are some clues during the history and physical exam that may point to bulimia?	Loss of dental enamel; unexplained hypokalemia; large fluctuations in weight; excessive exercise; esophageal problems (ie, bleeding)
What are some indications for admission for a patient who presents with bulimia?	Metabolic complications (ie, hypotension); suicidal ideation; persistent emesis

What is anorexia nervosa (AN)?	An eating disorder characterized by a preoccupying fear of obesity regardless of weight loss.
What are four diagnostic criteria of AN?	1. Preoccupying fear of gaining weight 2. Weight loss >15% of ideal body weight 3. Amenorrhea greater than three consecutive cycles 4. Distorted body image
What is the mortality rate of AN at 10 years?	Almost approaches 10%
What is characteristic of patients with AN who are in treatment?	Notorious for resistance to treatment and unmotivated
What are some clues during the history and physical exam that may point to AN?	Excessive exercise; unexplained weight loss or growth problems; activity or occupation (ie, dancer)
What are some considerations in the management of patients with AN?	Correct any underlying metabolic problems; initial evaluation may require psychiatric involvement as the illness is commonly associated with anxiety/depression, OCD; determine if outpatient treatment is possible

DEMENTIA AND DELIRIUM

Why are dementia and delirium important to consider?	Patients with dementia or delirium often have impaired ability to recognize their condition and may be susceptible to injury.
What is dementia?	Progressive and global impairment of cognitive function without alteration in consciousness.
What are some causes of irreversible dementia?	Alzheimer disease; vascular dementia (multi-infarct); Creutzfeldt-Jakob diseases; Parkinson disease
What are some of the signs and symptoms of dementia?	Multiple cognitive deficits that include memory impairment along with either or some of the following: apraxia, aphasia, and agnosia.

Is the onset of dementia typically acute?	No—gradual onset with disturbances in recent memory that can be exacerbated by illnesses or certain medications.
What are some causes of reversible dementia?	Medication; metabolic disorders; endocrine disorders; depression (pseudodementia)
What are some considerations in the treatment of dementia?	Eliminate medications that may exacerbate the condition; identify and correct any underlying metabolic or endocrine disorder; if dementia is irreversible, consider medication that may slow the progression
Is depression common among patients who have dementia?	Yes—depression rate among demented patients may be as high as 80%
What are some signs and symptoms of delirium?	Acute onset with often diurnal fluctuation of symptoms, cognitive impairment, and reduced ability to focus and sustain attention.
What are some important causes of delirium to consider?	Drugs and medications; heavy metals; CNS injury; infection; metabolic disturbances
What is the treatment for delirium?	Identify and treat the underlying cause; ensure the safety of a patient

INTOXICATION AND WITHDRAWAL

What is intoxication?	Ingestion of a drug or alcohol that often leads to impairment of judgment, perception, motor activity, and attention.
What are some signs and symptoms of intoxication?	Primarily manifests as impairment of judgment and motor activity with progression to delirium, coma, seizure, or even death with increasing amounts.
How is the diagnosis of intoxication typically made?	Clinically; less commonly with laboratory evaluation
What are some substances that cause psychostimulant intoxication?	Cocaine; methamphetamine; phenylpropanolamine

What are some signs and symptoms of psychostimulant intoxication?

Can have paranoid psychotic excitation, sympathetic autonomic response, and stereopathies (ie, nail biting).

What medication class is useful for patient with psychostimulant intoxication?

Benzodiazepines; antipsychotics (ie, haloperidol)

What are some considerations in the management of patients with psychostimulant intoxication?

Ensure safety of patient (ie, restraints); general supportive measures; treatment of the intoxicating agent; appropriate referral to psychiatry if needed

What are some signs and symptoms of alcohol intoxication?

Confusion, ataxia, agitation, slurred speech, hallucinations, and possible violent paranoid ideation.

What is an appropriate medication class if behavioral control is needed?

Antipsychotics; benzodiazepines

What is withdrawal?

Clinical syndrome that occurs with the cessation of a substance and can be reduced when the substance is taken again.

What is the most commonly encountered withdrawal syndrome?

Alcohol

What are the clinical stages of alcohol withdrawal from the time of last drink:

6-24 hours

Hypertension, tachycardia, nausea, anxiety, and sleep disturbances

24-72 hours

More severe autonomic disturbances and hallucinations and can take up to 6 days to resolve. Seizures can also occur during this time

3-5 days

Can progress to delirium tremens

What is delirium tremens?

Potentially fatal form of ethanol withdrawal

What are some signs and symptoms of delirium tremens?

Autonomic instability, global confusion, tremors, incontinence, and hallucinations with a substantial mortality if left untreated.

What is the treatment of acute alcohol withdrawal?	Establish supportive care; IV fluids along with thiamine, magnesium, and multivitamin; generally avoid giving glucose before thiamine as this may precipitate Wernicke encephalopathy; sedation with benzodiazepines is key
What are some indications for a head CT in an alcoholic who has seizures?	Focal seizures; status epilepticus; new-onset seizure

PSYCHOPHARMACOLOGY

Which class of medications is commonly used for short-term control of anxiety and agitation?	Benzodiazepines
What are some indications for the use of benzodiazepines?	Short-term management of anxiety; seizure control; alcohol withdrawal; induce muscle relaxation
Name two benzodiazepines commonly used in the ED setting for psychiatric emergencies:	1. Lorazepam 2. Diazepam
What are some side effects of benzodiazepines?	Impairment of motor coordination; respiratory depression; ataxia at higher doses; potential for addiction
Name two benzodiazepines that have potential for abuse:	1. Diazepam 2. Alprazolam
Is it possible to die from benzodiazepine withdrawal?	Yes; similar pathophysiology to alcohol withdrawal
What are some advantages of using lorazepam in the acute setting for behavioral emergencies?	Minimal cardiovascular depression; does not inhibit or induce cytochrome isoenzymes; no active metabolites
What is the primary concern of using high-dose benzodiazepines (especially IV route)?	Respiratory depression
Are overdoses of benzodiazepines commonly fatal?	No—unless concomitant ingestion with other sedatives such as alcohol.
What are some indications of neuroleptics?	Reduces aggression; reduces psychotic thinking; helps relieve anxiety

What is the primary mechanism of action of neuroleptics?	Antagonizes dopamine receptors in the mesolimbic area within the CNS
What are some side effects of neuroleptics?	Reflex tachycardia; orthostatic hypotension; can lower seizure threshold
What are some characteristics of haloperidol that make it an ideal neuroleptic to use in the ED?	Minimal cardiovascular effects; effective at reducing agitation; minimal sedation; rapid onset; synergistic with benzodiazepines
What side effect is common with haloperidol?	Dystonic reactions
What are some characteristics of atypical neuroleptics?	Effective for psychotic patients who are refractory to typical neuroleptics; effective for negative symptoms; less likely to cause tardive dyskinesia, but more likely to cause akathisia
Give some examples of atypical neuroleptics.	Olanzapine; quetiapine; clozapine
What are some examples of extrapyramidal symptoms seen with antipsychotics:	
Parkinsonism	Commonly within the first month of use; characterized by cogwheel rigidity, akinesia, masked facies, and bradykinesia; reducing the dose can help symptoms
Dystonias	Painful clonus of voluntary muscles; typically involves the face and neck; commonly within the first month of use; treatment is with diphenhydramine or benztropine
Akathisia	Internal sense of motor restlessness; most common form involves pacing and an inability to sit still; treat with diphenhydramine, benztropine, also propranolol
What is neuroleptic malignant syndrome (NMS)?	Rare, but life-threatening, idiosyncratic reaction to a neuroleptic medication
What are some signs and symptoms of NMS?	Characterized by fever, muscular rigidity, altered mental status, and autonomic dysfunction

Which types of neuroleptic are commonly associated with NMS?

Although potent neuroleptics (ie, haloperidol) are more commonly associated with NMS, all antipsychotic agents, typical or atypical, may precipitate the syndrome.

What is the diagnostic criterion of NMS?

High fever with severe muscle rigidity and two or more of the following:

Change in mental status; tachycardia; tremor; leukocytosis; metabolic acidosis; labile or high blood pressure; elevated CPK; lead-pipe rigidity of the extremities is a classic finding on examination

What is the treatment of NMS?

Commonly requires an ICU setting; stop all neuroleptics; benzodiazepines are the mainstay with supportive care as well as aggressive cooling for profound hyperthermia

Are there any emergent indications for the use of antidepressants in the ED?

No—they require weeks to take effect

What class of antidepressants was among the first to be used to treat depression?

Tricyclic antidepressants (TCAs)

Name some examples of TCAs:

Nortriptyline; amitriptyline; imipramine

Name one safety concern with TCAs:

Have a very low therapeutic index

What are some side effects of TCAs?

Anticholinergic, orthostatic hypotension, increased seizure risk, and have various cardiac effects.

What class of antidepressants has a high therapeutic index and largely replaced TCAs?

Selective serotonin reuptake inhibitors (SSRIs)

What are some examples of SSRIs?

Sertraline; citalopram; paroxetine

What are some indications for SSRIs?

Depression; anxiety; posttraumatic stress disorders; obsessive-compulsive disorders

What are some side effects of SSRIs?

Generally mild; notable drug interactions; toxic in only very high doses

What is serotonin syndrome?

It is an idiosyncratic reaction that can occur with interactions between serotonergic agents such as SSRIs.

What are some signs and symptoms of serotonin syndrome:

    Gastrointestinal

Nausea, emesis, and diarrhea

    Central nervous system

Hyperreflexia, tremor, and altered MS

    Autonomic instability

Hyperthermia, diaphoresis, and orthostasis

What is the treatment of serotonin syndrome?

Primarily supportive, also consider cyproheptadine

Name a class of antidepressants associated with hypertensive crisis with the ingestion of tyramine-containing foods:

Monamine oxidase inhibitors (MAOIs)

What are some tyramine-containing foods?

Aged cheese; wine; beer; fava beans

What are some signs and symptoms of MAOI-associated hypertensive crisis?

Hypertension, chest pain, severe headache, tachycardia, and diaphoresis.

What is the treatment of choice for hypertensive crisis?

Phentolamine

CLINICAL VIGNETTES—MAKE THE DIAGNOSIS

A 25-year-old woman presents to the Emergency Department with worsening mood over the last three months. She and her boyfriend broke up a few weeks ago, and she feels like she is having trouble sleeping and concentrating. She has lost weight, and has stopped going to her Aikido class, which used to be her favorite hobby. She is increasingly despondent, and has called out sick from work for the last week. Exam—vitals and exam within normal limits

    What is the most important issue to address during her emergency department stay?

    Risk for suicide: ask her directly about suicidal ideation, any specific plans, and the means with which to carry out her plan

    What other factors (organic) may be influencing or contributing to her depression?

    Drug or alcohol abuse, medication, systemic illness (undiagnosed diabetes, thyroid dysfunction, etc)

Two months after the initial presentation, the 25-year-old woman from Vignette #1 returns to the ED confused. She is brought in by her friends after having been found altered in her apartment this morning. Her friends explain that she had been doing very well since her last ED visit, having been started on Fluoxetine by her psychiatrist. Last week she injured her foot and had been prescribed tramadol for pain. Exam—febrile, confused, tachycardic. Evidence of clonus on neurological exam. What is the likely diagnosis and treatment?

Serotonin syndrome, treatment includes supportive care, aggressive IV fluids, airway monitoring, benzodiazepines as needed, possibly cyproheptadine (only available orally)

A 53-year-old man presents to the Emergency Department after a witness generalized seizure. He is now apparently back to his baseline mental status. He has a history of seizures in the past, but has never had medical workup for these events. He does relate a history of alcohol abuse—he drinks about 18-24 beers/day, but states he has not had a drink in two days as he is trying to quit. Exam—slightly hypertensive and tachycardic, coarse diffuse tremor noted. What class of medication would be the mainstay of choice for this evolving process?

Scheduled benzodiazepines. The patient most likely experienced a seizure related to alcohol withdrawal, but he should receive a full workup for in the ED as he has previously been undiagnosed.

A 41-year-old woman presents to the ED with dyspnea and chest pain. She has no significant medical history, but notes a strong family history of coronary artery disease. She smokes cigarettes. Tonight she developed sudden shortness of breath and felt extremely anxious. She now has developed chest pain and paresthesias in both hands. Upon presentation, she has a near syncopal episode in the waiting room. Exam—tachycardic, tachypneic, O2 sat normal, anxious appearing. Describe your differential diagnosis and initial management.

The above symptoms may well be related to a panic attack, but several other acute medical etiologies must be evaluated concurrently. Differential includes—acute coronary syndrome, pulmonary embolism, dysrhythmia, metabolic disturbance (hyperthyroidism), drug intoxication.

Treatment—while obtaining a workup to evaluate for other medical causes, consider calming reassurance and benzodiazepines.

CHAPTER 19

Stimulus Section

One of the new additions to the second edition is the stimulus section. Every year in February, virtually all emergency medicine residents sit down to take what is known as the in-service exam. It is administered from the makers of the actual qualifying examination all graduates take in order to qualify to take the oral examination, which is the final step in becoming board-certified. In addition to your standard multiple choice questions, the yearly in-service exam has a section referred to as the stimulus section. It is a booklet which contains various images, for example a radiograph or an ECG, and for each image there is an associated question/answer. In order to answer the question correctly, the test-taker must be able to ascertain what is being shown in the associated image. While most medical students probably do not take such an exam during their clerkship, they will no doubt come across various "stimulus" images during their rotations. It may be a physical exam finding with a unique rash or an attending may hand you an ECG and ask a related question. I have taken real-life cases with actual images collected over the years in hopes that this section will help prepare you for these "pimping" situations during your clerkship.

1. A 51-year-old woman with a history of pulmonary embolism and multiple lower extremity deep venous thromboses is admitted to the hospital with increased swelling of her right leg. A CT scan with intravenous contrast of her lower extremity reveals a clot extending above her Greenfield filter. A second filter is inserted and the patient is started on warfarin. A few days later the patient presents to an emergency department with a large lesion which was noted on her buttock and was said to resemble a burn. Later the lesion became necrotic and which required extensive debridement. What is the most likely diagnosis?

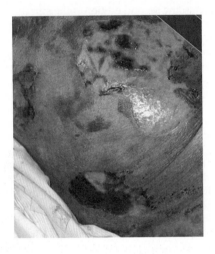

A. Hematoma

B. Steven-Johnson syndrome

C. Toxic epidermal necrolysis

D. Warfarin skin necrosis

E. Venous thrombosis

Answer D: Many cases of warfarin skin necrosis can be attributed to a relative deficiency of protein C or protein S. These factors are inhibitors of coagulation that are activated in the same vitamin K pathway as factors II, VII, IX, and X. Warfarin-induced coagulopathy results from a deficiency of coagulation factors II, VII, IX, and X. These factors (along with proteins S and C) must be activated in the liver by carboxylation of glutamic acid on their precursor proteins. This activation step is coupled to the oxidation of vitamin K and forms vitamin K 2,3-epoxide. Due to the relatively shorter half life of protein C and S compared to the coagulation factors, warfarin paradoxically increases clotting tendency initially. Warfarin skin necrosis usually occurs in women between their 4th and 6th day of therapy. Over the next day, petechiae will often appear and coalesce into ecchymotic areas. Ultimately thrombosis develops in subcutaneous veins and fat necrosis results. Patients can be given vitamin K_1 and fresh-frozen plasma to reverse the warfarin and provide a source of exogenous proteins S and C. Heparin, corticosteroids, and vasodilators have also been administered. Once a necrotic lesion occurs, tissue loss is inevitable. Local therapy with aggressive tissue debridement and wound repair may be indicated. Rechallenge with warfarin is considered inadvisable as the condition is likely to recur. Typically the initiation of warfarin is "bridged" with heparin to prophylactically avoid this hypercoagulable period.

2. A 71-year-old woman with a past medical history of a seizure disorder presents with a 2 to 3 day history of progressive rash, fever as well as weakness. She has been on phenobarbital for many years but due to some break-through seizures the patient was started on phenytoin which she has been on for a two-week period prior to the development of her symptoms. The patient is found to be febrile on examination but otherwise her heart rate and blood pressure are within normal limits. The patient has skin eruptions which can be characterized as a macular erythema that is pruritic and a confluent papular rash primarily involving her face and trunk. There is also tender lymphadenopathy on exam as well. What is the most likely diagnosis?

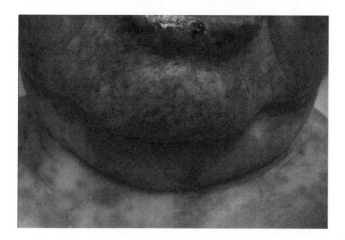

A. DRESS syndrome

B. Drug eruption

C. Meningococcemia

D. Stevens-Johnson syndrome

E. Toxic epidermal necrolysis

Answer A: The patient described above has a classic presentation for DRESS syndrome known as Drug Rash (or Reaction) with Eosinophilia and Systemic Symptoms formerly known as anticonvulsant hypersensitivity syndrome (AHS). AHS is traditionally associated with exposures to aromatic anticonvulsants such as phenytoin, carbamazepine, phenobarbital, and primidone. There are also reports of cases of DRESS with nonaromatic lamotrigine as a causative agent. DRESS occurs most frequently within the first 2 months of therapy and is not related to dose or concentration of the drug in question. The pathophysiology is related to accumulation of an arene oxide due to insufficient detoxification by the enzyme epoxide hydrolase with aromatic anticonvulsants. These reactive arene oxides bind to macromolecules and cause cellular apoptosis and necrosis. They also form neoantigens that may trigger an immunologic response. Interestingly, the same metabolite is believed to cause other serious dermatologic reactions, such as Stevens-Johnson syndrome and toxic epidermal necrolysis.

This syndrome is characterized by the triad of fever, rash, and internal organ involvement, most commonly the liver. A skin eruption characterized by macular erythema evolves into a pruritic and confluent papular rash primarily involving the face, trunk and later the extremities. The rash usually spares the mucous membranes which may help to distinguish DRESS from toxic epidermal necrolysis. Multiorgan involvement usually occurs 12 weeks into the syndrome. Liver disturbances range from mildly elevated aminotransferase concentrations to fulminant hepatic failure.

Prompt discontinuation of the suspected agent is essential to prevent symptom progression. Patients should be admitted to the hospital if there is some evidence that steroids may help to attenuate the response.

3. An 18-year-old man with a medical history of intravenous drug abuse as well as depression presents with a "seizure." The patient denies any history of seizures and is not currently on any antiepileptics. He mentions that for the past few days he has been "blacking-out" and had an episode when a neighbor called EMS for a suspected seizure where he passed out and was described to have "seizure-like" movements of his extremities. On arrival the patient is found to have normal vitals as well as normal capillary finger glucose. His medications include citalopram and methadone, but otherwise the patient has no other significant history. As you are interviewing the patient, he has a syncopal episode in front of you with myoclonic jerks. The patient was already on a monitor during which time the following rhythm is detected. What is this rhythm?

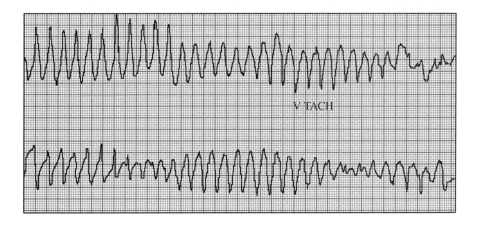

A. Atrial fibrillation

B. Brugada Syndrome

C. Premature ventricular tachycardia

D. Polymorphic ventricular tachycardia

E. Ventricular bigeminy

Answer D: The patient described above is actually presenting with syncope due to a cardiac disturbance as opposed to a seizure. While one should consider the many causes of syncope such as ectopic pregnancy or subarachnoid hemorrhage depending on the clinical context, a dysrhythmia should be high on the differential. One of the first screening tests that should be obtained with all cases of suspected syncope is an electrocardiogram (ECG). It is inexpensive and provides valuable information which may lead to the diagnosis of syncope such as a third degree heart block or ischemia. The patient was fortunate enough to be on a monitor during his syncopal episode. It is also important to realize that syncope may also cause myoclonic jerks that may appear like a "seizure" to others. A pitfall in this scenario would be to attribute his syncope to "seizures" when in fact it is due to an underlying cardiac problem which can be lethal if not detected.

The above rhythm strip shows polymorphic ventricular tachycardia also known as torsades de pointes with classic spiraling of QRS complexes around baseline. Torsades often occur in the setting of an existing prolonged QT interval, a reflection of abnormal ventricular repolarization. The normal range of QT duration must be corrected for sex, age, and heart rate. A QT interval of 500 ms or longer places the patient at an increased risk of torsades. Prolonged QT intervals can be congenital or acquired, with the latter being more common. Women have a greater risk of QT prolongation and torsades.

Acquired QT prolongation and torsades are often multifactorial, which may include interactions between drug therapy, myocardial ischemia, and electrolyte disturbances (hypokalemia and hypomagnesemia). Drugs (classes IA, IC, and III antiarrhythmic agents, plus many antibiotics, antifungals, antiemetics, antipsychotics, antiseizure medications, and a variety of other agents) can trigger prolonged QT intervals or torsades when new or in high concentrations, with abrupt infusion, or simply without warning.

Treatment of intermittent torsades in stable patients is based on correcting any metabolic or electrolyte abnormalities. Intravenous magnesium sulfate is also considered in treating paroxysmal torsades, but often used more for prophylaxis as it does not really terminate torsades once it occurs. Classes IA and IC agents may further prolong repolarization so are contraindicated. The class IB agents shorten repolarization, but their overall success rate is often low in these cases.

Patients who are unstable or in sustained torsades should be electrically cardioverted. As with any ventricular tachycardia; synchronization will usually not be possible. Treatment of all forms of catecholamine-induced torsades is based on slowing the heart rate, usually with beta-adrenergic blockers. Other agents, such as magnesium sulfate, calcium channel blockers, amiodarone, or phenytoin, have varying effectiveness and are second-line therapies.

The most likely cause in this patient is acquired as the patient is on two QT prolonging drugs. Methadone is a synthetic mu-opioid receptor agonist most commonly used for the treatment of chronic pain as well as a maintenance substitute for opioid dependence. At least in the United States, methadone is a racemic mixture of (R,S)-methadone. Methadone produces QT interval prolongation due to blockade of the hERG (human *ether-a-gogo* related gene) channel that mediates the rapidly activating delayed rectifier current.

4. A 55-year-old man with a history of hypertension, diabetes, and dyslipidemia presents with new onset right-sided weakness as well as slurred speech. The patient woke up in his normal state of health, however, during breakfast his wife noticed that the patient began having slurred speech which was soon followed by right-sided weakness. EMS was called and the patient was brought to the ED for further evaluation. On initial evaluation (2 h since the onset of symptoms) the patient was noted to have normal vitals as well as glucose of 189 mg/dL. Physical examination of the patient was remarkable for flaccid right-side of both the arm and leg along with obvious dysarthria. A non-contrast head CT was negative. At this time the patient is also seen by neurology. Given that the onset of symptoms was within the 3 hour window as well as clinical examination, the patient is given alteplase at the correct dose. Within ½ hour of alteplase administration the patient is noted to have altered mental status and a repeat non-contrast CT of the head is performed as shown. What is the best course of management at this point?

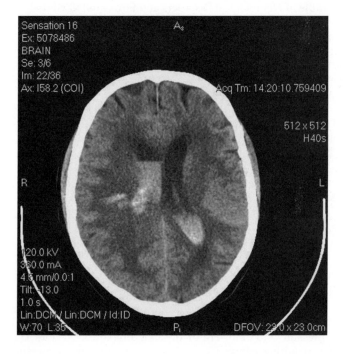

A. Aminocaproic acid
B. FACTOR VIIa, recombinant (NovoSeven)
C. Prothrombin complex (Bebulin VH)
D. Supportive care
E. Vitamin K

Answer D: The patient initially presented to the emergency department with an ischemic stroke most likely due to occlusion of the middle cerebral artery. A stroke can be defined as any vascular injury that reduces cerebral blood flow to a specific region of the brain, causing neurologic impairment which will depend on the area of the brain affected. The onset of symptoms may be sudden or stuttering, often with transient or permanent loss of neurologic function. Approximately 80% of all strokes are ischemic in origin with the remaining causes due to hemorrhages.

Management of a suspected stroke requires rapid recognition, evaluation, and treatment, often with early involvement with neurology. Prior to the use of lytic therapy, treatment mostly consisted of supportive care with proper regulation of blood pressure and glucose. The use of lytic therapy with agents such as alteplase is now considered the standard of care in many places despite potentially adverse effects as demonstrated by the case above. The use of intravenous t-PA has been approved by the U.S. Food and Drug Administration (FDA) for treatment of patients with acute ischemic stroke. These recommendations were based on the results of the National Institute of Neurological Disorders and Stroke (NINDS) trial.

Inclusion Criteria

1. Time of symptom onset well established to be less than 3 hours
2. Clinical diagnosis of ischemic stroke causing a measurable neurologic deficit (based on NIH stroke scale)
3. Age 18 years or older

Exclusion Criteria (some be considered relatively contraindications so consultation with neurology is paramount to determine if a patient is a candidate)

1. Noncontrast head CT with any evidence of intracranial hemorrhage
2. Rapidly resolving symptoms
3. High clinical suspicion of subarachnoid hemorrhage even with normal CT findings
4. Active internal bleeding (eg, gastrointestinal or urinary bleeding within last 21 days)
5. Known bleeding diathesis
6. Within 3 months of intracranial surgery, serious head trauma, or previous stroke
7. Within 14 days of major surgery or serious trauma
8. Recent arterial puncture at noncompressible site
9. History of intracranial hemorrhage, arteriovenous malformation, or aneurysm
10. Witnessed seizure at stroke onset
11. Systolic pressure >185 mm Hg or diastolic pressure >110 mm Hg at time of treatment, requiring aggressive treatment to reduce blood pressure to within these limits prior to administration of a lytic compound

Unfortunately the most devastating complication with the use of lytic agent is hemorrhage which in many cases lead to high morbidity and mortality. While there is no direct reversal agent, treatment is often supportive with aggressive control of airway as well as intracranial monitoring often in conjugation with neurosurgery. Aminocaproic acid is an analogue of the amino acid lysine, which makes it an effective inhibitor of certain proteolytic enzymes like plasmin, the enzyme responsible for fibrinolysis. While it is attractive in theory, the onset of action of most lytics is rapid which would render the use of aminocaproic acid ineffective. In contrast, effective antidotes do exist for other anti-coagulation medications, which are used in other clinical situations. The use of platelets should be considered for patients on aspirin and vitamin K, prothrombin complex (Bebulin VH), and factor VIIa, recombinant (NovoSeven) if the patient is on a vitamin K antagonist such as Coumadin. There is no evidence that these agents work in the absence of a vitamin K antagonist so should not be given empirically.

5. A 28-year-old woman with no past medical history is transferred to a tertiary referral center for the inability to remove the object visualized below by x-ray. The patient admitted to having her sexual partner insert a long object into her rectum which she was not able to remove. She states that the object was battery operated and still vibrating. She denies any abdominal pain as well as any emesis. Her vitals are normal on examination with an unremarkable exam. She has no tenderness, rebound, or guarding on examination but a faint buzzing noise can be heard on auscultation. What is the best management option to be considered in this case?

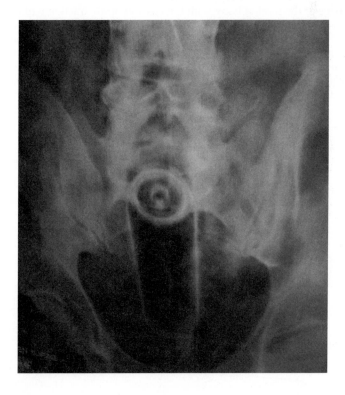

A. Discharge home with cathartics

B. Exploratory laparotomy

C. Conscious sedation for ED removal

D. CT scan of abdomen/pelvis

E. Surgical consultation

Answer E: The patient initially presented at an outside hospital during which time they were unable to remove the object after multiple attempts. Most objects are introduced directly into the anus, but some become lodged there after oral ingestion. The incidence of anorectal foreign bodies is increasing in incidence. Rectal foreign bodies can also be found in children, psychiatric patients, and victims of assault or as a result of iatrogenic injury. Complications of anorectal foreign body can include lacerations, intestinal obstruction, sepsis, and peritonitis. In most cases, removal can be done safely in the ED.

Treatment will depend primarily on the location and type of object that is inserted. As a general rule, objects that are low in the rectum and soft can be safely removed in the ED. For most cases, the removal is best performed with the patient awake (conscious sedation should be avoided if possible) so that patient can help with expulsion by performing Valsalva, although the use of a sedative such as a benzodiazepine can be used to help relax the patient.

There are several methods that are effective for removal. The easiest method is to grasp an edge of the foreign body with forceps and apply traction while the patient bears down. Another method is to use a foley catheter which can be placed beside the foreign body and the balloon inflated proximal to it. This breaks the suction of the rectal wall mucosa and provides a way to guide the object out of the rectal vault. In the event that this is unsuccessful, the next best option would be to have surgical involvement where the patient can be taken to the OR to be relaxed so the object can be removed in a controlled condition.

6. A 31-year-old man presents to the ED with complaints of general back pain. The patient has presented with general back pain to the ED four times over the past month. At these visits he was diagnosed with non-specific back pain and discharged with pain control as well as follow-up. In his most recent visit a week prior to this presentation he again complained of back pain during which time the patient was noted to have a normal physical exam. However, during this visit the patient now is complaining of "problems going to the bathroom" as well as tripping when he walks. His vitals are documented as normal with no temperature noted. His physical examination is positive for lower extremity weakness. He later admits to the use of intravenous drug which was not documented in previous visits. An MRI is obtained with the following results above. What is the most likely diagnosis?

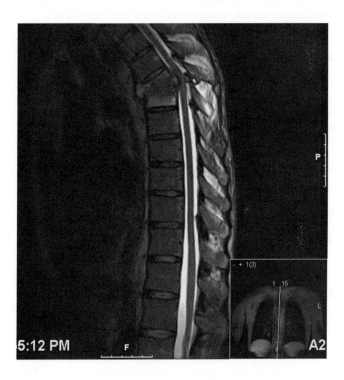

A. Cauda equina
B. Epidural abscess
C. Metastatic disease
D. Spinal fracture
E. Transverse myelitis

Answer B: The patient presents with an epidural abscess as a complication of his IV drug use. Lower back pain is a common presentation to the ED where most causes are typically benign in presentation. However, there are secondary causes of lower back pain that should always be considered such as epidural abscess or hematoma. Other causes should also be considered such as referred pain from another disease process such as a ruptured abdominal aneurysm.

Spinal epidural abscess is an infectious process usually confined to the adipose tissue of the dorsal epidural space. It is an uncommon disease, with an overall frequency of 0.2 to 1.2 per 10,000 hospital admissions. Major risk factors include IV drug use, diabetes, alcoholism, and immunosuppression. Although the disease may manifest in chronic or subacute, the acute presentation is seen most frequently in the ED. Thoracic and lumbar sites of infection are typically more common. The dura mater often limits the spread of an epidural infection, making subdural spread uncommon. Hematogenous spread of infection to the epidural space is the most common source. *Staphylococcus aureus* is the most common organism involved, being cultured in more than 50% of cases. Other frequently identified pathogens include *Pseudomonas aeruginosa* and *Escherichia coli*.

MRI is the imaging modality of choice and needs to be performed emergently if any spinal cord process is considered. While other tests such as a complete blood count may aid in the diagnosis of an epidural abscess, they are considered ancillary and should be used to rule out the diagnosis if the history and physical is suggestive. An erythrocyte sedimentation rate is often obtained, although not specific for epidural abscess, is virtually always elevated with this condition. Plain films usually are normal in appearance, unless evidence of osteomyelitis of an adjacent vertebral body is seen.

Urgent neurosurgical consultation for decompression usually is required. Antibiotics effective against the most common pathogens (particularly *S. aureus*) should be started empirically. Outcome is related to the speed of diagnosis before the development of myelopathic signs. The disease is fatal in 18 to 23% of cases, and patients with neurologic deficit rarely improve if surgical intervention is delayed more than 12 to 36 hours after onset of paralysis. Patients operated on before development of neurologic symptoms have an almost universally good outcome, but this can be a difficult diagnosis to make if one does not have a clinical suspicion.

7. A 23-year-old man with no known past medical history presents with 1 day of diffuse abdominal pain. He mentions that he recently returned from South America yesterday after an uneventful visit. He states that the pain began soon after arriving in the United States and endorses associated nausea, as well as non-bilious and non-bloody emesis. He also states that he has been unable to pass any flatus as well. The patient denies any surgical history as well as any unusual food and drank only bottled water while in South America. The patient appears nervous on examination and despite attempting to be stoic he does appear to be in discomfort. Vitals are normal and examination is significant only for generalized abdominal pain. An abdominal radiograph (shown here) is obtained with the following results. What is the best management strategy based on the radiograph?

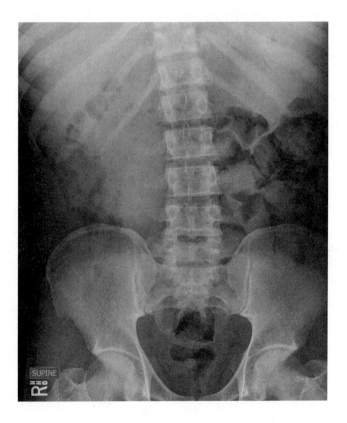

A. Admission with surgical consultation

B. Bowel regiment and discharge

C. Further imaging with CT of the abdomen

D. Naloxone drip

E. Whole-bowel irrigation

Answer A: The patient is most likely a body packer. The abdominal radiograph obtained above displays packets of some drug of abuse (typically cocaine or heroin). It is important to distinguish between a body packer versus a body stuffer, as the outcome and management is drastically different.

A body packer often ingests large amounts of well-wrapped drug in an attempt to smuggle cocaine or heroin across international borders. It is also often the case that the majority of these packets do not open as they are often well prepared. However, when they rupture, the amount of drug contained is often lethal despite aggressive supportive care, in particular, with cocaine. The presence of mechanical bowel obstruction or *any* sign of packet rupture is considered an absolute indication for surgery. In asymptomatic patients, whole bowel irrigation with Polyethylene Glycol-Electrolyte Lavage Solution (PEG-ELS) is initiated and single- or multiple-dose activated charcoal therapy may also be considered. The general agreement is that *any* evidence of cocaine rupture (tachycardia, agitation, positive cocaine urine screen, etc) is an indication for surgical removal. However, in the setting of opioid packets, a naloxone drip can be considered with GI decontamination, but many would advocate surgical removal.

In contrast, a body stuffer ingests drug in an attempt to avoid detection or prosecution. The drug is normally unwrapped or wrapped for transport, and therefore often readily available for gastrointestinal absorption. While diagnostic imaging can be considered, it is not very sensitive of specific given the small ingestion as opposed to a body packer. If symptoms of cocaine toxicity develop, they usually manifest within a few hours of ingestion, although the onset of toxicity may be more delayed with crack-vial ingestion. Although it is generally accepted that life-threatening toxicity is uncommon as a result of delayed and incomplete absorption of a relatively small dose, serious toxicity and death are reported. There is also evidence that amphetamine stuffers may have potential bad outcome so admission for observation should be considered.

Decontamination with multiple-dose oral-activated charcoal therapy should be sufficient in most cases as cocaine is very well adsorbed to activated charcoal. Whole-bowel irrigation (WBI) with PEG-ELS can also be considered but often requires patient cooperation which may be difficult as this particular patient population ingested the packets to avoid the police. They are often reluctant to have the packets pass if they are under police custody so may refuse any intervention.

Answer B, C, D may be considered and would be appropriate, but ultimately all these patients should be admitted with early surgery involvement so they can also follow the patient for possible surgical intervention.

8. A 23-year-old man with no past medical history presents with a 3 to 4 day history of progressive substernal chest pain. He states that he started to develop intermittent chest pain while he was working out in the gym a few days prior to his presentation. He mentions that the pain was becoming more constant and now developed shortness of breath when he exerted himself with an activity. He denies any fever, chill, no sick contacts, and no productive coughing and denies a positional component. He denies any history of drug use but does admit to using anabolic steroids. An ECG is obtained and is displayed here. What is the ideal management choice given the history and ECG obtained?

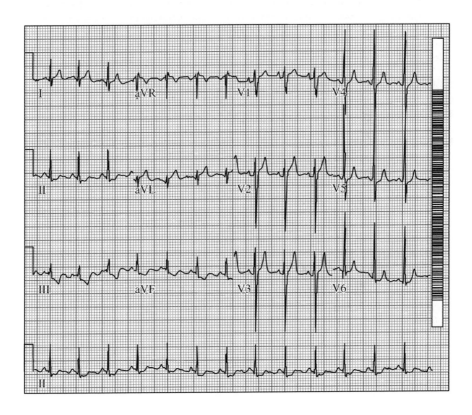

A. Admit for chest pain evaluation with cardiology consultation

B. Cardiac catheterization

C. CT of the chest with intravenous contrast

D. NSAIDs and discharge for follow-up

E. Thrombolytic therapy

Answer A: The patient has evidence of ischemia by ECG with ST depression in the inferior leads that is concerning for a NSTEMI. Patient is a young male with no obvious traditional risk factors such as diabetes or hypertension so not considering cardiac ischemia would be considered a pitfall. It is becoming recognized that younger patients are also susceptible to cardiac ischemia such as those with a history of cocaine use as well as anabolic steroid use as demonstrated with the case above.

In sports, the general purpose of taking androgens is to increase the anabolic effects and to avoid the unwanted side effects of feminization, such as gynecomastia, or masculinizing secondary sexual characteristics such as facial hair and deepening voice. Creating a substance that completely dissociates the desired from the undesired effects has not been possible. Therefore, athletes are directed on the use of agents to manipulate the metabolic pathways of androgen metabolism and decrease unwanted side effects by combining xenobiotics with antiestrogenic or antiandrogenic activity.

Without question, supraphysiologic doses of testosterone, when combined with strength training, increase muscle strength and size. The most common musculoskeletal complications of steroid use are tendon and ligament rupture.

Hepatic subcapsular hematoma with hemorrhage is reported. Peliosis hepatis, a condition of blood-filled sinuses in the liver that may result in fatal hepatic rupture, occurs most commonly with alkylated androgens and may not improve when androgen use is stopped. This condition is not associated with the dose or duration of treatment. Cyproterone acetate is a chlorinated progesterone derivative that inhibits 5α-reductase and reportedly causes hepatotoxicity.

Cardiac complications include acute myocardial infarction and sudden cardiac arrest. Autopsy examination of the heart may reveal biventricular hypertrophy, extensive myocardial fibrosis, and contraction-band necrosis. Myofibrillar disorganization and hypertrophy of the interventricular septum and left ventricle are present. Intense training and use of anabolic-androgen steroids (AAS) impair diastolic function by increasing left ventricular wall thickness. Animal models and in vitro myocardial cell studies show similar pathologic changes.

Bibliography

Marx J, Hockberger R, Walls R. Rosen's Emergency Medicine: Concepts and Clinical Practice. 7th ed. Philadelphia: Mosby, 2009.

Nelson LS, Lewin NA, Howland MA, et al. Goldfrank's Toxicologic Emergencies. 9th ed. New York: McGraw-Hill, 2010.

Roberts JR, Hedges JR. Clinical Procedures in Emergency Medicine. 5th ed. Philadelphia: Saunders, 2009.

Schwartz DT. Emergency Radiology: Case Studies. New York: McGraw-Hill, 2007.

Tintinalli JE, Kelen GD, Stapczynski JS, et al. Tintinalli's Emergency Medicine: A Comprehensive Study Guide. 6th ed. New York: McGraw-Hill, 2004.

Index

Page numbers followed by *f* or *t* indicate figures or tables, respectively.